An additional chapter - *The use of bright light in the treatment of insomnia,* by Drs. Leon Lack and Helen Wright - is available for free download.

Download your PDF at:

http://www.elsevierdirect.com/product.jsp?isbn=9780123815224

Behavioral Treatments for Sleep Disorders

A Comprehensive Primer of Behavioral Sleep Medicine Interventions

Behavioral Treatments for Sleep Disorders

A Comprehensive Primer of Behavioral Sleep Medicine Interventions

Edited by

Michael Perlis, PhD
Associate Professor, Psychiatry
Department of Psychiatry, University of Pennsylvania
Director, Center for Sleep and Respiratory Neurobiology
University of Pennsylvania
School of Nursing University of Pennsylvania

Mark Aloia, PhD, C.BSM
Associate Professor, Medicine
National Jewish Health
Director of Sleep Research
National Jewish Health

Brett Kuhn, PhD, C.BSM
Associate Professor, Pediatrics and Psychology
Munroe-Meyer Institute for Genetics and Rehabilitation
University of Nebraska Medical Center
Director, Behavioral Sleep Medicine Services
Children's Sleep Disorders Center: In Affiliation with
University of Nebraska Medical Center

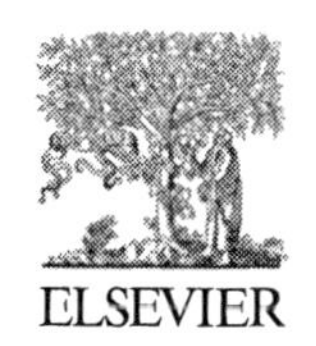

AMSTERDAM • BOSTON • HEIDELBERG • LONDON
NEW YORK • OXFORD • PARIS • SAN DIEGO
SAN FRANCISCO • SINGAPORE • SYDNEY • TOKYO

Academic Press is an imprint of Elsevier

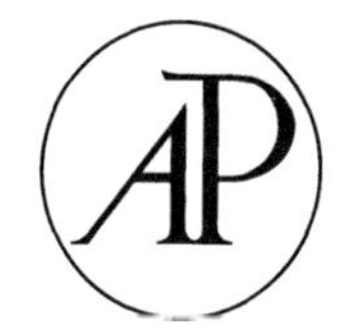

Academic Press is an imprint of Elsevier
32 Jamestown Road, London NW1 7BY, UK
30 Corporate Drive, Suite 400, Burlington, MA 01803, USA
525 B Street, Suite 1800, San Diego, CA 92101-4495, USA

First edition 2011

British Library Cataloguing-in-Publication Data
A catalogue record for this book is available from the British Library

Library of Congress Cataloging-in-Publication Data
A catalog record for this book is available from the Library of Congress

ISBN : 978-0-12-381522-4

For information on all Academic Press publications
visit our website at www.elsevierdirect.com

Transferred to Digital Printing 2011

Michael L. Perlis, PhD

Associate Professor of Psychiatry, University of Pennsylvania
Adjunct Associate Professor of Nursing, University of Pennsylvania
Director of the Upenn Behavioral Sleep Medicine Program;
Philadelphia, PA, USA

Visiting Professor/Adjunct Faculty, University of Glasgow
Visiting Professor/Adjunct Faculty, University of Freiburg

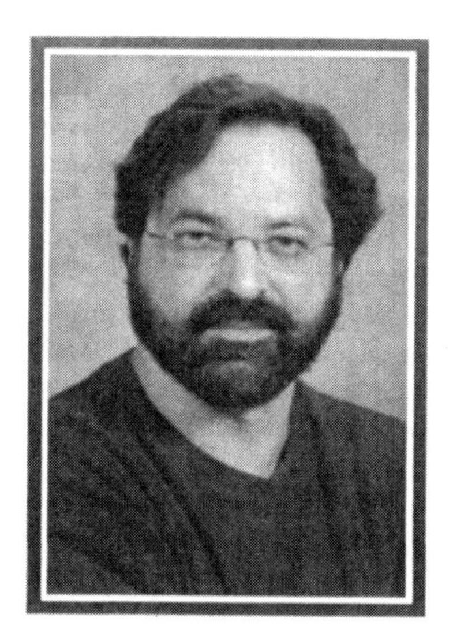

Dr Perlis' areas of research include neurocognitive phenomena in insomnia, the cognitive and/or behavior effects of sedative hypnotics and the development of alternative treatment approaches for insomnia. His clinical expertise is in the area of Behavioral Sleep Medicine, and he is a coauthor of the first textbook in this field (*Treating Sleep Disorders: The Principles and Practice of Behavioral Sleep Medicine*, Wiley & Sons) and the senior author of a published CBT-I treatment manual.

In addition to his academic endeavors, he has served on the editorial boards of *Sleep*, the *Journal of Sleep Research*, and the *Journal of Behavioral Sleep Medicine*; as a founding member of the American Academy of Sleep Medicine Presidential Committee on Behavioral Sleep Medicine (2000–2004); as the section chair for Behavioral Sleep Medicine (2003–2004); as a member of the program committee for the first Behavioral Sleep Medicine Conference (Spring 2009); as a founding member of the Society of Behavioral Sleep Medicine; and as the SBSM's first president (2010–2011).

Mark S. Aloia, PhD, C.BSM

Associate Professor of Medicine, National Jewish Health
Adjunct Associate Professor of Psychology, University of Colorado at Denver
Adjunct Associate Professor of Nursing, University of Colorado Health Sciences Center
Director of Sleep Research, National Jewish Health
Director of Clinical Research, Philips/Respironics, Inc.

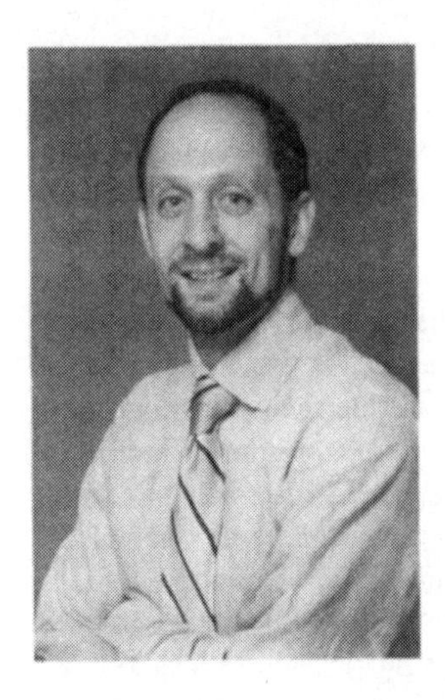

Dr Aloia's areas of research include the study of behavioral methods to improve adherence to treatment and the neuropsychological consequences of chronic disease. He has received several NIH grants to study adherence to treatment for Obstructive Sleep Apnea, and has contributed to the growing literature on neuroimaging in sleep apnea.

Dr Aloia has served on the editorial boards of *Sleep*, *Behavioral Sleep Medicine*, and *Health Psychology*. He has been a standing member on an NIH review panel, and is committed to the development of future scientists as a teacher and mentor. He currently holds his primary academic position as an Associate Professor of Medicine at National Jewish Health in Denver, where he also serves as the Director of Sleep Research. Dr Aloia also holds adjunct appointments in Psychology at the University of Colorado at Denver and in the Department of Nursing at the University of Colorado Health Sciences Center. Outside of academia, Dr Aloia serves as the Director of Clinical Research for Philips/Respironics, Inc.

Brett R. Kuhn, PhD, C.BSM

Associate Professor, Munroe-Meyer Institute for Genetics and Rehabilitation Pediatrics and Psychology, University of Nebraska Medical Center
Director, Behavioral Sleep Medicine Services,
Children's Sleep Disorders Center, In affiliation with
University of Nebraska Medical Center

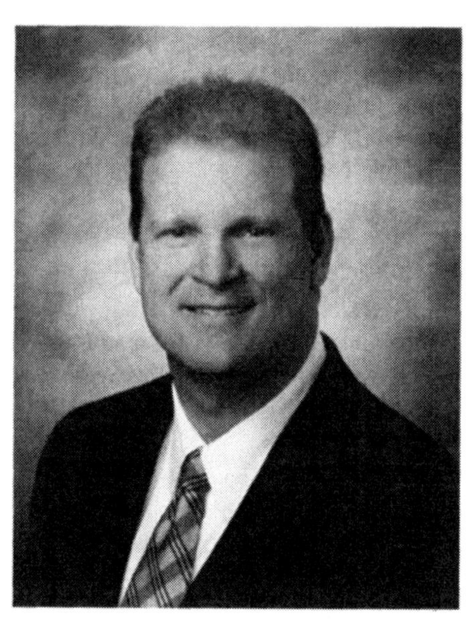

Dr Kuhn is a licensed psychologist, and is certified in behavioral sleep medicine (C.BSM) by the American Academy of Sleep Medicine (AASM). He served on the AASM committee to help create the national standards of practice for children with bedtime resistance and night-time awakenings. Dr Kuhn currently directs behavioral sleep medicine services at the Children's Sleep Disorders Center in Omaha, where he also supervises medical residents, sleep medicine fellows, and psychology interns in the assessment and treatment of pediatric sleep disorders. Dr Kuhn has nearly 20 years of experience working in clinical settings with children and their parents. He has published a number of professional journal articles and book chapters on children's behavioral health issues, including sleep problems, elimination disorders, and disruptive behavior.

To Dick Bootzin and Don Posner – Where would I be without you?
I know only one thing for sure: It was seeing the world through your eyes that "precipitated and perpetuates" (pun intended) my interest in Behavioral Sleep Medicine.

To Donna Giles and Michael Thase – If not for you, there by the "crates of cod go I" ... Thank you.

To Sean Drummond, Michael Smith, Phil Gehrman, Jay Ellis, Ken Lichstein, Dieter Rieman, and Collin Espie – Thank you for your friendship and collegiality – on any given day you guys are the wind, the rudder, or both. How lucky am I?

To Dwight Evans, David Dinges, and Allan Pack – Thank you for inviting me to be a part of Penn. I cherish the opportunity to work here and all that can be accomplished as a crew member on this great ship.

To my parents (Edie and Marvin Perlis), my sister and brother (Sue Marx and Jeff Perlis) and my wife and daughter (Ariana and Mia Huberman Perlis) there would be no home port and no crew to sail with … without you.

Michael L. Perlis

I would like to thank Donn Posner and Donna Giles for their mentorship in sleep.

This book is dedicated to my wife, Jill, and our star sleepers, Jake & Zane. They fulfill my life, inspire me and keep me going.

Mark S. Aloia

To my parents (Bob and Gwynne Kuhn), who wisely led me to the path without pushing me down it.

To my girls (wife Tami, and daughters Kelsi, Kristen, and Karlie), who make the path worth walking each day.

To the professors and psychologists who served as mentors and friends (Ken Nikels, Bill Wozniak, Dan and Cheryl McNeil, Frank Collins, Stan Shoemaker, Joe Evans, Keith Allen and Bill Warzak among others). Thank you for helping me carve my career path and for showing me the behavioral way.

Finally, thank you Meg Floress and Brandy Roane for assisting me in reviewing and editing the chapters for this book.

Brett R. Kuhn

Contents

Contributors

Mark S. Aloia, National Jewish Health, Division of Psychosocial Medicine, Denver, CO

Delwyn Bartlett, Medical Psychology, Sleep & Circadian Group, Woolcock Institute of Medical Research, Glebe, and University of Sydney, NSW, Australia

Lynda Bélanger, Université Laval, Québec City, Canada

Richard R. Bootzin, Departments of Psychology and Psychiatry; Sleep Research Laboratory; and Insomnia Clinic, Arizona Health Sciences Center; University of Arizona, Tucson, AZ, USA

Helen J. Burgess, Biological Rhythms Research Laboratory, Rush University Medical Center, Chicago, IL, USA

Daniel J. Buysse, Department of Psychiatry, University of Pittsburgh School of Medicine, Pittsburgh, PA, USA

Kelly Byars, Department of Clinical Psychology, Cincinnati Children's Hospital Medical Center, Cincinnati, OH, USA

Edward R. Christophersen, University of Missouri at Kansas City School of Medicine and Staff Psychologist, Children's Mercy Hospital and Clinics, Kansas, MO, USA

Shannon L. O'Connor Christian, National Jewish Health, Division of Psychosocial Medicine, Denver, CO, USA

Ronald E. Dahl, Department of Psychology, University of Pittsburgh, Pittsburgh, PA

Robert Didden, Behavioural Science Institute/Department of Special Education, Radboud University, Nijmegen, The Netherlands

Jack D. Edinger, Department of Veterans Affairs, Medical Center and Duke University Medical Center, Durham, NC, USA

Polina Eidelman, Golden Bear Sleep and Mood Research Clinic, Psychology Department, University of California, Berkeley, CA, USA

Colin A Espie, University of Glasgow Sleep Centre, Sackler Institute of Psychobiological Research, University of Glasgow, Scotland, UK

Karyn G. France, Health Sciences Centre, University of Canterbury, Christchurch, New Zealand

Patrick C. Friman, Director of Boys Town Center for Behavioral Health, University of Nebraska Medical Center, Boys Town, NE, USA

Phil Gehrman, Department of Psychiatry, University of Pennsylvania, Philadelphia, PA, USA; Center for Sleep and Respiratory Neurobiology, University of Pennsylvania, Philadelpia, PA, USA

Anne Germain, Department of Psychiatry, University of Pittsburgh School of Medicine, Pittsburgh, PA, USA

Paul B. Glovinsky, St Peter's Sleep Center, Washington Avenue Extension, Albany, NY; Cognitive Neuroscience Program, The City College of New York, New York, NY, USA

Melanie A. Gold, Division of Adolescent Medicine, Department of Pediatrics, University of Pittsburgh School of Medicine, Pittsburgh, PA, USA; Student Health Services, Division of Student Affairs, University of Pittsburgh Student Health Service, Pittsburgh, PA, USA

Kathryn Harnett McConahay, Pediatric Associates, Kansas City, MO, USA

Jodie Harris, Adelaide Institute for Sleep Health, Repatriation General Hospital, Adelaide, South Australia

Allison G. Harvey, Golden Bear Sleep and Mood Research Clinic, Psychology Department, University of California, Berkeley, CA, USA

Tiffany Kodak, Department of Pediatrics, Center for Autism Spectrum Disorders, Munroe-Meyer Institute, University of Nebraska Medical Center, Omaha, NE, USA

Barry Krakow, Sleep & Human Health Institute, Maimonides Sleep Arts & Sciences, Ltd, Albuquerque, NM, USA

Brett R. Kuhn, Monroe-Meyer Institute Department of Pediatric Psychology, University of Nebraska Medical Center, Children's Sleep Disorders Center, Omaha, NE, USA

Leon Lack, Department of Psychology, Flinders University, Adelaide, South Australia

Giulio E. Lancioni, Department of Psychology, University of Bari, Bari, Italy

Kenneth L. Lichstein, Department of Psychology, University of Alabama, Tuscaloosa, AL, USA

Rachel Manber, Department of Psychology and Behavioral Sciences, Stanford University, CA, USA

Christina S. McCrae, Department of Clinical Psychology, University of Florida, Gainesville, FL, USA

Susan M. McCurry, Department of Psychosocial and Community Health, University of Washington, Seattle, WA, USA

Melanie K. Means, Department of Veterans Affairs Medical Center and Duke University Medical Center, Durham, NC, USA

Lisa J. Meltzer, Sleep Center, Children's Hospital of Philadelphia, Philadelphia, PA; Department of Pediatrics, University of Pennsylvania School of Medicine, Philadelphia, PA, USA; Department of Pediatrics, National Jewish Health, Denver, CO, USA

William L. Mikulas, Department of Psychology, University of West Florida, Pensacola, FL, USA

Jodi A. Mindell, Department of Psychology, Saint Joseph's University, Philadelphia, PA; Sleep Center, Children's Hospital of Philadelphia, Philadelphia, PA, USA

Charles M. Morin, Université Laval, Québec City, Canada

Arie Oksenberg, Sleep Disorders Unit, Loewenstein Hospital-Rehabilitation Center Raanana, Israel

Jason C. Ong, Johnston R. Bowman Center, Rush University Medical Center, Chicago, IL, USA

Michael L. Perlis, Department of Psychiatry, University of Pennsylvania; Center for Sleep and Respiratory Neurobiology, University of Pennsylvania; School of Nursing, University of Pennsylvania, Philadelphia, PA, USA

Cathleen C. Piazza, Munroe-Meyer Institute and Department of Pediatrics, University of Nebraska Medical Center, Omaha, NE, USA

Donn Posner, Department of Psychiatry, Brown University, Providence, RI; The Sleep Disorders Center of Lifespan Hospitals, Providence, RI, USA

Ann E. Rogers, Emory University, Atlanta, GA, USA

Connie J. Schnoes, Father Flanagan's Boys' Home, Boys Town, NE, USA

Jeff Sigafoos, School of Educational Psychology & Pedagogy, Victoria University of Wellington, Karori, Wellington, New Zealand

Keith J. Slifer, Pediatric Psychology Program, Department of Behavioral Psychology, Kennedy Krieger Institute, Baltimore, MD, USA; Departments of Psychiatry and Behavioral Sciences and Pediatrics, Johns Hopkins University School of Medicine, Baltimore, MD, USA

Arthur J. Spielman, Cognitive Neuroscience Program, The City College of New York, New York, NY; Center for Sleep Disorders Medicine and Research, New York Methodist Hospital, Brooklyn, NY; Center for Sleep Medicine, Weill Cornell Medical College, Cornell University, New York, NY, USA

Carl Stepnowsky, University of California, San Diego, CA; VA San Diego Healthcare System, San Diego, CA, USA

Brian Symon, Kensington Park, Adelaide, South Australia

Lisa Talbot, Golden Bear Sleep and Mood Research Clinic, Psychology Department, University of California, Berkeley, CA, USA

Daniel J. Taylor, Department of Psychology, University of North Texas, Denton, TX, USA

S. Justin Thomas, Department of Psychology, University of Alabama, Tuscaloosa, AL, USA

William J. Warzak, Munroe-Meyer Institute for Genetics and Rehabilitation, Department of Pediatrics, University of Nebraska Medical Center, Omaha, Nebraska, USA

Chien-Ming Yang, Department of Psychology/The Research Center for Mind, Brain, & Learning, National Cheng-Chi University, Taipei, Taiwan

Abbreviations

AASM	American Academy of Sleep Medicine
ADHD	Attention Deficit Hyperactivity Disorder
AHI	Apnea Hypopnea Index
BBTI	Brief Behavioral Treatment of Insomnia
BIC	Behavioral Insomnia of Childhood
BiPAP	Bilevel Positive Airway Pressure
BSM	Behavioral Sleep Medicine
BZRA	Benzodiazepine Receptor Agonist
CBT	Cognitive Behavioral Treatment
CBT-I	Cognitive Behavioral Treatment of Insomnia
CDSMP	Chronic Disease Self-Management Program
COPD	Chronic Obstructive Pulmonary Disease
CPAP	Continuous Positive Airway Pressure
CR	Conditioned Response
CS	Conditioned Stimulus
CT	Cognitive Therapy
DBAS	Dysfunctional Beliefs and Attitudes about Sleep
EBT	Evidence-Based psychological Treatments
ED	Education
EEG	Electroencephalography
EMD	Excuse-Me Drill
EXT	Extinction
GERD	Gastroesophageal reflux disease
GSES	Glasgow Sleep Effort Scale
ICSD-2	International Classification of Sleep Disorders, 2nd edition
IRT	Imagery Rehearsal Therapy
ISI	Insomnia Severity Index
ISR	Intensive Sleep Retraining
MBSR	Mindfulness-Based Stress Reduction Program
MBTI	Mindfulness-Based Therapy for Insomnia
MET	Motivational Enhancement Therapy
MI	Motivational Interviewing
MR	Mental Retardation
MSLT	Multiple Sleep Latency Test
NIH	National Institute of Health
NREM	Non-Rapid Eye Movement
OSA	Obstructive Sleep Apnea

PAP	Positive Airway Pressure
PERB	Post-Extinction Response Burst
PI	Paradoxical Intention
PLM index	Periodic Limb Movement Index
PMR	Progressive Muscle Relaxation
PSG	Polysomnography
PSQI	Pittsburgh Sleep Quality Index
PTSD	Post-Traumatic Stress Disorder
RCT	Randomized Controlled Trial
REM	Rapid Eye Movement
SA	Scheduled Awakenings
SAMI	Sleep Associated Monitoring Index
SASMP	Sleep Apnea Self-Management Program
SBSM	Society of Behavioral Sleep Medicine
SC	Standard Care
SCT	Stimulus Control Therapy
SE	Sleep Efficiency
SHEP	Shoulder-Head Elevation Pillow
SHI	Sleep Hygiene Index
SIDS	Sudden Infant Death Syndrome
SL	Sleep Latency
SOA	Sleep Onset Association
SOL	Sleep Onset Latency
SRBQ	Sleep-Related Behaviours Questionnaire
SRT	Sleep Restriction Therapy
SSS	Stanford Sleepiness Scale
ST	Sleep Terrors
STQ	Sleep Timing Questionnaire
SW	Sleepwalking
TASB	Thoracic Anti-Supine Band
TIB	Time in Bed
T_{min}	Core body temperature rhythm minimum
TST	Total Sleep Time
UCR	Unconditioned Response
UCS	Unconditioned Stimulus
WASO	Wake After Sleep Onset

Introduction

Michael L. Perlis
Department of Psychiatry and Nursing, University of Pennsylvania School of Medicine, Philadelphia, PA

Mark S. Aloia
National Jewish Health, Division of Psychosocial Medicine, Denver, CO

Brett R. Kuhn
Behavioral Sleep Medicine Services, Children's Sleep Disorders Center, Children's Hospital & Medical Center, Omaha, NE

Over the past two to three decades there has been a proliferation of Behavioral Sleep Medicine (BSM) treatment regimens. While the best known, and best validated, BSM treatments are those that serve as the core interventions for Cognitive Behavioral Therapy for Insomnia (i.e., CBT-I: Stimulus Control, Sleep Restriction, and Sleep Hygiene), there are literally dozens of new and established non-pharmacologic interventions for virtually all of the major sleep disorders.

One of the major obstacles to the widespread dissemination and implementation of these interventions is that the details of the protocols themselves tend to be known, and researched by, only behavioral sleep experts. Thus, the major impetus for this textbook was to bring together in one text all of the major BSM interventions and to provide this information in the most straightforward manner possible.

Each chapter within this volume utilizes a common format including the following components:

Protocol name (e.g., SRT)
Gross indication (e.g., Insomnia)
Specific indications (e.g., type of DX or subtype)
Contraindications
Rationale for intervention
Step-by-step description of procedures (How to)
Possible modifications/variants
Proof of concept/supporting data/evidence base
Recommended reading

The content of this book is intended to be informative for at least three groups of readers:

1. Practicing Behavioral Sleep Medicine clinicians who wish to extend their current practices to include part or all of the full spectrum of available BSM treatments
2. Clinicians and clinical students from other fields who wish to begin the process of incorporating BSM interventions in to their practices
3. Clinical researchers who require basic protocol descriptions to conduct efficacy, effectiveness, and/or comparative studies on BSM interventions.

For the first two groups of would-be "end users" we strongly suggest that training in this area works best using an apprenticeship model, and accordingly recommend that a series of mentored or peer-supervised experiences be used to augment the materials presented in this manual. For individuals within established BSM programs, arranging for mentorship and peer supervision may be easily accomplished. For community-based clinicians, arranging for mentorship and peer supervision may be be more challenging, but can likely be accomplished by telephone consultation with established Behavioral Sleep Medicine specialists.

Finally, it is our hope that this book is of substantial interest to the behavioral therapists who, while regularly confronted with patients who have sleep disorders, do not have formal training in Sleep Medicine. To these individuals, we would encourage you to gain a passing familiarity with the foundational knowledge that can be gained from the following texts:

Principles & Practice of Sleep Medicine (M. Kryger, R. Roth & Dement, eds), 4th edn. Elsevier Saunders Co., Philadelphia, PA, 2005.
Sleep Disorders Medicine (S. Chokroverty, ed.), 2nd edn. Butterworth-Heinemann, Boston, MA, 1999.

The courses, webinars, and slide sets that are made available by the American Academy of Sleep Medicine (AASM, www.aasmnet.org) and the newly formed Society of Behavioral Sleep Medicine (SBSM, www.sbsm-net.org) may also be found to be useful educational tools.

We hope you find this book useful, and better yet, enjoyable.

One final note: this manual is intended to be narrowly focused on the provision of Behavioral Sleep Medicine interventions. The text should not be used as a guide for "self help" or by clinicians without the proper background training, and/or without the proper consultation from individuals with a dedicated expertise in Sleep Medicine and Behavioral Therapy.

Part I

BSM Treatment Protocols for Insomia

Introduction

Michael L. Perlis
Department of Psychiatry and Nursing, University of Pennsylvania School of Medicine, Philadelphia, PA

Though Behavioral Sleep Medicine as a field is in its infancy (perhaps more accurately "in gestation") [1–3], the state of the science with respect to insomnia might be best likened to the fourth decade of life: the organism is fully mature but much remains to be learned, said, and done.

With respect to the maturity of the insomnia area, at this point in time there is a well-defined infrastructure that includes (1) a variety of conceptual models, (2) standardized definitions, (3) a general approach to assessment, (4) well-established therapies that are evidence based (with respect to both efficacy and effectiveness), (5) published treatment manuals and courses available for treatment dissemination and implementation, and (6) a new generation of treatments that hold the promise of even better clinical outcomes than those obtained presently. These issues are briefly reviewed below, followed by a short commentary about future directions for the insomnia field.

STATE OF THE SCIENCE

Conceptual Models

This aspect of behavioral sleep medicine is perhaps the most developed, starting with, in the early era sleep research and sleep medicine (1970s and 1980s), the Bootzin Stimulus Control Perspective [4] and the Spielman Three Factor Model [5]. Since the 1990s there has been a proliferation of theoretical perspectives on the etiology and pathophysiology of insomnia that includes ten human models and three animal models [6]. Taken together, these perspectives provide a rich panoramic view of the factors that (1) may serve to "predispose, precipitate, and perpetuate" insomnia as a disorder, (2) may account for the efficacy of the current treatment modalities, and/or (3) may serve as targets for the development of new therapies.

Standardized Definitions

Insomnia is, without a doubt, the first of the sleep disorders to be described as either a symptom or a disease. References to this form of sleeplessness may be found in the oldest documents known to man, including *The Iliad*, *The Epic of Gilgamesh*, the *Torah*, the *New Testament* and the *Koran*. Presently, insomnia is described in each of the major nosologies that define human disease and mental illness, including the ICD-9, DSM-IV-TR, and the ICSD-2. These diagnostic classifications have been augmented with the delineation of formal research diagnostic criteria [7]. Perhaps the most significant accomplishment within this area in recent times has been the effort to challenge the validity and utility of the diagnostic classifications of "primary and secondary" insomnia [8,9]. At this juncture, many appear ready to doff the concept of "secondary" insomnia in favor of the concept of "comorbid" insomnia.

Standardized Assessment Methods

What exists presently is the general agreement that:

- prospective assessment with sleep diaries is required;
- an evaluation of depressive and anxiety disorders is necessary;
- it may be helpful to retrospectively assess insomnia severity (e.g., the ISI), and insomnia timing and frequency (e.g., the TPQ [10]); and
- it may be useful to assess the factors that are thought to moderate, if not mediate, illness severity, including such factors as sleep hygiene infractions (e.g., the SHI [11]), dysfunctional beliefs about sleep (e.g., the DBAS [12]), sleep effort (e.g. the GSES [13]), and the selective attention to sleep "threats" (e.g., the SAMI [14]).

Efficacy and Effectiveness Data

Most would agree that the first case series studies, if not full-blown clinical trials, occurred in the 1930s as tests of the efficacy of progressive muscle relaxation (PMR). Since that time approximately 200 trials have been conducted on either single interventions (Stimulus Control, PMR, and Sleep Restriction) or multicomponent interventions that may be characterized as Cognitive Behavioral Therapy for Insomnia (or CBT-I). This extensive literature has been quantitatively summarized using meta-analytic statistics on at least three occasions [15–17], and there is at least one comparative meta-analysis that evaluates the relative efficacy of CBT-I as compared to benzodiazepine receptor agonists (BZRAs) [18]. The data from this literature suggest, consistent with the conclusions of the NIH State of the Science Conference [19], that (1) CBT-I is highly efficacious, (2) BZRAs and CBT-I produce comparable outcomes in the short term, and (3) CBT-I appears to have more durable effects when active treatment is discontinued.

Beyond the issue of efficacy is the issue of effectiveness. That is, are the clinical outcomes observed in clinical trials comparable to investigations of treatment outcome in (1) patients with insomnia comorbid with other medical and/or psychiatric illnesses (e.g., Edinger, Savard, Currie, Jungquist, Lichstein, and their colleagues [20–25]), and/or (2) studies of patients who are treated in clinical care settings (e.g., Perlis and colleagues [26,27])? To date there have been more than 20 studies in patient samples who suffer such co-morbidities as cancer, chronic pain, depression, and PTSD. The data from these studies not only show CBT-I to be effective, but also show that the clinical outcomes are, by and large, comparable to those found with patients with primary insomnia. In some cases, the effects are actually larger [21,24]. As noted above, there has also been a variety of clinical case series studies. The effect sizes for these studies also appear comparable to those obtained in randomized clinical trials. Taken together, these findings clearly suggest that CBT-I is more than ready for mass dissemination and implementation.

Treatment Dissemination and Implementation

Significant advances have been made in recent years within this domain, particularly with respect to the issues of training and credentialing. First, there are at least three published treatment manuals that delineate how to conduct CBT-I [28–30]. Second, there are several multi-day courses that are available on an annual or biannual basis. One such course, which is largely an introduction to Behavioral Sleep Medicine, has been available through the American Academy of Sleep Medicine (AASM) since 2004, and will continue to be available through the newly formed Society of Behavioral Sleep Medicine (SBSM) for the foreseeable future; another such course, which is a dedicated training seminar in CBT-I, has been offered annually since 2006 through the University of Rochester, and is currently offered through the University of Pennsylvania. Third, in 2005 and 2006 the BSM committee of the AASM established training opportunities via the credentialing of BSM fellowships and mini fellowships. Fourth, as result of the vision and generosity of the AASM, there is (as of 2004) a credentialing board for BSM that is underwritten by the academy and administered by the American Board of Sleep Medicine.

New Treatments

In recent years, there has been a substantial resurgence in the effort to develop new treatments. In many ways, it is this spirit and the fruits of these labors that give rise to the impetus for this book: the need to collect into one place a description of each of the procedures that not only comprise CBT-I but also the therapies that have recently been developed. With respect to insomnia, these new therapies include the following:

1. The use of bright light as adjuvant therapy (see Chapter 17)
2. Sleep re-training (see Chapter 13)
3. Utilization of cognitive therapy including behavioral experiments to treat dysfunctional beliefs and safety behaviors (see Chapters 7–10)
4. Adaptation of cognitive therapy for catastrophic thinking from exercises intended for patients with anxiety disorders to patients with insomnia (see Chapter 12)
5. Application of mindfulness and meditation as methods to enhance coping with insomnia (see Chapters 4 and 14).

FUTURE DIRECTIONS

While much has been accomplished, there can be no question that much remains to be done.

Conceptual Models

The existing theories need to be put to the test with experiments that allow for falsification. The animal models need to be assessed for their validity (although less so, ironic as it may be, for the *Drosophila* model [6,31]). New animal models need to be developed that focus on the factors delineated in the human models and, conversely, findings from animal models need to be examined in human models.

Standardized Definitions

The existing nosologies need to be critically evaluated so as to allow for proper phenotyping of the disorder. Such an effort will require a thoroughgoing assessment of the validity and utility of the existing insomnia types (e.g., psychophysiologic insomnia, paradoxical insomnia, idiopathic insomnia), subtypes (e.g., early, middle and late insomnia), and whether the phenomenon of non-restorative sleep in the absence of problems initiating and maintaining sleep should be considered a form of insomnia. Further, an empirical assessment needs to be conducted not only on the distinction between acute and chronic insomnia but also on the other clinical characteristics of the disorder (with an eye towards establishing quantitative criteria), including illness frequency, duration and severity.

Standardized Assessment Methods

Perhaps the best single effort to accomplish the task of standardizing the assessment of insomnia (at least for research purposes) was undertaken at the 2005

Pittsburgh Consensus Conference [32]. The recommendations from this conference, though very useful, have not been adopted as "the standard" for clinical practice by either the AASM or the SBSM. Revisiting the findings from this conference will represent an ideal point of departure towards the identification of minimum standards for assessment for the initial evaluation process, progress over the course of therapy, and for the determination of pre-post change.

Efficacy and Effectiveness Data

The established therapies (primarily CBT-I) need to be evaluated in deconstruction studies to determine what components are maximally effective (in general) and for whom (for each of the types and subtypes of insomnia). Studies are also needed to test the effectiveness of CBT-I in "real world" conditions in terms of different provider types (e.g. psychologist, physician, nurse practitioner), settings (e.g., sleep disorders center, private practice), and patient types (e.g. the full range of comorbidities).

Treatment Dissemination and Implementation

One of the major challenges for the field, though perhaps developmentally appropriate, is the problem of how to disseminate and implement CBT-I at the national and international levels. That is, how does one go about (1) making the public aware of the CBT-I treatment option, (2) making the relevant professional disciplines aware of CBT-I as a treatment option, and (3) putting into place the requisite training and credentialing processes? These represent truly daunting questions, and are currently the major focus of the SBSM.

New Treatments

In general, CBT-I produces about a 50 percent reduction in sleep initiation and maintenance problems [15–18]. Though this represents a powerful clinical effect (the corresponding effect sizes ranging from 0.46 (TST) to 1.05/1.03 (SL and WASO respectively)), it also clearly indicates that work remains to be done [33], and in at least one of two ways. First, strategies need to be developed that extend the average treatment response to more patients. Second, adjuvant therapies need to be developed to boost clinical outcomes to the next level where a large percentage of patients reach remission and/or recovery. To date, research and development has focused primarily on the latter proposition, and includes several of the protocols delineated in the present volume.

In sum, we hope this brief review has been helpful in setting a context for the therapies detailed in this section.

REFERENCES

[1] E.J. Stepanski, Perlis ML, Behavioral sleep medicine. An emerging subspecialty in health psychology and sleep medicine, J. Psychosom Res. 49 (2000) 343–347.

[2] M. Perlis, M.T. Smith, How can we make CBT-I and other BSM services widely available? Clin. Sleep Med. 4 (1) (2008) 11–13.

[3] W. Pigeon, V.M. Crabtree, M. Scherer, The future of behavioral sleep medicine, Clin. Sleep Med. 3 (1) (2008) 73–79.

[4] Bootzin R.R. Stimulus control treatment for insomnia. Proceedings, 80th Annual Convention, APA 1972;395–396.

[5] A Spielman, L. Caruso, A behavioral perspective, Psychiatr. Clin. North Am. (1987).

[6] M. Perlis, P.J. Shaw, G. Cano, C.A. Espie, Models of insomnia, in: M. Kryger, T. Roth, W.C. Dement, (Eds.), Principles and Practice of Sleep Medicine, Saunders-Elsevier, Philadelphia, PA, 2010 TBA.

[7] J.D. Edinger, M.H. Bonnet, R.R. Bootzin, et al., Derivation of research diagnostic criteria for insomnia: report of an American Academy of Sleep Medicine Work Group, Sleep 27 (2004) 1567–1596.

[8] C.S. McCrae, K.L. Lichstein, Secondary insomnia: diagnostic challenges and intervention opportunities, Sleep Med. Rev. 5 (2001) 47–61.

[9] K.L. Lichstein, Secondary insomnia: a myth dismissed, Sleep Med. Rev. 10 (2006) 3–5.

[10] T.H. Monk, D.J. Buysse, K.S. Kennedy, et al., Measuring sleep habits without using a diary: the sleep timing questionnaire, Sleep 26 (2003) 208–212.

[11] D.F. Mastin, J. Bryson, R. Corwyn, Assessment of sleep hygiene using the Sleep Hygiene Index, J. Behav. Med. 29 (2006) 223–227.

[12] C.M. Morin, J. Stone, D. Trinkle, et al., Dysfunctional beliefs and attitudes about sleep among older adults with and without insomnia complaints, Psychol. Aging 8 (1993) 463–467.

[13] N.M. Broomfield, C.A. Espie, Toward a valid, reliable measure of sleep effort, J. Sleep Res. (2010) in press.

[14] C.N. Semler, A.G. Harvey, Monitoring for sleep-related threat: a pilot study of the Sleep Associated Monitoring Index (SAMI), Psychosom. Med. 66 (2004) 242–250.

[15] M.R. Irwin, J.C. Cole, P.M. Nicassio, Comparative meta-analysis of behavioral interventions for insomnia and their efficacy in middle-aged adults and in older adults 55+ years of age, Health Psychol. 25 (2006) 3–14.

[16] C.M. Morin, J.P. Culbert, S.M. Schwartz, Nonpharmacological interventions for insomnia: a meta-analysis of treatment efficacy, Am. J. Psychiatry 151 (1994) 1172–1180.

[17] D.R. Murtagh, K.M. Greenwood, Identifying effective psychological treatments for insomnia: a meta-analysis, J. Consult. Clin. Psychol. 63 (1995) 79–89.

[18] M.T. Smith, M.L. Perlis, A. Park, et al., Behavioral treatment vs pharmacotherapy for insomnia – a comparative meta-analysis, Am. J. Psychiatry 159 (2002) 5–11.

[19] NIH State-of-the-Science Conference Statement on Manifestations and Management of Chronic Insomnia in Adults, 2005.

[20] J.D. Edinger, M.K. Olsen, K.M. Stechuchak, et al., Cognitive behavioral therapy for patients with primary insomnia or insomnia associated predominantly with mixed psychiatric disorders: a randomized clinical trial, Sleep 32 (2009) 499–510.

[21] J. Savard, S. Simard, H. Ivers, C.M. Morin, A randomized study on the efficacy of cognitive-behavioral therapy for insomnia secondary to breast cancer: i – sleep and psychological effects, J. Clin. Oncol. 23 (2005) 6083–6096.

[22] S.R. Currie, K.G. Wilson, A.J. Pontefract, L. deLaplante, Cognitive-behavioral treatment of insomnia secondary to chronic pain, J. Consult. Clin. Psychol. 68 (2000) 407–416.

[23] J.D. Edinger, W.K. Wohlgemuth, A.D. Krystal, J.R. Rice, Behavioral insomnia therapy for fibromyalgia patients – a randomized clinical trial, Arch. Intern. Med. 165 (2005) 2527–2535.

[24] C.R. Jungquist, C. O'Brien, S. Matteson-Rusby, et al., The efficacy of cognitive-behavioral therapy for insomnia in patients with chronic pain, Sleep Med. 11 (2010) 302–309.
[25] K.L. Lichstein, N.M. Wilson, C.T. Johnson, Psychological treatment of secondary insomnia, Psychol. Aging 15 (2000) 232–240.
[26] M. Perlis, M. Aloia, A. Millikan, et al., Behavioral treatment of insomnia: a clinical case series study, J. Behav. Med. 23 (2000) 149–161.
[27] M.L. Perlis, M. Sharpe, M.T. Smith, et al., Behavioral treatment of insomnia: treatment outcome and the relevance of medical and psychiatric morbidity, J. Behav. Med. 24 (2001) 281–296.
[28] J. Edinger, C.E. Carney, Overcoming Insomnia: A Cognitive-Behavioral Therapy Approach Therapist Guide, Oxford University Press, New York, NY, 2008.
[29] C.M. Morin, C.A. Espie, Insomnia: A Clinician's Guide to Assessment and Treatment, Springer, Philadelphia, PA, 2003.
[30] M. Perlis, C. Jungquist, M.T. Smith, D. Posner, The Cognitive Behavioral Treatment of Insomnia: A Treatment Manual, Springer, New York, NY, 2005.
[31] L. Seugnet, Y. Suzuki, M. Thimgan, et al., Identifying sleep regulatory genes using a *Drosophila* model of insomnia, J. Neurosci. 29 (2009) 7148–7157.
[32] D.J. Buysse, S. Ancoli-Israel, J.D. Edinger, et al., Recommendations for a standard research assessment of insomnia, Sleep 29 (2006) 1155–1173.
[33] A.G. Harvey, N.K.J. Tang, Cognitive behaviour therapy for insomnia: Can we rest yet? Sleep. Med. Rev. 7 (2003) 237–262.

Chapter 1

Sleep Restriction Therapy

Arthur J. Spielman
Cognitive Neuroscience Program, The City College of New York, New York, NY
Center for Sleep Disorders Medicine and Research, New York Methodist Hospital, Brooklyn, NY
Center for Sleep Medicine, Weill Cornell Medical College, Cornell University, New York, NY

Chien-Ming Yang
Department of Psychology/The Research Center for Mind, Brain, & Learning, National Cheng-Chi University, Taipei, Taiwan

Paul B. Glovinsky
St Peter's Sleep Center, Washington Avenue Extension, Albany, NY
Cognitive Neuroscience Program, The City College of New York, New York, NY

PROTOCOL NAME

Sleep Restriction Therapy (SRT).

GROSS INDICATION

Sleep restriction therapy is indicated for the treatment of insomnia, including trouble sleeping during the beginning, middle or end of the time spent in bed [1].

SPECIFIC INDICATION

SRT is indicated for sleep difficulties in which the subjective sleep efficiency (sleep time/time in bed × 100%), based on a 1- to 2-week sleep log or retrospective report, is less than 85 percent (or less than 80 percent in older individuals).

There are also individuals who exhibit relatively high sleep efficiency and yet remain amenable to SRT. For example, there are those who do not get enough sleep on weekdays because they wake up too early. Having learned through experience that if they do resume sleep, it will be right before their alarms ring, they just end the night and get out of bed after, say, 5 hours. However, on non-workdays these individuals tend to stay in bed long enough to fall back asleep and sleep late into the day. Averaged across the entire week their sleep efficiency may still be above 85 percent; nonetheless, such sleepers can benefit from SRT.

Behavioral Treatments for Sleep Disorders. DOI: 10.1016/B978-0-12-381522-4.00001-8

There is no systematic evidence that SRT is the treatment of choice for a particular insomnia diagnosis (e.g., psychophysiologic vs idiopathic vs paradoxical insomnia).

CONTRAINDICATIONS

The increased sleep propensity produced by SRT (especially at the start of treatment) will make patients sleepy. Therefore, individuals who need to maintain optimal vigilance to avoid serious accidents should not engage in SRT. For example, long-haul truck drivers, long-distance bus drivers, air traffic controllers, operators of heavy machinery, and some assembly-line workers would be placed at unacceptably increased risk because of the sleepiness produced by SRT. Similarly, individuals with conditions that are exacerbated by sleepiness or deep sleep, such as epilepsy, parasomnias, and sleep disordered breathing, should not engage in SRT.

Individuals who fall asleep quickly and have short, compact sleep prior to a terminal early morning awakening (even on non-workdays and holidays) are unlikely to benefit from SRT. In these cases restricting time in bed will (1) not reduce sleep latency, (2) not reduce the number or duration of awakenings, and (3) not likely increase the duration of sleep. Judgment will be necessary when patients report that they stay in bed "completely awake" just to rest. The ability to perceive sleep is imperfect (sometimes to a significant degree, as in paradoxical insomnia, previously called sleep-state misperception), and individuals may be unaware that they are getting some sleep after the major sleep period. In cases where some light or unappreciated sleep does occur at the end of the night, SRT may be of benefit.

Some individuals may be very sensitive to the side effects of SRT and therefore find the restrictions too demanding. Intolerance may develop to even a short period of fatigue, sleepiness, memory impairment, irritability, or diminished concentration. Despite the likelihood of improved sleep depth and efficiency at the start of SRT, this intolerance of daytime deficits may preclude adherence to SRT for a sufficient duration to consolidate gains.

RATIONALE FOR INTERVENTION

One of the most reliable ways to strengthen the homeostatic sleep drive and thereby increase the propensity for sleep during upcoming nights is to limit the amount of sleep currently being accumulated [2,3]. Restricting time in bed over a number of nights is a simple way to limit sleep accumulation. Sleep restriction also redresses such indicators of poor sleep as elevated amounts of light Stage N1 sleep, prolonged sleep latencies, and excessive wakefulness after sleep onset. Rapid sleep onset and a well-consolidated night of quality sleep, core goals of insomnia treatment, are achieved rapidly and reliably at the start of SRT. However, other treatment objectives are deferred, such as accruing sufficient sleep to function well during the day. As treatment proceeds through adjustments in time in bed, a balance is sought whereby better daytime functioning is restored while sufficient sleep quality is maintained.

According to the 3P model of insomnia [4,5], behavioral practices and cognitive tendencies that perpetuate sleep disturbance are often the most promising targets for intervention. Many of these perpetuating factors, such as spending too much time in bed, anticipatory anxiety about the prospects for sleep, and inordinate concern about daytime performance deficits, are addressed by SRT. As noted above, SRT quickly changes the experience of insomnia, replacing sleep that has been haphazard and light with deeper, more consolidated sleep. There is little doubt that it is an "active treatment," even if it does have significant side effects. Patients can rest assured that their sleep problem is being addressed, and this translates into less worry about what the night will bring. While they can no longer expect a luxuriously long night of sleep, there is also less likelihood of virtually sleepless nights. Patients learn that they can at least muddle through the day on what sleep they reliably accumulate, lowering the stakes regarding sleep loss. Finally, hyperarousal (whether a trait-like predisposing factor or reactive to events) is directly dampened by sleep loss.

Another reason SRT is effective is that it tightens regulatory control of sleep by the endogenous circadian pacemaker. Patients with chronic insomnia often display widely varying times of retiring to and rising from bed, with consequent variability in the timing of light exposure, social interaction, physical activity, and other stimuli that entrain the circadian system. The output of the endogenous oscillator is weakened as it continually responds to these shifting patterns, leading in turn to increased variability in the propensity to fall asleep and wake up. By closely regulating the time of "lights out" and "lights on" SRT gradually returns sleep regulation to effective circadian control, resulting in more reliably timed phases of sleep and wakefulness.

STEP BY STEP DESCRIPTION OF PROCEDURES

In the original SRT study we followed a rigid protocol with few procedures [1]. After a 2-week sleep log we set the initial TIB equal to the average estimated sleep time. Regardless of reported sleep time, no individuals were assigned less than 4 hours and 30 minutes of TIB. Time to get up in the morning was set to the time subjects needed to be up on work days. Based on information provided to a telephone answering machine for 8 weeks, a 5-day window was analyzed for sleep efficiency and changes were made to TIB according to the following rules:

- If SE was ≥90 percent (85 percent in seniors), TIB was increased by 15 minutes
- If SE was <85 percent (80 percent in seniors), TIB was decreased to the average estimated sleep time
- If TIB was between 85 and <90 percent, no changes were made

- In addition, subjects were not permitted to lie down or nap at times other than the assigned TIB.

We have modified our approach to SRT, as will be detailed below, for the following reasons. In order to limit the sleep deprivation at the start of treatment, we set the lower limit of TIB at 5 hours and allow for a 30-minute increase in TIB to quickly forestall severe sleepiness. To promote the most and best quality sleep at the start of treatment, we no longer set the wake-up time no later than the earliest time subjects need to be up (usually for work) on any day of the week. As will be seen in the examples below (see I, Example 3), the timing of the sleep period now takes into account the time of the night when sleep is the most likely to be experienced as deep and refreshing. In later clinical applications we did not end treatment after 8 weeks but when TIB is sufficient to sustain daytime functional capacity without leaving the individual too vulnerable to a recurrence of insomnia (see III below).

Initiation of SRT

SRT begins by estimating three key features of sleep: (1) typical sleep duration; (2) workday wake-up time; and (3) the portion of the night likely to contain the best sleep. These features are best assessed via a representative 1- to 2-week graphic sleep diary (by averaging estimated total sleep times and logged workday wake-up times, and perusal of the patterning of sleep segments within a night) along with a clinical interview. TIB at the start of treatment is set equal to the average sleep duration. (The minimum amount of TIB should not be less than 5 hours.) Wake-up time on SRT should be no later than the average logged workday wake-up time. However, the specific bedtime period assigned will depend on the individual's sleep pattern. If, for example, a patient's verbal report and sleep log show that the best sleep is obtained in the first two-thirds of the night, with erratic sleep thereafter, the assigned wake-up time should be earlier than the average logged workday wake-up time.

Example 1

For example, the 1-week sleep diary reveals the following:

Average bedtime to rising time	11 pm to 6:30 am
Average TIB	7 hours and 30 minutes
Average sleep latency	15 minutes
Average nightly sleep time	5 hours and 45 minutes
Average workday wake-up time	6:15 am

The latter 2 hours of sleep are described as "light" and interrupted frequently on the log.

The SRT prescription for the initial sleep schedule is as follows:

Allowed TIB	5 hours and 45 minutes
Bedtime	11 pm
Wake-up time	4:45 am, 7 days per week

The patient is asked to continue logging sleep on the new schedule and follow-up in 1 week. The prescribed TIB, 5 hours and 45 minutes, is determined from the calculated average nightly sleep time. The decision to have the patient wake-up at 4:45 am is based on the report of poor sleep in the latter 2 hours of the night.

Example 2

Suppose the sleep latency in the above example had been 1 hour and 15 minutes, with 30 minutes of wakefulness after sleep onset typically distributed in two awakenings. The initial SRT sleep schedule would then be:

Allowed TIB	5 hours and 45 minutes
Bedtime	12:30 am
Wake-up time	6:15am, 7 days per week

In this case, TIB is assigned later in the night to reduce sleep onset latency. Wake-up time on SRT is set equal to the average workday wake-up time; working back 5 hours and 45 minutes yielded the assigned bedtime.

Example 3

Suppose the sleep log in the above examples revealed wakefulness interspersed fairly evenly throughout the night, with a moderately long sleep latency of 35 minutes, a couple of awakenings of 15–20 minutes' duration, and a terminal awakening of about 30 minutes. The initial SRT sleep schedule would then be:

Allowed TIB	5 hours and 45 minutes
Bedtime	12:00 am
Wake-up time	5:45 am

Now, the nightly average of 1 hour and 45 minutes of wakefulness in bed (calculated from the sleep log) is addressed by assigning both a later bedtime and an earlier wake-up time, with the aim of consolidating sleep in between.

SRT Procedures During the "Middle Phase" of Treatment

According to the standard SRT procedure, sleep efficiency (SE) is calculated each week from a sleep diary:

- If SE is ≥90 percent, then TIB is increased by 15 or 30 minutes. The clinician/researcher uses judgment (or a rule) to decide on whether TIB is increased by 15 or 30 minutes. In older individuals, the SE cut point for increasing TIB is ≥85 percent.
- If SE is between 85 percent and <90 percent, then TIB is not changed. (In older individuals, the range is between 80 percent and <85 percent.)
- If SE is <85 percent, then TIB is reduced by 15 or 30 minutes. (In older individuals, the cut point is <80 percent.)

Example 4

A 74-year-old woman presents with sleep maintenance insomnia. Her 2-week sleep log shows accumulation of an average of 6 hours of sleep within an average TIB of 8 hours and 30 minutes. She is started on SRT, with bedtime set between midnight and 6 am. She returns with a 1-week sleep log showing an average subjective sleep time of 5 hours and 15 minutes, with relatively short sleep latencies but a persistent tendency to awaken too early in the morning. Her new assigned SRT sleep schedule would be:

Allowed TIB	6 hours and 15 minutes
Bedtime	11:45 pm
Wake-up time	6:00 am

This elderly patient's sleep efficiency of 87.5 percent (5.25/6.00 × 100%) qualifies her for an extra 15 minutes of sleep, which were added to the beginning of the night given that she has more difficulty maintaining sleep toward morning.

In cases of paradoxical insomnia, patients may report very limited sleep time – for example, 3 hours per night on average. As SRT does not permit reduction of TIB below 5 hours, these patients may not progress in SRT. A decision must be made in such cases to persist with TIB set at 5 hours or to discontinue SRT.

Completing SRT

We have previously shown that SRT is amenable to analysis within a cost/benefits model [6]. This model is useful in determining when to end treatment. Maximizing sleep efficiency cannot be the sole endpoint, since sleep efficiency will tend to be highest when time in bed is cut to the prescribed minimum of 5 hours, yielding very sleepy and likely noncompliant patients. In our model, satisfying nocturnal sleep and good daytime functioning are seen as primary "benefits" whereas the time spent in bed in order to accumulate sleep and vulnerability to insomnia are "costs".

Prior to treatment, costs are high and benefits low, in that patients are spending a lot of time in bed, only to garner broken, unreliable and non-refreshing sleep. Daytime functioning is poor, marred not only by the effects of sleep loss but also by anticipatory anxiety over what the next night will bring. At the start of SRT there is a dramatic lowering of costs, as much less time is spent in bed, and susceptibility to very poor nights of sleep is reduced due to an increased homeostatic sleep drive. There is often a concurrent reduction in benefits, however, in that typically less sleep is accumulated, leading to increased sleepiness and deficits in mood, attention, and other aspects of daytime functioning.

As treatment progresses, there is generally an increase in both costs and benefits (e.g., less time is spent in bed, but more sleep is obtained, with only slightly increased susceptibility to insomnia). The increase in benefits rises at a greater rate than the increase in costs. As the titration proceeds, a point of maximal net benefit is reached. Time in bed is restricted enough to maintain a reliable pattern of well-consolidated sleep, but not so much as to yield significant daytime deficits.

This is the desired endpoint of treatment, and the schedule the patient should strive to maintain on his or her own. If time in bed were to be further increased – perhaps approaching its baseline value – there would likely not be much additional benefit in terms of extra sleep, since the bulk of the patient's homeostatic sleep need has now been addressed, whereas the risk of reintroducing variable, broken sleep would be elevated.

Example 5

The 74-year-old woman introduced in Example 4 qualified for three additional 15-minute increments to TIB, which were added to the beginning of the night to yield the following SRT schedule:

Allowed TIB	7 hours
Bedtime	11:00 pm
Wake-up time	6:00 am

Subsequent logs showed estimated sleep time hovering near 5 hours and 45 minutes, yielding sleep efficiencies between 80 percent and 85 percent and therefore not qualifying for either an increase or a decrease in time in bed. The patient reported good daytime functioning. She was getting nearly as much sleep as prior to treatment, but in a much more efficient and predictable manner, with less worry about what would happen each night. Therefore, SRT was ended, and she was advised to maintain an 11 pm to 6 am bedtime schedule going forward.

POSSIBLE MODIFICATIONS/VARIANTS

Investigators and clinicians have modified the original SRT procedure or created treatments that share essential features with SRT. The initial prescribed TIB in the SRT approach may be experienced by the patient as a severe deprivation and result in significant daytime sleepiness. In addition, given that sleep efficiency is rarely 100 percent, the initial TIB prescribed within SRT introduces some degree of sleep deprivation. One modification of the SRT procedure that takes this into account sets the initial TIB equal to the average amount of sleep reported plus 30 minutes [7]. This is a sensible and modest change to SRT; it eases the patient into a restricted bedtime schedule. Similarly, allowing or prescribing a daytime nap has been used to limit daytime sleepiness at the start of treatment [8]. Another change from the original SRT procedure that we wholeheartedly endorse is basing all changes in TIB on 7 days of data rather than the 5 days used in the original study.

Another approach that avoids the shock of a radically reduced TIB is called sleep compression [9–11]. While sharing the assumption that individuals with insomnia benefit from a reduction of TIB, this intervention starts with a modest reduction in TIB compared to SRT. During the first session, patients were advised to reduce TIB by half of the difference between baseline TIB and baseline TST. During the second and third sessions, TIB was further reduced by one-quarter of the difference between baseline TIB and baseline TST. For a complete description of sleep compression, please see Chapter 5. This approach is consistent with the clinical wisdom to "start where the patient is". We have frequently suggested that when SRT is used clinically it is important to negotiate initial TIB with the patient so that resistance is minimized [12].

We have been impressed with how rarely we have had to reduce TIB after the initial restriction. Therefore, we have implemented a modification of SRT in which, following the initial restricted schedule (determined as usual from the average reported sleep time across a baseline week), we do not further reduce TIB. Instead, we increase TIB by either 15 or 30 minutes on a weekly basis regardless of reported sleep efficiency [12,13]. This approach is necessary in individuals with paradoxical insomnia who do not report sufficiently greater sleep efficiency on a significantly restricted schedule to trigger extra allotments of TIB.

PROOF OF CONCEPT

The treatment efficacy of SRT has been tested in a number of studies with different patient populations. There are only a few studies in which the effectiveness of SRT is assessed as a stand-alone treatment. Spielman and colleagues [1] administered SRT to 35 adults with psychophysiological insomnia and insomnia co-morbid with psychiatric disorders in eight weekly individual sessions. Treatment outcomes, as measured by subjective sleep onset latency (SOL), total sleep time (TST), sleep efficiency (SE), and ratings on insomnia symptoms were all improved after treatment as well as at a 36-week follow-up. Although initially restricted, TST eventually increased from 320 minutes to 343 minutes and SE improved from 67 percent to 87 percent. This study did not employ a control group; therefore, its findings cannot be attributed directly to the treatment.

Subsequently, several studies modified the SRT procedures for elderly patients with insomnia, with more flexibility in the prescription of TIB [14–16], gradual sleep compression instead of abrupt cut-down of TST [8,10,11], and/or installing a mandatory or optional daytime nap [8,15]. These procedures were intended primarily to enhance the patients' tolerance of sleep restriction and/or to reduce daytime sleepiness due to partial sleep deprivation. In comparison to various control treatments (waiting-list control, relaxation training, sleep hygiene education, and a placebo desensitization procedure), SRT in these studies was found to increase SE and TST, and decrease wake after sleep onset (WASO). The outcome on SOL was not as consistent as the other measures. Treatment effects were at least partially maintained at short-term (2-month) and long-term (up to 2 years) follow-up.

For example, Friedman and colleagues [14] compared modified SRT with progressive muscle relaxation training. Subjects' tolerance was taken into consideration in the assignment of the prescribed TIB at the start of treatment to increase compliance. Also, TIB was not reduced for failure to reach criterion to avoid drop-out. The results showed that both treatments were effective in increasing TST, and reducing SOL and WASO. However, SRT was more effective in increasing SE and TST than relaxation training. Lichstein and colleagues [11] compared sleep compression (see above for the shared assumptions with SRT) that reduced TIB gradually in 5 weeks with relaxation training and placebo desensitization procedures; treatment effects were significant for sleep-log derived variables but not for those derived from a polysomnogram. It was found that both treatments produced significant improvement in SOL and WASO at post-treatment, but WASO benefits were maintained only in the sleep compression group at 1-year follow-up. Relaxation did better than sleep compression in enhancing TST.

The effective deployment of SRT in an inpatient setting was described in a case report. A 49-year-old woman with insomnia co-morbid with major depression and chronic pain was treated with SRT with the assistance of nursing staff. The SRT was administered in a modified form by starting with 4 hours in bed for 3 nights, increasing to 5 hours for the subsequent 3 nights. TIB was further increased to 6 hours per night after SE achieved 85 percent, and increased to 7 hours for 2 weeks prior to discharge. TST was improved from 2 hours 30 minutes to over 6 hours after about 2 weeks of treatment, and the improvements were maintained at 4-month follow-up [17]. Sleep compression has also been found effective when delivered by self-help video, although additional meetings with a therapist did enhance the treatment outcomes [10].

Based on a review of the research evidence, the Practice Parameters for the Psychological and Behavioral Treatment of Insomnia [18] and the Clinical Guideline for the Evaluation and Management of Chronic Insomnia in Adults [19] published by the American Academy of Sleep Medicine rated SRT as a Guideline treatment, meaning that SRT is a patient-care strategy with a moderate degree of clinical certainty [20]. Although SRT is effective as a stand-alone treatment, clinically it is typically incorporated into the multi-component treatment known as cognitive behavior therapy for insomnia (CBT-I). The most common combination involves an educational component (sleep hygiene), a behavioral component (stimulus control, SRT, relaxation), and a cognitive component (cognitive restructuring). One study comparing different components of CBT-I reported that while relaxation was more effective for sleep onset problems, a combination of stimulus control and SRT had more benefits for sleep maintenance variables [21]. Both the 2006 Practice Parameter [18] and the 2008 Clinical Guideline [19] papers that rated CBT as a Standard explicitly include SRT as one of the three behavioral components of this approach. The review paper accompanying the Practice Parameters paper [20] showed that SRT was more commonly a part of CBT than relaxation therapy. In all twelve of the studies cited, SRT was a component of CBT.

REFERENCES

[1] A.J. Spielman, P. Saskin, M.J. Thorpy, Treatment of chronic insomnia by restriction of time in bed, Sleep 10 (1) (1987) 45–56.

[2] W. Webb, H. Agnew, Sleep: Effects of a restricted regime, Science 150 (1965) 1745–1747.

[3] W. Webb, H. Agnew, The effects of a chronic limitation of sleep length, Psychophysiology 11 (1974) 265–274.

[4] A.J. Spielman, Assessment of insomnia, Clin. Psychol. Rev. 6 (1986) 11–25.

[5] A.J. Spielman, L. Caruso, P. Glovinsky, A behavioral perspective on insomnia treatment, Psychiatr. Clin. N. Am. 10 (4) (1987) 541–553.

[6] A.J. Spielman, C.M. Yang, P.B. Glovinsky, in: Buysse, Sateia, (Eds.), Sleep Restriction Therapy, Informa, 2010 (in press).

[7] J.D. Edinger, C.E. Carney, Overcoming Insomnia: A Cognitive-Behavioral Therapy Approach – Therapist Guide, Oxford University Press, Inc, New York, NY, 2008.

[8] J.O. Brooks, III, L. Friedman, D.L. Bliwise, J.A. Yesavage, Use of the wrist actigraph to study insomnia in older adults, Sleep 16 (2) (1993) 51–55.

[9] B.W. Riedel, K.L. Lichstein, W.O. Dwyer, Sleep compression and sleep education for older insomniacs: self-help versus therapist guidance, Psychol. Aging 10 (1995) 54–63.

[10] B.W. Riedel, K.L. Lichstein, Strategies for evaluating adherence to sleep restriction treatment for insomnia, Behav. Res. Ther. 39 (2001) 201–212.

[11] K.L. Lichstein, B.W. Riedel, N.M. Wilson, et al., Relaxation and sleep compression for late-life insomnia: a placebo-controlled trial, J. Consult. Clin. Psychol. 69 (2) (2001) 227–239.

[12] P.B. Glovinsky, A.J. Spielman, Sleep restriction therapy, in: P. Hauri, (Ed.), Case Studies in Insomnia, Plenum, New York, NY, 1991, pp. 49–63.
[13] M.L. Rubinstein, S.A. Rothenberg, S. Maheswaran, Modified sleep restriction therapy in middle-aged and elderly chronic insomniacs, Sleep Res. 19 (1990) 276.
[14] L. Friedman, D.L. Bliwise, J.A. Yesavage, S.A. Salom, A preliminary study comparing sleep restriction and relaxation treatment for insomnia in older adults, J. Gerontol. 46 (1991) 1–8.
[15] L. Friedman, K. Benson, A. Noda, et al., An actigraphic comparison of sleep restriction and sleep hygiene treatments for insomnia in older adults, J. Geriatr. Psych. Neurol. 13 (1) (2000) 17–27.
[16] T.J. Hoelscher, J.D. Edinger, Treatment of sleep-maintenance insomnia in older adults: sleep period reduction, sleep education, and modified stimulus control, Psychol. Aging 3 (3) (1988) 258–263.
[17] C.M. Morin, R.A. Kowatch, G. O'Shanick, Sleep restriction for the inpatient treatment of insomnia, Sleep 13 (2) (1990) 183–186.
[18] T. Morgenthaler, M. Kramer, C. Alessi, et al., Practice parameters for the psychological and behavioral treatment of insomnia: an update. An American Academy of Sleep Medicine report standards of practice, Sleep 29 (11) (2006) 1415–1419.
[19] S. Schutte-Rodin, L. Broch, D. Buysse, et al., Clinical guideline for the evaluation and management of chronic insomnia in adults, J. Clin. Sleep Med. 4 (5) (2008).
[20] C.M. Morin, R.R. Bootzin, D.J. Buysse, et al., Psychological and behavioral treatment of insomnia: update of the recent evidence (1998–2004), Sleep 29 (11) (2006) 1398–1414.
[21] W.F. Waters, M.J. Hurry, P.G. Binks, et al., Behavioral and hypnotic treatments for insomnia subtypes, Behav. Sleep Med. 1 (2) (2003) 81–101.

Chapter 2

Stimulus Control Therapy

Richard R. Bootzin
Departments of Psychology and Psychiatry; Sleep Research Laboratory; and Insomnia Clinic, Arizona Health Sciences Center; University of Arizona, Tucson, AZ

Michael L. Perlis
Department of Psychiatry and Nursing, University of Pennsylvania School of Medicine, Philadelphia, PA

PROTOCOL NAME

Stimulus Control Therapy (SCT).

GROSS INDICATION

Stimulus control therapy is indicated for the treatment of acute and/or chronic insomnia.

SPECIFIC INDICATION

SCT has been found to be effective for the treatment of all types of insomnia. There is no evidence to suggest that this form of therapy is differentially effective for one or another type of insomnia (psychophysiologic vs idiopathic vs paradoxical insomnia) or for any of the phenotypes/subtypes of insomnia (initial vs middle vs late insomnia). This said, the SCT instructions are formulated to be particularly effective for sleep onset problems, whether they occur at the beginning or middle of the night.

CONTRAINDICATIONS

While there is no evidence to show "where and when" this form of therapy is contraindicated, modifications of the instructions may be necessary in the following cases:

- patients who are disabled and cannot easily get out of bed unassisted;
- patients who cannot safely get out of bed owing to risk of slips and falls;
- patients who do not have the cognitive capacity due to dementia or mental retardation to follow the stimulus control instructions.

Behavioral Treatments for Sleep Disorders. DOI: 10.1016/B978-0-12-381522-4.00002-X

RATIONALE FOR INTERVENTION

SCT for the treatment of insomnia was proposed by Bootzin [1]. The instructions were expanded during the next few years [2,3] and have remained unchanged to the present. SCT for insomnia is based on a learning analysis of sleep in which falling asleep is conceptualized as an instrumental act emitted to produce reinforcement (i.e., sleep) [2,3]. Cues, both external and internal to the individual [4], that are associated with the onset of sleep become discriminative stimuli for the occurrence of reinforcement. Consequently, difficulty in falling asleep may be due to inadequate stimulus control. Strong discriminative stimuli for sleep may not have been established, or discriminative stimuli for activities that interfere with sleep may be present [2–4].

In addition to the importance of discriminative stimuli, Pavlovian conditioning in which cues are associated with emotional reactions is also important. The bed and bedroom can become cues for the distress and frustration of trying to fall asleep [3]. Internal cues, such as mind racing, anticipatory anxiety, and physiological arousal, thus become cues for further arousal and sleep disruptions [5]. The goal of SCT is to reduce cues associated with arousal as well as cues that are discriminative stimuli for activities that are incompatible with sleep [4–6].

Stimulus control therapy was designed to help individuals suffering from insomnia to strengthen the bed and bedroom as cues for sleep, to weaken the bed and bedroom as cues for arousal, and to develop a consistent sleep–wake schedule to help maintain improvement [2,3].

STEP BY STEP DESCRIPTION OF PROCEDURES

There are essentially three steps to the process:

1. Introduce the exercise
2. Detail the stimulus control instructions
3. Make a plan for what to do during the night.

Introduce the Exercise

The dialogue below is intended to be an example of how one might introduce the concept of stimulus control. It represents one of many approaches. The value of this particular example is that it emphasizes the learning aspect of stimulus control instructions. See Figure 2.1 for an example of the diagram referenced below.

Therapist: I'm going to suggest that you try stimulus control therapy which is based on the idea of strengthening the cues of bed and bedroom for sleep and weakening the cues for activities that interfere with falling asleep. But first, let me ask you a

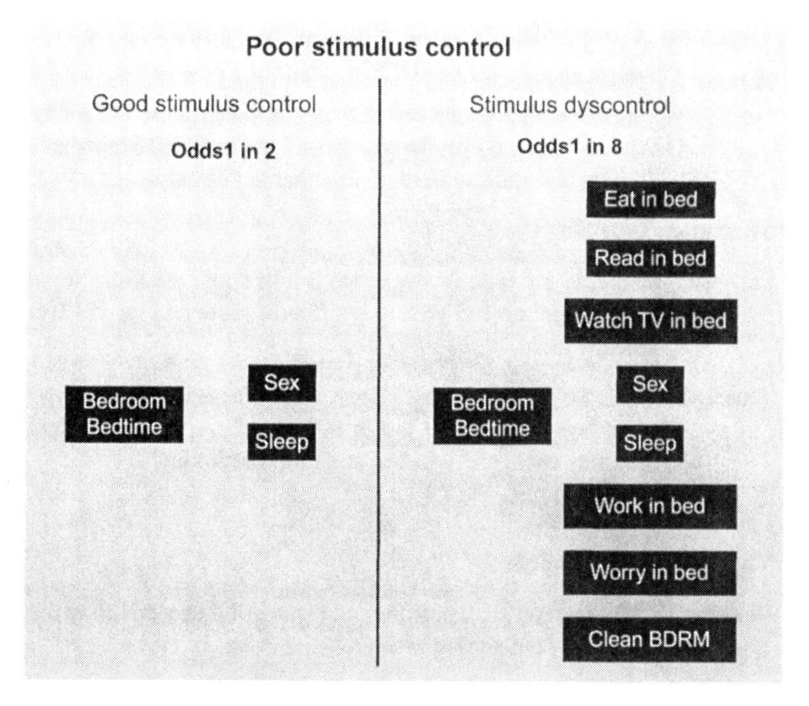

FIGURE 2.1 Poor stimulus control.

question that I often ask college students. If you were studying for an exam, what would happen if you studied in bed?

Patient: It's been a while since I've been a student, but I'd guess that I'd study for a while but would probably fall asleep.

Therapist: Yes. Exactly right. The cues for sleeping in bed are stronger than the cues for studying. So what would happen if you studied at the kitchen table?

Patient: I guess the same idea would apply. I'd study for a while, but I imagine that I'd think about having a snack and would stop to get one.

Therapist: Yes. The cues for activities that interfere with studying, like having a snack, are stronger at the kitchen table than the cues for studying. So let's switch to sleep. Tell me a bit about when you're awake at night. What you do?

Patient: I try to stay in bed, relax, and pray to God that I get enough sleep to be able to function tomorrow.

Therapist: I know what you mean. What else do you do?

Patient: Sometimes I do things to keep my mind off the fact that I am not sleeping, maybe read, maybe watch some TV, sometimes I work on my laptop or surf the Internet. Sometimes I'll lie bed and meditate – I have heard this helps.

Therapist: Anything else?

Patient: Sure. If my wife is awake we'll talk about the kids. Some times I get up and go into a different room and see if I feel sleepy there.

Therapist: OK. So let's draw this. For a good sleeper, someone who just lays down and is out in 60 seconds … what behaviors do they engage in – in bed and in the bedroom?

Patient: Sleep.

Therapist: Anything else?

Patient: Maybe read … but if they are out in 60 seconds they are probably not getting much reading done.

Therapist: I bet that's true. Anything else?

Patient: Well … Sex … I guess.

Therapist: As you'll see in the instructions, sex is the one activity other than sleeping that is allowed in bed. Usually I tell patients that the reason we allow sex in bed is that we're just not very creative about where we have sex. The dining room table just doesn't seem that appealing. So let's say that it's sleep or sex in bed.

Therapist: In your case … you do more than sleep and sex in the bedroom in the effort to stay "ready for sleep". You read, work, surf the Internet, talk with your wife, meditate … and frankly you probably spend a fair amount of time in bed worrying about not sleeping.

Patient: You betchya.

Therapist: OK. So if we count these up … there's at least eight things you do in the bed and bedroom when you can't sleep. And although we can't calculate the exact odds of falling asleep, we know it has to be less if there are eight activities of which seven compete with sleep than if there are only two. So how can you make it more likely that you would fall asleep?

Patient: Don't do anything in the bed/bedroom besides sleep and sex.

Therapist: Exactly.

Patient: What am I supposed to do when I am awake?

Therapist: Anything you like (but that is not going to be too arousing) – and not in the bedroom. I recommend against doing work or being on the computer. There is more light from even a laptop because we sit closer to the computer than we would watching TV.

Patient: So when I am awake, I am supposed to get up and go into another room?

Therapist: Exactly.

Patient: How do I know when to get up and go into another room?

Therapist: The original formulation of this recommends that one stay in bed for no more than 15 minutes. Our sense of this is its better not to use a time-based rule but rather simply get out of bed when you realize that you are awake and/or that you are feeling frustrated about not being asleep.

Patient: How long do I have to stay out of bed?!

Therapist: The original formulation states that you should stay out of bed until you're sleepy. For some people, self monitoring for sleepiness puts on too much pressure. It's often easier to start by deciding ahead of time to stay awake for 30 or 60 minutes.

Patient: Why those time intervals?

Therapist: Good question. Because these time increments line up with the duration of what's usually on TV (which is what many people do when they are out of bed).

Patient: What if I get sleepy?

Therapist: Try and stay awake to the time you selected.

Patient: What if I get sleepy. Do I sleep on the couch?

Therapist: I am glad you asked that. If we're attempting to create a strong pairing between *sleep & sleepiness* and the *bed & bedroom…* would it be helpful in the long run to sleep on the couch?

Patient: I suppose not. What if I am awake a lot of times across the night?

Therapist: I am glad you asked that too. If we're attempting to weaken the association between *wakefulness* and the *bed & bedroom*, should you miss an opportunity to break that association by staying in bed some of the time?

Patient: I suppose not. But this means I may be up and down like a yoyo during the night.

Therapist: That may well happen. And on the nights that it happens it's bound to be unpleasant ... It's a trade off ... You'll be a yoyo for a few days, at worst a couple of weeks, and then you can expect to be better. It took a long time for your insomnia to develop, you have to give it a few weeks to get better.

Patient: Sounds reasonable.

Therapist: Let's review the rules and the reasons for each rule. We'll also discuss what you can do during the night that will make this, if not something to look forward to, than at least bearable for the next week or two.

An alternative or adjunctive approach to the above introduction might be to orient the patient to the Pavlovian conditioning aspect of stimulus control. This latter approach is particularly useful for patients who report "being terribly sleepy at the end of the day" and then find themselves "instantly awake as they cross the threshold into the bedroom".

The SCT instructions [2,3] are:

1. Lie down to go to sleep only when you are sleepy.
2. Do not use your bed for anything except sleep; that is, do not read, watch television, eat, or worry in bed. Sexual activity is the only exception to this rule. On such occasions, the instructions are to be followed afterward when you intend to go to sleep.
3. If you find yourself unable to fall asleep, get up and go into another room. Stay up as long as you wish and then return to the bedroom to sleep. Although we do not want you to watch the clock, we want you to get out of bed if you do not fall asleep immediately. Remember, the goal is to associate your bed with falling asleep *quickly*! If you are in bed more than about 10 minutes without falling asleep and have not gotten up, you are not following this instruction.
4. If you still cannot fall asleep, repeat step (3). Do this as often as is necessary throughout the night.
5. Set your alarm and get up at the same time every morning irrespective of how much sleep you got during the night. This will help your body acquire a consistent sleep rhythm.
6. Do not nap during the day.

Rationale for the Specific SCT Instructions

In our experience, it is not sufficient to just hand a patient with insomnia the list of SCT instructions. It is desirable to discuss the rationale for each instruction [5,6].

Instruction 1: The first instruction is intended to help individuals become more aware of their body's cues for sleepiness. Frequently, individuals with insomnia decide to go to bed at a specific time because of a calculation of how much sleep they feel they must get before awakening in the morning. This may produce increasing anxiety as sleeplessness persists, and can result in excessive time in bed for the amount of sleep that is obtained. Initially, individuals with insomnia rarely rely on internal cues of sleepiness as a signal to go to bed. Instruction 1 should be viewed as an aspirational goal to be achieved gradually over the first few weeks, rather than as an imperative to be started immediately [4]. Becoming sensitive to internal cues of sleepiness aids patients to determine an appropriate time to go to bed based on sleepiness, not on the clock.

Instruction 2: This instruction is the first of two core elements of SCT. It is intended to help strengthen the cues of the bed and bedroom with falling asleep, and weaken the cues of bed and bedroom with arousal and wakefulness. Often individuals with insomnia engage in activities in bed that interfere with falling asleep, such as reading, watching television, playing games on computers or the Internet, talking on the phone, text-messaging, checking email, or working. Engaging in these behaviors establishes the bed and bedroom as conditioned stimuli for wakefulness, not sleep. Patients are typically asked to engage in activities associated with arousal in a different room in the house *before* going into the bedroom. This helps individuals with insomnia create a new bedtime routine that is better suited to facilitate sleep onset [6].

Instructions 3 and 4: The third and fourth instructions reflect the second core element of SCT. Instructing patients to get out of bed if they are not sleeping limits them from being awake in bed, and further strengthens the association between the bed and bedroom and falling sleep. While SCT is focused primarily on sleep onset problems, Instruction 4 is incorporated for use with sleep maintenance issues. Getting out of bed to engage in other activities when unable to sleep strengthens a perception of control over insomnia. This makes the problem less distressing and more manageable for the patient [6].

Instruction 5: The goal of Instruction 5 is to establish a consistent sleep rhythm [5]. This is accomplished by setting a consistent wake-up time for all 7 days of the week, with less than 1 hour of discrepancy between days off and workdays [6]. Many people with insomnia stay in bed later in the morning in the hope of catching up on the sleep they missed the night before. However, irregular schedules weaken the association between the cues of the bed and bedroom and sleep. Maintaining consistent sleep schedules has been found to reduce daytime fatigue and sleepiness [7]. Consequently, a consistent schedule helps both strengthen cues for sleep and reduce daytime problems associated with sleep disturbance.

Instruction 6: The rationale for the final instruction about not napping to is ensure that those with insomnia use the sleep deprivation from the prior night to facilitate falling asleep quickly on the next night [5]. This strengthens the cues of the bed and bedroom with falling asleep, and provides a success experience for the patient to help maintain compliance with the instructions. It should be emphasized that we are not opposed to all naps. Instruction 6 is intended to increase the likelihood that SCT will successfully change a dysfunctional sleep pattern. With some individuals, such as the elderly, however, it may be wise to have a brief nap (30 minutes or less) scheduled at the same time every day [5,6]. It is the irregularity of napping that produces and maintains irregular sleep schedules.

POSSIBLE MODIFICATIONS/VARIANTS

There are two variants that have been used in successfully implementing SCT [6]. First, how long should someone with insomnia be in bed before getting out of bed? The instructions place a premium on getting out of bed quickly – within 10 minutes. However, some individuals with insomnia become anxious with such a recommendation, and constantly check the clock to determine if it is time to get out of bed. To avoid clock-checking, patients are typically instructed to turn the face of the clock away from them. If time pressure produces increased anxiety, Instruction 3 is often modified to put emphasis on the internal cues of frustration and distress rather than on how much time has passed [6]. Thus, the patient is instructed to get out of bed at the first signs of frustration at not having fallen asleep. It is important to stress, however, that it is not permissible to stay in bed for long periods of time while waiting to fall asleep (such as 60 minutes or longer) even if not frustrated. The goal of the SCT instructions remains to associate the bed and bedroom with falling asleep *quickly*. Research has indicated that a quarter-hour rule (staying in bed for no more than 15 minutes before falling asleep) is manageable and effective in producing improved sleep in those with insomnia [8].

A second variant is that once patients have gotten out of bed, what activities are permissible, and how long should they stay awake before going back to bed? A good clinical rule of thumb for when to return to sleep is that patients should stay out of bed long enough to feel that they might successfully be able to fall asleep if they returned to bed [6]. This is an opportunity to practice paying attention to internal cues of sleepiness and using them as a guide. Generally, this means staying awake for at least 15 or more minutes before trying to go to sleep again.

Regarding what activities are permissible when out of bed in the middle of the night, patients should be encouraged to do something relaxing and enjoyable. Because of the increasing evidence that even room light can alter sleep–wake circadian schedules [9], we have placed additional emphasis on keeping lights dim when out of bed during the night. Reading with a reading light and watching television from a distance is acceptable. We discourage patients from doing anything on the computer – even checking email – since the amount of light from the monitor when sitting close to it is brighter than most individuals realize, and activities done on the computer are usually arousing [6]. Finally, many adults with sleep maintenance problems elect to start the day at 4 am or 5 am rather than trying to return to the bed for additional sleep. This is not a wise strategy, since even 30 or 60 minutes of additional sleep increases alertness and reduces fatigue during the day. As long as the usual final wake-up time is maintained, returning to bed is recommended when there are 45 minutes or more until wake-up time [6].

PROOF OF CONCEPT/SUPPORTING DATA/EVIDENCE BASE

There have been numerous reviews and meta-analyses of the effectiveness of cognitive behavioral treatments for chronic insomnia. Practice guidelines have been used to identify which treatments have sufficient evidence of efficacy to be recommended for use. In 1999, a review [10] and practice guidelines [11] identified SCT as the only psychological and behavioral treatment to meet the highest standard for recommendation. In 2006, the American Academy of Sleep Medicine (AASM) published an update of both the review [12] and evidence-based practice parameters for psychological and behavioral treatment of insomnia [13]. Most of the newly added studies in the review investigated multi-component cognitive behavioral treatments in which SCT is a core component. Nevertheless, the AASM identified individual treatment components that met their standard for recommendation, and SCT continued to be identified as an "effective and recommended therapy in the treatment of chronic insomnia" [13, p. 1417].

A commonly employed multi-component package combines stimulus control instructions, sleep restriction, sleep education, and cognitive therapy. This combination of interventions lends itself well to clinical settings in which patients with diverse insomnia symptoms are seen. Case series studies have found this treatment combination to be as effective in clinical settings as in controlled outcome studies [14–17].

REFERENCES

[1] R.R. Bootzin, Stimulus control treatment for Insomnia. Proceedings, 80th Annual Convention, APA (1972) 395–396.

[2] R. Bootzin, Effects of self-control procedures for insomnia, in: R Stuart, (Ed.), Behavioral Self-Management: Strategies and Outcomes, Brunner/Mazel, New York, NY, 1977.

[3] R.R. Bootzin, P. Nicassio, Behavioral treatments for insomnia, in: M. Hersen, R. Eisler, P. Miller (Eds.), Progress in Behavior Modification, Vol. 6, Academic Press, New York, NY, 1978, pp. 1–45.

[4] N.M. Blampied, R.R. Bootzin, Sleep – a behavioral account, in: G.J. Madden (Ed.), APA Handbook of Behavioral Analysis, in press.

[5] R.R. Bootzin, D.R. Epstein, Stimulus control instructions, in: K.L. Lichstein, C.M. Morin, (Eds.), Treatment of Late-Life Insomnia, Sage, Thousand Oaks, CA, 2000, pp. 167–187.

[6] R.R. Bootzin, L.J. Smith, P.L. Franzen, S.L. Shapiro, Stimulus control therapy, in: D.J. Sateia, D.J. Buysse (Eds.), Insomnia: Diagnosis and Treatment. Informa Healthcare, 2010, pp. 268–276.

[7] R. Manber, R.R. Bootzin, C. Acebo, M.C. Carscadon, The effects of regularizing sleep–wake schedules on daytime sleepiness, Sleep 19 (1996) 432–441.

[8] M. Malaffo, C.A. Espie, Insomnia: the quarter of an hour rule (QHR), a single component of stimulus control, improves sleep, Sleep (2006) A257.

[9] J.M. Zeitzer, D.J. Dijk, R.E. Kronauer, et al., Sensitivity of the human circadian pacemaker to nocturnal light: melatonin phase resetting and suppression, J. Physiol. 526 (Pt.3) (2000) 695–702.

[10] C.M. Morin, P.J. Hauri, C.A. Espie, et al., Nonpharmacologic treatment of chronic insomnia: an American Academy of Sleep Medicine Review, Sleep 22 (1999) 1134–1156.

[11] A.L. Chesson, W.M. Anderson, M. Littner, et al., Practice parameters for the nonpharmacologic treatment of chronic insomnia. Standards of Practice Committee of the American Academy of Sleep Medicine, Sleep 22 (8) (1999) 1128–1133.

[12] C.M. Morin, R.R. Bootzin, D.J. Buysse, et al., Psychological and behavioral treatment of insomnia: update of the recent evidence (1998–2004), Sleep 29 (11) (2006) 1398–1414.

[13] T. Morgenthaler, M. Kramer, C. Alessi, et al., Practice parameters for the psychological and behavioral treatment of insomnia: an update. An American Academy of Sleep Medicine Report, Sleep 29 (11) (2006) 1415–1419.

[14] M.J. Chambers, S.D. Alexander, Assessment and prediction of outcome for a brief behavioral insomnia treatment program, J. Behav. Ther. Exp. Psychiatry 23 (1992) 289–297.

[15] C.M. Morin, J. Stone, K. McDonald, et al., Psychological management of insomnia: a clinical replication series with 100 patients, Behav. Ther. 25 (1994) 291–309.

[16] M. Perlis, M. Aloia, A. Millikan, et al., Behavioral treatment of insomnia: a clinical case series study, J. Behav. Med. 23 (2000) 149–161.

[17] M.L. Perlis, M. Sharpe, M.T. Smith, et al., Behavioral treatment of insomnia: treatment outcome and the relevance of medical and psychiatric morbidity, J. Behav. Med. 24 (2001) 281–296.

Chapter 3

Sleep Hygiene

Donn Posner
Department of Psychiatry, Brown University, Providence, RI
The Sleep Disorders Center of Lifespan Hospitals, Providence, RI

Philip R. Gehrman
Department of Psychiatry, University of Pennsylvania, Philadelphia, PA

PROTOCOL NAME

Sleep hygiene.

GROSS INDICATION

Sleep hygiene is indicated for patients who engage in habits, consume substances, and/or set up sleep environments that are not conducive to initiating or maintaining sleep.

SPECIFIC INDICATION

To date, there is no evidence to suggest that this form of therapy is differentially effective for one or another type of insomnia (psychophysiologic vs idiopathic vs paradoxical insomnia) or for any of the phenotypes/subtypes of insomnia (initial vs middle vs late insomnia). This said, it stands to reason that sleep hygiene factors are an important precipitating or perpetuating factor for "inadequate sleep hygiene insomnia" and, conversely, are of little relevance for "idiopathic insomnia".

CONTRAINDICATIONS

While it is generally held that sleep hygiene is a benign intervention for which there are no contraindications, it may be that specific rules, in specific patients, may not be carried out safely. For example:

- physical activity may not be possible for patients with physical limitations;
- evening snacking may not be appropriate for patients with GERD or other disorders that require restrictive diets;
- rapid smoking cessation in heavy smokers may prove to be as deleterious to sleep as smoking itself;

Behavioral Treatments for Sleep Disorders. DOI: 10.1016/B978-0-12-381522-4.00003-1

- the use of white noise or ear plugs may not be possible for patients who serve as caregivers;
- fully light-attenuating the sleep environment may not be ideal for elderly patients who are at risk for disorientation and/or falls.

RATIONALE FOR INTERVENTION

Although the earliest systematic reference to sleep hygiene was made by Kleitman [1], who in 1939 reviewed evidence regarding factors such as sleep duration, bedtime rituals, sleep surface, ambient temperature, sleep satiety, and body position, his work was discursive and bears little resemblance to the list of dos and don'ts that exist today as sleep hygiene instructions. Peter Hauri [2] is thought to have been the first person to codify the various sleep hygiene imperatives, and summarizes them thus:

Sleep Hygiene Education is intended to provide information about lifestyle (diet, exercise, substance use) and environmental factors (light, noise, temperature) that may interfere with or promote better sleep. Sleep hygiene also may include general sleep-facilitating recommendations, such as allowing enough time to relax before bedtime, and information about the benefits of maintaining a regular sleep schedule.

The role, and perhaps the relevance, of sleep hygiene have varied with time. Decades ago, prior to the widespread dissemination of sleep hygiene instructions, it is entirely plausible that some insomnias were precipitated and perpetuated by poor sleep hygiene. That is, it is entirely plausible that patients seeking clinical help might have reported that they were, for example, drinking three cups of coffee, eating heavy meals, and/or engaging in strenuous exercise before bed. In such cases, altering these behaviors might have resolved the sleep complaint. In the present era, this seems less likely. More often than not patients, long before they seek professional help, are already aware of sleep hygiene and have addressed their most egregious infractions. In fact, it is far more likely that patients have always practiced moderately good sleep hygiene and, following the development of chronic insomnia, simply fail to see the relevance of minor sleep hygiene infractions as disease/disorder moderators (as opposed to causal factors). In the present era, the rationale for sleep hygiene has less to do with fixing the problem and more to do with (1) optimizing clinical outcomes, and (2) making the patient less vulnerable to relapse or recurrence. In the case of the former, good sleep hygiene might be the difference between a patient being able to achieve 6 hours and 45 minutes or 7 hours of sleep, as opposed to 6 hours and 30 minutes if they were still engaging in poor sleep habits. In the case of the latter, addressing each sleep hygiene infraction may serve to decrease the patient's overall vulnerability to relapse and/or recurrence by decreasing their predisposition for insomnia.

STEP BY STEP DESCRIPTION OF PROCEDURES

Procedures

As surprising as it may be, there is a variety of approaches to the delivery of sleep hygiene, the most common being the provision of sleep hygiene instructions as a one-page handout. A second approach is (with or without a handout) to review all the sleep hygiene instructions with the patient using a didactic or Socratic approach. A third approach includes using a paper and pencil instrument to assess (1) the extent to which sleep hygiene issues are operational and (2) which issues in particular are relevant.

The "handout" approach is not recommended for several reasons. First, it is likely that the patient has already been exposed to sleep hygiene in this manner. Had it been effective, no further treatment would be required. Second, to the extent that sleep hygiene is effective, its potency may have less to do with the facts themselves and more to do with the patient's increased understanding of sleep–wake regulation and how to use this knowledge to promote adherence to both the sleep hygiene rules and the other components of CBT-I. Third, to the extent that monotherapy with sleep hygiene is *ineffective*, there is the risk that the patient and/or clinician may generalize this treatment failure to CBT-I. That is, many view sleep hygiene as one and the same as CBT-I, and when sleep hygiene is found to be ineffective the conclusions are that (1) behavior therapy isn't effective, and (2) the only recourse is medical treatment.

The other extreme (*vis-à-vis* approaches to the delivery of sleep hygiene) is to devote a whole session to this component of CBT-I, where considerable amounts of time are dedicated to explaining the general concept (strengths and limitations), the various imperatives, the rationales for the imperatives, the applicability of the rules to the individual patient, and the interventions' relevance for therapy in general and for relapse prevention in specific. The whole session approach usually contains the following steps.

Step 1. Explain the concept of sleep hygiene, emphasizing that these factors are:

- not likely to be causal;
- likely contribute to the development of insomnia;
- (when addressed) may allow for an augmentation of clinical gains;
- (when addressed) may have prophylactic value re. recurrence.

Step 2. Have the patient read each imperative, pausing between the rules to allow the therapist to elaborate.

Step 3. Have the therapist address:

- the relevance of the rule for the patient;
- the underlying concept and related science;
- the specific plan for the patient.

The manner in which sleep hygiene is introduced will vary with the style of each clinician. Our preferred approach to covering the core points is exemplified by the dialogue below.

Therapist: Before we go over the list of rules, I would like to discuss the ways in which changes you make with regard to these rules can be useful for you. My guess is that you have already seen some of these rules elsewhere. Rules about diet, exercise, caffeine – Yes?

Patient: Oh yeah, I've gone over that stuff plenty, and then my mother kept telling me to drink warm milk before bed.

Therapist: And did any of that ever make a difference for you.

Patient: Nope – my sleep (or lack thereof) never seems to change.

Therapist: Well I am going to give you the same list, and if you change rule (4) tonight my guess is that it is not going to help. In fact we have data that says that using sleep hygiene alone to fix your sleep is unlikely to work.

Patient: Then why should we bother to go over it?

Therapist: I am glad you asked that question. As I have said, I think that changes here can be useful, but perhaps not in the way that you are thinking. To begin with, your sleep habits are not terrible; in fact, they are pretty decent. I do think you are doing some things that could be done differently, but I will bet now that none of these small infractions of the sleep hygiene rules has caused your sleep problem. Do you remember what we said was probably a contributing factor to your insomnia?

Patient: Yes; it was when my company was laying off some workers and I wasn't sure if I was going to be next.

Therapist: Right, that was the start. It was not likely the coffee you were drinking or the fact that you are not much of an exerciser. Nevertheless, what we can say about those factors is that perhaps they made you more vulnerable to a sleep problem to begin with. I like to think of each of these factors as if they are rungs in a ladder of arousability and that with each rung you climb – that is, rule you break – you increase your vulnerability to a sleep problem.

Patient: You mean if I had been exercising and drinking less coffee at the time of the layoffs that I wouldn't have had insomnia?

Therapist: I suppose that is possible, but it's also possible that it would have happened anyway. As we talked about: once you started having bad nights you began to get very frustrated about your sleeplessness and began going to bed earlier in order to compensate. As we discussed, this set up a vicious cycle of insomnia that you found near impossible to escape.

Under these circumstances, with all that worry and frustration about sleep, and constantly falling asleep on the couch after dinner, does it seem likely that stopping that decaf cup of coffee in the afternoon was going to make a difference?

Patient: I guess not.

Therapist: I would guess that when it didn't, you not only concluded that sleep hygiene doesn't work but also that caffeine doesn't affect you.

Patient: Exactly – I figured coffee didn't make a difference to me.

Therapist: Right, but caffeine is a stimulant for you just like it is for everyone else, and must therefore be having some effect. So as we are addressing your sleep in other ways by restricting your schedule and getting you out of bed when you don't sleep, it may be useful to remove as many of those rungs in the arousability ladder as possible so that we make you less vulnerable to a sleep problem and so that the work we are already doing does not encounter any obstacles. Also once you are sleeping better, what do you think it might mean to you in the future if you have fewer poor habits or rungs in the ladder?

Patient: That I will be less arousable at night?

Therapist: Right, and therefore less prone to relapse. Now with that in mind, let's go over the list together to see what rungs are in your ladder and how we might get them out.

As noted above regarding the introduction to sleep hygiene, the method for the review of the imperatives may vary with the style of each clinician. Some may prefer a purely didactic approach (the patient reads the rule and the therapist explains the rule). Some may prefer a more Socratic approach, where, after reading the rule, the patient is queried about how the infraction might lead to poor sleep. Ultimately (and regardless of style), when adopting this approach it is important to go over each rule individually so as to (1) acknowledge or dispute its general validity, (2) ascertain its relevance for the patient, (3) explain the concepts and findings that undergird the imperative, and (4) provide for a plan to implement the relevant rules. Further, it is useful to periodically reiterate (every three to five rules) the essential message that no one rule, or even the combination of all the rules, will necessarily eliminate the insomnia. An example dialogue is provided below.

Therapist: So, having a light carbohydrate snack before bed can help to eliminate a blood sugar drop during the night which could have an impact on your sleep (e.g., cause an awakening that might otherwise not occur).

Patient: Yeah, that's not a problem for me because I never wake up hungry.

Therapist: Right. Hunger may not be *the* reason that you are waking. What may be true in your case is that your blood sugar dropping is increasing your vulnerability to waking. Just as when you noted that you don't tend to have to use the bathroom in the middle of the night. Nevertheless, with regard to increasing vulnerability, even a semi-full bladder might contribute to waking if there are enough other changes taking place in your body at the same time. Each of these factors we are discussing are the rungs in a ladder of increasing arousability. With each rung you may be getting closer to the waking threshold, even if stepping on that rung did not specifically cause you to reach, and exceed, the waking threshold.

Patient: So you are saying that changing these things together may have more of an impact on my sleep than just changing one at a time, like I have done in the past?

Therapist: Yes, exactly. Plus it is also more likely to have an impact on vulnerability if you are consistently applying these rules over time as opposed to just 1 night. If you eat the proper snack and drink less liquid tonight, do you think you will sleep better tonight?

Patient: Probably not.

Therapist: Exactly. When talking about vulnerability to sleep disruption, it is more likely that several changes made over a period of time will result in more positive benefit for you sleep ability in the future.

The final approach represents a compromise between the other two more extreme approaches. As noted above, paper and pencil instruments may be used to assess the extent to which sleep hygiene issues are operational, and which issues in particular represent problems for the patient. To our knowledge, there are three sleep hygiene assessment instruments:

1. The Sleep Hygiene Awareness and Practice Scale (Lacks and Rotert, 1986)
2. The Sleep Hygiene Self-Test (Blake and Gomez, 1998)
3. The Sleep Hygiene Index (Mastin et al., 2006).

The benefit of this approach is that it allows (1) for a quantitative assessment of this aspect of illness severity (and a measure of its change with treatment), (2) for a tailored approach to treatment (although one which can be applied systematically as part of research), and (3) (on average) for less time to be devoted to this component of treatment with, presumably, the same end results.

Sleep Hygiene Rules

The actual rules for sleep hygiene vary widely from text to text. Some compendiums have dozens of rules that often include abbreviated forms of other therapies, including stimulus control and sleep restriction procedures, chronotherapy, and phototherapy. While these treatments may be useful in their unexpurgated form, there is no evidence that these interventions as sleep hygiene rules have any effectiveness. Finally, when sleep hygiene is conducted (as it should be) as part of a multi-component treatment regimen, there is no need for this redundancy. Accordingly, it seems ideal to use *a limited set of rules including those that are not explained or detailed as part of other procedures.* What follows is a list of generally accepted rules. Following the simple imperative, a specific rationale for the rule is provided, along with caveats/considerations, and recommendations for therapist "talking points" and possible alternative approaches. The text below (imperative and rationale) is written as it would be shared with the patient.

Exercise in the Late Afternoon or Early Evening

Rationale: While it is unclear whether exercise can help you fall asleep more quickly and/or get more sleep overall, there is good evidence that aerobic exercise can deepen sleep. Deeper sleep may be more restorative, and also protective against awakenings related to noise, pain, hot flashes, etc.

Caveats/considerations: Patients who do not have an established exercise regimen, and/or who have medical issues, should be advised to proceed carefully regarding the initiation of an exercise program, ideally instituting the regimen in consultation with their primary care clinician and/or professional trainer. Timing of the exercise program is also important, as it is generally held that afternoon exercise is optimal and that exercise immediately before bed may be counter productive.

"Talking points": The therapist may use this opportunity to address issues related to temperature regulation, the timing of sleep, and the density of slow wave sleep.

Alternative approaches: There are data to suggest that "passive heating" (aka a warm bath) taken an hour or two before bedtime may yield the same effects as aerobic exercise. This is thought to be the case because both similarly affect core body temperature and have the result of increasing slow wave sleep. If this approach is considered, the patient (and/or therapist) should discuss this possibility with the primary care clinician, as warm temperatures may make some medical conditions worse. Also, some elderly individuals may be at risk for slips and falls entering and exiting the tub.

Do Not Take Naps During the Day

Rationale: Naps are likely to increase your problems falling or staying asleep owing to their influence on the mechanisms that determine sleep timing, duration, and depth.

Caveats/considerations: Some patients, such as retirees, may have the opportunity and desire to take regular naps. While ill advised from the "night sleep" perspective, napping may provide such patients with a boost or "second wind" for later in the day. A patient who elects to nap should be warned that occasional napping may lead to regular napping via conditioning, altered sleep–wake timing, and altered sleep homeostasis.

"Talking points": The therapist may use this opportunity to address issues related to the two-process model of sleep–wake regulation (circadian timing and sleep homeostasis).

Alternative approaches: Allow napping given a sensible approach. Napping earlier in the day may be less impactful on night-time sleep. Further, the patient should be counseled to: (1) nap for relatively brief periods of time (30–60 minutes), and (2) delay bedtime for an amount of time equivalent to the period spent in bed during the day. For example, if the patient naps and is in bed for 60 minutes and reports sleeping 30 minutes, bedtime should be delayed by 60 minutes.

Eat a Light Snack Before Bedtime

Rationale: A snack can be helpful about 1 hour before bedtime. Carbohydrates (i.e., crackers, bread, cereal, fruit) are best for a good night's sleep. It is a good idea to avoid chocolate or heavily sweetened foods. Such snacking may help to avoid a blood sugar drop during the night that can disrupt sleep.

Caveats/considerations: As stated earlier, this may be contraindicated in patients with GERD or other digestive disorders or patients on restricted diets.

Avoid Liquids Before Bedtime

Rationale: Liquids close to bedtime will fill your bladder and result in discomfort while you sleep, causing you to wake more frequently.

Caveats/considerations: Patients who wish to drink small amounts of liquid may do so by restricting intake to less than 6–7 ounces in the 4 hours prior to bedtime, and by making sure they void before going to bed. As stated earlier, there may be medical problems or conditions that require patients to be better hydrated, and this should supersede any sleep habit instruction. There should also be awareness of the fact that some conditions (e.g., enlarged prostate) and some medications (e.g., diuretics) may necessitate middle of the night voiding regardless of how much liquid restriction takes place.

Some patients, such as those on continuous positive airway pressure (CPAP), report waking in the night with a dry mouth. These patients should be encouraged to take a few sips of water in the middle of the night, perhaps even to have a small cup ready next to their bed to avoid having to get up. However, they should be dissuaded from drinking large amounts.

If patients do wake in the night with even a mild sense of bladder distension, they should be encouraged to get up and void. Attempts to go back to sleep with bladder distension are likely to fail or will result in repeated arousals.

Avoid Caffeinated Products within 6 Hours of Bedtime

Rationale: Caffeine works as a stimulant in your body and can keep you awake.

Caveats/considerations: It is unlikely that caffeine in the morning is going to have much if any impact on night-time sleep, even in the most sensitive of patients. In addition, there is some evidence that stimulants, used judiciously in the earlier part of the day, may actually provide some benefit, especially to those patients engaged in sleep restriction therapy, in that it can help them to remain more awake and alert during the day. Permission to use caffeine may actually serve to decrease patients' anxiety about not sleeping at night, and this may aid in promoting better sleep. On the other hand, the length of time before bed that caffeine should be curtailed before it is an issue will vary from patient to patient, and this is one rule that will require tailoring.

Although decaffeinated products contain much less caffeine than their caffeinated counterparts, it is possible that small amounts of caffeine in the evening, especially in the most sensitive individuals, may still serve to be an irritant to sleep onset. This is an example of how a modest infraction may serve as a predisposing factor to sleep problems even if it is not a direct cause.

Patients should be encouraged to read product labels and make sure that they are not inadvertently consuming caffeine late in the day. It can be illustrative to point out that many lighter-colored sodas and some aspirin brands contain caffeine.

Avoid Alcohol as a Hypnotic

Rationale: Although alcohol use before bedtime can help some people to fall asleep more easily, it has been shown that use of alcohol to promote sleep (i.e., larger quantities than is typical for the individual) results in more fragmented sleep, more awakenings during the night, and/or early morning awakenings.

Caveats/considerations: While some may tolerate a glass or two of wine at dinner, others may find that this makes their sleep more fitful, while still others may find that this promotes the occurrence of early morning awakenings.

Quite apart from its effect on sleep maintenance, another possible reason to curtail or eliminate alcohol consumption is that while in active behavioral treatment, one of the greatest difficulties that patients have is to remain awake until the prescribed bedtime. Drinking alcohol will only serve to make this task more difficult. So the patient may be encouraged to temporarily suspend alcohol consumption during active treatment so that they can stay awake at night.

Avoid Nicotine

Rationale: Nicotine is a stimulant, and it has been demonstrated that chronic cigarette smokers have experienced significantly improved sleep when they quit.

Caveats/considerations: It is possible that during the early stages nicotine withdrawal may actually exacerbate sleep disruption, especially in the patients who are most addicted. Patients should therefore be educated about the effects of nicotine on sleep, and then encouraged to work on sleep and smoking cessation at different times.

One thing that could be tried during active sleep treatment would be to have patients experiment with changing the times of smoking to see what changes might benefit sleep. For example, patients could be encouraged not to smoke in the middle of the night when they can't sleep, as such smoking might be training them to wake at night to smoke. A consistent change in this regard might at least alter that pattern without having to go through full smoking cessation. Further, smoking cessation techniques might aide in this process (e.g., the use of a nicotine patch) and represent a reasonable first step in smoking cessation.

Use Ear Plugs or White Noise to Mitigate Noise

Rationale: Irregular noises, even quiet ones, can be disruptive to sleep. White noise, such as the sound of a fan or humidifier, can drown out other more disruptive noises, leading to less broken sleep.

Caveats/considerations: As previously noted, caution may be needed in situations where a patient is a caregiver (e.g., for an elderly Alzheimer's parent) and may need to hear what is happening in other parts of the house. It should generally be noted that this scenario would not be ideal for a good night's sleep to begin with, and may be part of the problem.

There many types of white-noise machines on the market that have a variety of settings. While some settings (e.g., waterfall or tropical rainforest) may provide a decent white noise, others (e.g., forest birds or thunderstorm), while being relaxing sounds, are not essentially white noises in that they are not constant and meaningless. Such sound could serve to actually disrupt sleep or at least keep the patient from sleeping as deeply.

Avoid Co-Sleeping with One's Pets

Rationale: Pets will frequently move around and/or jump on and off the bed, causing movement and noise which can be disruptive to sleep.

Caveats/considerations: There is no real caution to this, except that the therapist should expect to meet strong resistance from some patients regarding this recommendation. At times it is helpful to engage in some problem solving regarding how a patient can teach a pet to sleep alongside the bed or in another room.

Make the Sleep Environment Comfortable and Conducive to Sleep

Rationale: Make sure you have a comfortable mattress, and keep your bedroom generally cool and dark.

Caveats/considerations:

- Bedding. Many patients have not bought new bedding for decades. This is problematic to the extent that sleeping on worn-out pillows and mattresses may contribute to sleep disturbance by promoting levels of discomfort and/or pain that, if not precipitating frank awakenings, shallow sleep and increase one's vulnerability to awakenings. A decent rule of thumb is to replace pillows regularly (every 1–3 years) and mattresses once every one to two decades. Patients should, if able, be encouraged to invest in their sleep comfort, and counseled that such investments may, in and of themselves, yield dividends.
- Temperature. There is no "right temperature for sleep", but the general rule is "sleep loves the cold". Further, it is easier to keep the room temperature cold and to regulate the patient's own temperature by covering up with blankets than it is to keep the room warm and to find some way to cool down when feeling too hot.
- Light. Light attenuation in the bedroom in the morning is generally desirable, especially for those patients who are larks in their circadian pattern and tend to wake early or suffer from "terminal" insomnia.

Keep a Regular Sleep Schedule by Setting an Alarm in the Morning

Rationale: Keeping a consistent wake time will promote better circadian cycling, and setting an alarm will prevent giving your insomnia the function of waking you in the morning.

Caveats/considerations: Some patients will balk at the idea of setting a regular wake time 7 days per week. It would be worth noting that setting strict times may be more crucial during the treatment phase while trying to strengthen the circadian control of sleep and wakefulness. Once it is well established, maintaining a good schedule may not require as strict a protocol and may allow for 1 or 2 days of modest changes in wake time (sleeping in) as long as the patient is still maintaining standard wake times the rest of the week.

Some patients are also likely to resist setting an alarm, feeling that this increases their anxiety and will keep them awake. The concern is that by not setting an alarm the patient is setting up an anxious expectation about when wake time is coming, thus necessitating a lighter or more fragmented sleep so that he or she does not miss the desired wake time. Setting an alarm every morning will allow patients to become reliant on the alarm to wake them, and not their poor sleep.

"Wrapping Up"

When wrapping up, patients should be reminded that in many ways they are doing this to decrease their vulnerability to insomnia, improve the chances of therapy working, and get the most efficient sleep that they can. As such, they can be encouraged to practice all of the sleep hygiene rules as faithfully as possible and to do so consistently, at least for the time that therapy is taking place. However, once they are sleeping well and have determined optimal amounts of sleep, then it may be possible to consider looking at some rules individually and seeing whether an experiment in which they begin again to break a specific rule results in any adverse changes to their overall sleep. For example, while patients might be advised to stop drinking alcohol during the weeks that therapy takes place, once they are sleeping well they certainly do not need to remain teetotal. Given no history of substance abuse, it may be fine to drink occasionally or even to have a glass of wine per night. Some may find their improved sleep is not appreciably changed, while others may find that even one drink may actually fragment their sleep. In the latter case, it will then be up to individual patients to decide whether or not it is worth it for them to drink. The important point is that by having eliminated the alcohol entirely, the patients will then more easily be able to tell how alcohol affects their sleep as they add this habit back into the routine. The same can be said for snacking before bed, drinking more liquid in the evening, having chocolate in the evening, etc.

POSSIBLE MODIFICATIONS/VARIANTS

Noted above.

PROOF OF CONCEPT/SUPPORTING DATA/EVIDENCE BASE

It is generally held that sleep hygiene is not effective as a monotherapy. This common belief may be a bit of an overgeneralization from the existing facts which are more consistent with the 2006 AASM Standards of Practice Committee [3] conclusion that there is "insufficient evidence to recommend sleep hygiene as a single therapy" (p. 221).

The state of the science, with respect to sleep hygiene, is simply this:

1. There are only a few studies that evaluate the efficacy of sleep hygiene as a single treatment, and in these cases there is no standard for what sleep hygiene is (i.e., what rules are covered) or how it is administered (e.g., handout vs full session review). Thus it remains possible that some form of sleep hygiene may produce significant clinical gains.
2. The clinical gains obtained with sleep hygiene are thought to be marginal as many investigators use this intervention as a *control condition* for CBT-I randomized clinical trials. In such studies it has been reliably shown that CBT-I produces significantly greater magnitude results than does sleep hygiene. This said, it may be that sleep hygiene, when used as a control condition, utilizes such an abbreviated form of the treatment that

it is indeed akin to an inert-monitor only condition. Thus, once again, it remains possible that some form of sleep hygiene may produce reasonable clinical gains.

3. There are at least two investigations showing that patients with insomnia do not differ from good sleepers with respect to sleep hygiene infractions [4,5].

Finally, it should be noted that some, if not many, of the components of sleep hygiene are based on empirical evidence (e.g., the effects of diurnal napping on nocturnal sleep) and/or are grounded on well established theory (e.g., sleep–wake regulation as delineated in Borbley's Two Process Model [6]). For an excellent summary of these findings, the reader is referred to Stepanski and Wyatt's 2003 review on sleep hygiene [7]. The fact that some of the sleep hygiene rules are scientifically "well justified" suggests, once again, that sleep hygiene (given adequate coverage, a reasonable form of delivery, and the obtention of patient compliance with the rules that derive from the hard science) should produce significant clinical gains.

In sum, the most reasonable conclusion about sleep hygiene is this: it is a useful addition to a multi-component CBT-I protocol in that engaging in improved sleep hygiene may enhance outcomes or at least remove obstacles to progress.

REFERENCES

[1] N. Kleitman, Sleep and Wakefulness, Chicago University Press, Chicago, IL, 1987 (original version 1939).

[2] P.J. Hauri, Sleep Disorders, Upjohn, Kalamazoo, MI, 2004.

[3] T. Morgenthaler, M. Kramer, C. Alessi, et al., Practice parameters for the psychological and behavioral treatment of insomnia: an update. An American Academy of Sleep Medicine Report, Sleep 29 (2006) 1415–1419.

[4] L.A. Gellis, K.L. Lichstein, Sleep hygiene practices of good and poor sleepers in the United States: an internet-based study, Behav. Ther. 40 (2009) 1–9.

[5] C.S. McCrae, M.A. Rowe, N.D. Dautovich, et al., Sleep hygiene practices in two community dwelling samples of older adults, Sleep 29 (2006) 1551–1560.

[6] A.A. Borbely, A two process model of sleep regulation, Hum. Neurobiol. 1 (1982) 195–204.

[7] E.J. Stepanski, J.K. Wyatt, Use of sleep hygiene in the treatment of insomnia, Sleep Med. Rev. 7 (2003) 215–225.

RECOMMENDED READING

P.J. Hauri, Case Studies in Insomnia, Plenum Medical Book Company, New York, NY, 2003.

V.P. Zarcone, Sleep hygiene, in: M.H. Kryger, T. Roth, W.C. Dement, (Eds.), Principles and Practice of Sleep Medicine, WB Saunders Company, Philadelphia, PA, 1989.

Chapter 4

Relaxation for Insomnia

Kenneth L. Lichstein
Department of Psychology, University of Alabama, Tuscaloosa, AL

Daniel J. Taylor
Department of Psychology, University of North Texas, Denton, TX

Christina S. McCrae
Department of Clinical Psychology, University of Florida, Gainesville, FL

S. Justin Thomas
Department of Psychology, University of Alabama, Tuscaloosa, AL

PROTOCOL NAME

Relaxation for insomnia.

GROSS INDICATION

Relaxation methods are used when heightened somatic and/or cognitive arousal interferes with sleep. As most people with insomnia experience some form of arousal, relaxation techniques are appropriate for most people with insomnia.

SPECIFIC INDICATION

Research suggests that relaxation is more effective for sleep onset insomnia than sleep maintenance insomnia [1].

CONTRAINDICATIONS

There are no serious contraindications for relaxation therapy. Patients who do not have time to practice will not profit from this approach. A small percentage of patients will experience paradoxical increased anxiety during relaxation.

RATIONALE FOR INTERVENTION

There are dozens of methods of relaxation that may be collectively referred to as quiescent self inquiry. The variants of relaxation are numerous. Beginning

Behavioral Treatments for Sleep Disorders. DOI: 10.1016/B978-0-12-381522-4.00004-3

with meditative forms of Hindu yoga dating to some 5000 years ago, continuing with autogenics and progressive relaxation introduced about 100 years ago, through more recent methods such as guided imagery, passive body focusing, and some aspects of mindfulness, and including machine guided relaxation (i.e., biofeedback), the core processes and effects of relaxation have changed little over the millennia.

All methods that fall beneath the relaxation umbrella conform to Benson's [2] relaxation response, yielding physiological and experiential calm. If some form of somatic and/or cognitive arousal is delaying and/or disrupting sleep, then relaxation works to diminish those barriers. Research suggests that cognitive arousal is more salient to insomnia than somatic arousal, and the mental calm accompanying well-practiced relaxation directly addresses this irritant.

STEP BY STEP DESCRIPTION OF PROCEDURES

The Relaxation Response

The four procedural elements comprising Benson's [2] approach to relaxation are: (1) a quiet environment, (2) an object to dwell upon, (3) a passive attitude, and (4) a comfortable position. The virtue of the first and last of these is perhaps obvious. It would be difficult to attain physiological/experiential calm in a noisy, distracting environment, or when assuming a posture that was uncomfortable and physically distracting. A completely quiet environment is not necessary; indeed, many enjoy music during relaxation. Individual preference will dictate which sounds are conducive and which simply noise. Similarly, the lotus position (legs intertwined while sitting) is often adopted by experienced meditators, but would be inimical to relaxation in many others. Lying down, reclining in a padded chair, or sitting up are all acceptable relaxation poses. Some find slow or rhythmic movement is nurturing of relaxation. Rather than stipulating acceptable sound and posture prescriptions, we encourage patients to define a pleasing environment.

The second element, an object to dwell upon, refers to a "mental device" that consumes attention and displaces daily concerns. This device must be repetitive and monotonous; the more boring the better. It can take many different forms and again, individual tailoring is useful. Benson recommended slowly repeating in one's mind or aloud the neutral, secular word "one", but Eastern-sounding words such as "om" or "shirim" would do as well. Eyes may be closed, or one's gaze can be fixed on a flower, a candle, a vase, one's breath, etc., replacing the repetition of a word or phrase. Images of pleasant nature scenes or personally meaningful objects can be the mental device.

Benson believes the third element, passive attitude, is the most important relaxation ingredient. It is the most indispensable, and it is the most likely to help sustain the relaxation effect beyond the boundaries of the relaxation practice session. Famed sexologists William Masters and Virginia Johnson cautioned that you cannot will an erection; an erection will occur only when it is not the focus of attention. So it is with relaxation. The harder you try to relax, the less likely it is to occur. A relaxed, passive attitude is essential to achieving a relaxed state. The first challenge to most people is how to manage the near universal experience of mind-wandering, and this provides a valuable opportunity to cultivate a relaxed attitude. Don't struggle for control over your mind. Allow your mind to wander, and in time it will wander back to the relaxation task. Acceptance of mind-wandering is a helpful gauge of how well the patient has embraced a passive attitude. Regular relaxation practice will both profit from and cultivate a relaxed attitude. Patients should be encouraged to maintain a relaxed attitude throughout the day, and this will translate into a more relaxed (Type B) personality.

Relaxation Practice

It matters little which relaxation method is used. Practice is critical, and if the patient practices regularly, therapeutic benefits are likely to emerge. We invest a fair amount of time in

- explaining the importance of practice and
- scheduling practice.

We prescribe at least two relaxation practices a day: one during the day and one at bedtime. Relaxation can also be practiced during middle-of-the-night awakenings.

The daytime practice is for skill development. It should be done during a low-stress time. Patients are more skillful at being anxious than at being relaxed. If daytime practice is done at a high-stress time, the novice relaxation skill will be at a competitive disadvantage with anxiety. The skill will be slow to develop, and patients will complain relaxation does not work.

The night-time practice is the therapeutic dose. It should be done when the patient gets into bed with the intent of going to sleep. It may be helpful to allow a couple of weeks of relaxation practice during the day before commencing night-time practice, to protect the skill development period.

Patients often have difficulty adhering to the daily daytime practice. We invest time in discussing its importance and planning for its occurrence. When encouraged, patients can be creative in creating 5–10 minutes of practice time early in the morning, at work, or early evening. We will often contract with patients to practice certain times, certain days. We may use the Premack Principle, making more preferred activities contingent on less preferred activities – for example, the patient agrees to practice relaxation before he or she starts watching television in the evening.

Relaxation Procedures

For the past two decades, our research and clinical work has mainly relied on a hybrid passive relaxation procedure (given verbatim in Lichstein [3]). The procedure has four components: relaxed attitude; slow, deep breathing; passive body focusing; and autogenic phrases. The entire induction takes about 10 minutes. All the components are physically non-demanding, so issues of exacerbating painful areas are avoided. The procedures are simple and easily mastered. Because the four components are independent, patients are encouraged to emphasize those parts with which they feel most comfortable, resulting in a naturally occurring tailoring process.

Relaxed attitude. Description of relaxed attitude concerning mind wandering and distracting sensations/noises; advice is given not to force relaxation (45 seconds).

Deep breaths. Patients are asked to take five deep breaths, hold each for 5 seconds, and softly say "relax" as they exhale (1 minute 30 seconds).

Body focusing. Patients are directed to focus on a body-part sequence that covers the whole body: arms, face, trunk, and legs; the patient dwells on each part for about 45 seconds and seeks out relaxing feelings in each (5 minutes).

Autogenic phrases. Patients are instructed to focus on sensations of heaviness and warmth in their arms and legs (2 minutes).

POSSIBLE MODIFICATIONS/VARIANTS

The possible modifications and variants of relaxation are likely infinite. In this section, we attempt to focus on those variants and modifications that are most commonly used. The methods of relaxation that have received the most attention in the insomnia literature are progressive muscle relaxation (PMR), autogenic training, meditation, and imagery. New evidence is emerging on the use of mindfulness-based stress reduction for the treatment of insomnia, so this intervention will also be discussed. Other relaxation methods, such as diaphragmatic breathing, hypnosis, and transcendental meditation, may be used clinically, but they have no empirical backing as treatments of insomnia, and thus will not be discussed here, to conserve space.

Progressive Muscle Relaxation (PMR)

The protocol for PMR varies somewhat between delivery methods, but globally involves alternately tensing and relaxing different muscle groups throughout the body [4,5]. Patients are trained to focus on and compare feelings of relaxation with the tension that was present before the relaxation procedure. Different practitioners utilize different durations (e.g., tense for 5–15 seconds and relax for 20–45 seconds). No comparative studies have been performed to help determine which tensing and relaxing durations are most beneficial, so it is ultimately up to the therapist and perhaps the patient. This technique typically takes 10–30 minutes. Some therapists go through each body part individually multiple times. Others focus on individual body parts early in therapy, focus on body regions in the middle sessions, and finally focus on the whole body by the final sessions, so the patients can achieve relaxation more rapidly.

Homework typically involves practicing the relaxation at home during the day, just prior to bedtime, and sometimes during night-time awakenings. Some therapists do not like to assign the bedtime practice, because they feel it produces performance anxiety, but there is no evidence to support this belief. Patients are typically asked to do the bedtime relaxation in bed, so that if they fall asleep during the procedure, they do not have to move back to their bedroom. In addition, it might be useful to perform the daytime practice in the bedroom, in an attempt to facilitate classical conditioning. Multiple scripts for progressive muscle relaxation are available both online and within treatment texts (see, for example, Lichstein [6], Morin and Espie [7], and Smith [8]).

Autogenic Training

One variant of relaxation that is often included in other forms of relaxation training is autogenic training. In this method, the patient visualizes a peaceful scene and repeats autogenic phrases intended to deepen the relaxation response. The patient typically repeats phrases focused on each arm and leg which include "heaviness" and "warmth" (e.g., my left arm is heavy … my left arm is warm … my left arm is heavy …, etc.). From there the patient moves on to focusing on cardiac regulation, respiration, abdominal warmth, and cooling of the forehead. In the original form, the patient took 6 months to learn this method, with one to two sessions to learn each component (e.g., left arm). Briefer methods [6] have been developed which focus on the same or similar areas, but for a shorter period of time (i.e., 30 seconds for each component).

Meditation

Meditation is a difficult concept to define, because a multitude of meditation techniques exist. We present two variants.

Yoga

Kundalini Yoga was popularized by Yogi Bhajan in the late 1960s as a means of general life enhancement and to explore altered states of consciousness without the use of drugs. Yoga involves the awareness of breath (pranayama) and thought processes, in addition to a series of postures (asanas) designed to stretch and strengthen the body. Yoga, as traditionally practiced, is often combined with aspects of PMR (especially in "corpse pose") and meditation. As one can see, many of these elements overlap with the relaxation techniques already discussed.

The following Kundalini yoga treatment has been used for insomnia [9]:

1. Meditation on long, slow abdominal breathing (1–3 minutes).
2. Arms extended upwards at a 60° angle with the palms flat and facing upwards with meditation on the breath (1–3 minutes).

3. Arms extended horizontally to the sides with the wrists bent upwards and the palms facing away with meditation on the breath (1–3 minutes).
4. Hands clasped together at the sternum with the arms pushing the palms together with meditation on the breath (1–3 minutes).
5. A breathing meditation called "Shabad Kriya" (30 minutes).
   - Palms are resting in lap, facing upward, with right over left and thumbs touching
   - Eyes are one-tenth open and gaze downwards past the tip of the nose
   - Inhalation is in 4 segments or "sniffs", followed by breath retention for 16 counts, and exhalation in 2 segments (ratio of inhale : hold : exhale is 4 : 16 : 2)
   - During inhalation, the mantra "Sa, Ta, Na, Ma" is mentally recited with each segment
   - During breath retention, this mantra is mentally repeated four times
   - During the exhalation the mantra "Wahe Guru" is mentally recited concurrently with each exhale segment
   - Overall breathing frequency should be as slow as is comfortable, while maintaining the specified ratio of inhale : hold : exhale.

Participants are instructed to perform the treatment in the evening, preferably just before bedtime. If, on occasion, the subject's evening schedule makes it difficult to incorporate the treatment, participants are to practice the treatment at another time of day.

Mindfulness

The Mindfulness-Based Therapy for Insomnia (MBTI [10]) method is discussed elsewhere in this text, but deserves some mention at this point. This form of therapy combines common behavioral treatments of insomnia (e.g., stimulus control) with mindfulness meditation practices and exercises. Based on the Mindfulness-Based Stress Reduction Program (MBSR [11,12]), each session combines formal mindfulness meditation, followed by didactics, and group dialogue to teach the principles of mindfulness. The major point of emphasis in the mindfulness meditation component is a focus on present thoughts, actions, body functions, feelings, etc., without judgment. A point of emphasis in MBTI is using the principles of acceptance and letting go to work with negative emotional reactions to disturbed sleep. In this way, the procedure is much like other meditation.

Imagery

Imagery is employed in most forms of relaxation training, but has received little supportive research as a single treatment. Guided imagery is generally a reminiscent task, as patients tend to choose images of places from their past which were relaxing. Future orientation tends to be discouraged, as it is thought to be less relaxing and more activating. Generally, a pleasant nature scene is ideal. Patients are asked to close their eyes, find a comfortable position, and select an image that they find relaxing, that they have actually experienced, and that is relatively fresh in their memory. They are then guided through making the image as realistic as possible by focusing on the details of the scene and using the five senses (i.e., vision, hearing, smell, taste, and touch).

Note that not everyone is good at imagery, so caution must be used with this technique.

Biofeedback

Biofeedback is a specific form of relaxation treatment that differs from those mentioned above because it actually provides sensory feedback (usually visual or auditory), either mechanically (i.e., thermometers) or, more frequently, with computers and amplifiers, to help patients learn how to control physiological parameters (such as finger temperature or muscle tension) in order to reduce somatic arousal [13]. For instance, frontalis electromyography (EMG) biofeedback, the most commonly studied form of biofeedback, teaches subjects to reduce muscle tension in the muscles of the forehead and face. Biofeedback seems to help patients attain states of mental and physical relaxation, and become more aware of their own bodily sensations and responses to stressors. Biofeedback actively involves the patient in the therapeutic process, and provides immediate measures of progress. One difficulty with evaluating the effectiveness of biofeedback is that it is often paired with some form of relaxation exercise, making it difficult to parse out the independent effects of each. In addition, improvements appear to be comparable to PMR, which takes less time for the patient to learn and requires no expensive equipment.

PROOF OF CONCEPT/SUPPORTING DATA/EVIDENCE BASE

Relaxation is commonly used as a form of therapy for disorders in which arousal (cognitive and physiological) plays an important role (e.g., anxiety, chronic pain, insomnia). There is considerable evidence (more than 50 studies) to support its use as a monotherapy, as part of CBT-I, and as part of multicomponent therapies for insomnia. In 2006, an American Academy of Sleep Medicine Task Force concluded that this evidence was sufficient to recommend relaxation training (e.g., PMR, autogenics) as a standard treatment for insomnia [13]. Because relaxation is an umbrella term that refers to a family of therapeutic techniques (PMR, passive relaxation, autogenics, biofeedback, imagery training, meditation), the amount of evidence supporting a specific technique varies with the bulk of studies examining PMR or similar techniques (e.g., passive relaxation) [14,15]. Over the past 30+ years, two notable trends have emerged in the literature. Specifically, research prior to 1997 [14] tended to examine relaxation as a stand-alone treatment and included a wider range of techniques, including PMR, biofeedback, guided imagery, and meditation, while more recent research [15] tends to focus on PMR or similar techniques and to examine relaxation as just one component of either CBT-I or multi-component interventions.

As a stand-alone technique, controlled studies (placebo, wait list, and/or no treatment) have shown that relaxation (regardless of technique) produces improvements in sleep quality ratings as well as 20- to 30-minute improvements in self-reported sleep onset latency, wake time after sleep onset, and total sleep time from baseline to post-treatment [14,15]. In studies that included follow-up evaluations, these improvements were generally well maintained. Imagery training is a notable exception, as research examining this technique has produced mixed results. Polysomnography was included as an objective outcome measure in only a handful of studies, and findings support little to no improvement on objective sleep measures. Some studies have also included measures of daytime functioning. However, improvements have been documented primarily for subjective sleep outcomes. Most experts would agree that this is not surprising, given that insomnia (similar to chronic pain) is largely a subjective sleep disorder by nature.

Trials that included relaxation as part of CBT-I or a multi-component treatment have largely produced results similar to, and in some cases slightly better than, those of trials evaluating relaxation as a stand-alone treatment. Although this evidence may make it tempting to conclude that relaxation alone may be able to replace CBT-I and multi-component treatment for insomnia, it is important to note that dismantling studies have yet to be conducted. Therefore, no conclusions can be drawn regarding the active element of CBT-I or multi-component interventions. Additionally, some evidence suggests that, when used as stand-alone techniques, stimulus control and sleep restriction may be more effective than relaxation.

A handful of recent studies (see, for example, Lichstein [16]) have utilized relaxation (either alone or combined with other techniques) in protocols including medication withdrawal. Those studies have documented reductions and even the complete elimination of hypnotic medication in some patients. One such study compared relaxation and medication withdrawal to medication withdrawal alone, and found sleep efficiency improved in medicated and non-medicated patients [16]. Not surprisingly, there was a worsening of all other measures during withdrawal that was not attenuated by relaxation. However, only medicated patients who were receiving relaxation reported improvements in sleep quality and fewer withdrawal symptoms.

REFERENCES

[1] C.M. Morin, J.P. Culbert, S.M. Schwartz, Nonpharmacological interventions for insomnia: a meta-analysis of treatment efficacy, Am. J. Psych. 151 (1994) 1172–1180.

[2] H. Benson, The Relaxation Response, William Morrow, New York, NY, 1975.

[3] K.L. Lichstein, Relaxation, in: K.L. Lichstein, C.M. Morin, (Eds.), Treatment of Late-life Insomnia, Sage, Thousand Oaks, CA, 2000, pp. 185–206.
[4] B. Bernstein, T. Borkovec, Progressive Relaxation Training, Research Press, Champagne, IL, 1973.
[5] E. Jacobson, Progressive Relaxation: A Physiological and Clinical Investigation of Muscular States and their Significance in Psychology and Medical Practice, University of Chicago Press, Chicago, IL, 1929.
[6] K.L. Lichstein, Clinical Relaxation Strategies, Wiley, New York, NY, 1988.
[7] C.M. Morin, C.A. Espie, Insomnia: A Clinical Guide to Assessment and Treatment, Kluwer Academic/Plenum Publishers, New York, NY, 2003.
[8] J.C. Smith, Relaxation, Meditation & Mindfulness, Springer, New York, NY, 2005.
[9] S.B.S. Khalsa, Treatment of chronic insomnia with Yoga: a preliminary study with sleep–wake diaries, Appl. Psychophysiol. Biofeedback 29 (2004) 269–278.
[10] J.C. Ong, S.L. Shapiro, R. Manber, Mindfulness meditation and CBT for insomnia: a naturalistic 12-month follow-up, Explore: J. Sci. Healing 5 (2009) 30–36.
[11] J. Kabat-Zinn, Full Catastrophe Living: Using the Wisdom of Your Body and Mind to Face Stress, Pain, and Illness, Delacorte Press, New York, NY, 1990.
[12] S. Santorelli, Heal Thyself: Lessons on Mindfulness in Medicine, Crown, New York, NY, 1999.
[13] T. Morgenthaler, M. Kramer, C. Alessi, et al., Practice parameters for the psychological and behavioral treatment of insomnia: an update. An American Academy of Sleep Medicine report, Sleep 29 (2006) 1415–1419.
[14] C.M. Morin, P.J. Hauri, C.A. Espie, et al., Nonpharmacologic treatment of chronic insomnia. An American Academy of Sleep Medicine review, Sleep 22 (8) (1999) 1134–1156.
[15] C.M. Morin, R.R. Bootzin, D.J. Buysse, et al., Psychological and behavioral treatment of insomnia: update of the recent evidence (1998–2004), Sleep 29 (2006) 1398–1414.
[16] K.L. Lichstein, R.S. Johnson, Relaxation for insomnia and hypnotic medication use in older women, Psychol. Aging 8 (1) (1993) 103–111.

RECOMMENDED READING

H. Benson, The Relaxation Response, William Morrow, New York, NY, 1975.
B. Bernstein, T. Borkovec, Progressive Relaxation Training, Research Press, Champagne, IL, 1973.
E. Jacobson, Progressive Relaxation: A Physiological and Clinical Investigation of Muscular States and their Significance in Psychology and Medical Practice, University of Chicago Press, Chicago, IL, 1929.
J. Kabat-Zinn, Full Catastrophe Living: Using the Wisdom of Your Body and Mind to Face Stress, Pain, and Illness, Delacorte Press, New York, 1990.
K.L. Lichstein, Clinical Relaxation Strategies, Wiley, New York, NY, 1988.
K.L. Lichstein, Relaxation, in: K.L. Lichstein, C.M. Morin, (Eds.), Treatment of Late-life Insomnia, Sage, Thousand Oaks, CA, 2000, pp. 185–206.
T. Morgenthaler, M. Kramer, C. Alessi, et al., Practice parameters for the psychological and behavioral treatment of insomnia: an update. An American Academy of Sleep Medicine report, Sleep 29 (2006) 1415–1419.
C.M. Morin, C.A. Espie, Insomnia: A Clinical Guide to Assessment and Treatment, Kluwer Academic/Plenum Publishers, New York, NY, 2003.

C.M. Morin, J.P. Culbert, S.M. Schwartz, Nonpharmacological interventions for insomnia: a meta-analysis of treatment efficacy, Am. J. Psychiatry 151 (1994) 1172–1180.
C.M. Morin, R.R. Bootzin, D.J. Buysse, et al., Psychological and behavioral treatment of insomnia: update of the recent evidence (1998–2004), Sleep 29 (2006) 1398–1414.
S. Santorelli, Heal Thyself: Lessons on Mindfulness in Medicine, Crown, New York, NY, 1999.
J.C. Smith, Relaxation, Meditation & Mindfulness, Springer, New York, NY, 2005.

Chapter 5

Sleep Compression

Kenneth L. Lichstein, S. Justin Thomas
Department of Psychology, University of Alabama, Tuscaloosa, AL

Susan M. McCurry
Department of Psychosocial and Community Health, University of Washington, Seattle, WA

PROTOCOL NAME

Sleep compression.

GROSS INDICATION

Sleep compression is ideal for those who exhibit sleep continuity disturbance but not substantial daytime deficits.

SPECIFIC INDICATION

Poor sleep accompanied by little daytime impairment suggests that enough sleep has been obtained to satisfy biologic need. Decreasing wake time in bed, not increasing sleep, becomes the primary therapeutic goal.

There is insufficient experience with this method to recommend its preferred use with a type of insomnia (e.g., primary vs comorbid, midlife vs late life) or with a particular pattern of wakefulness (e.g., onset vs maintenance). However, sleep compression does use an incremental approach to decreasing time in bed, as compared to abrupt contraction in the method of sleep restriction, and sleep compression may be better tolerated by individuals who are experiencing daytime fatigue or mild sleepiness, or who may be sensitive to abrupt alteration of their time in bed pattern.

CONTRAINDICATIONS

There are no serious contraindications for sleep compression. Temporary, increased daytime sleepiness that sometimes occurs with the introduction of the similar procedure of sleep restriction has not been observed with sleep compression.

Behavioral Treatments for Sleep Disorders. DOI: 10.1016/B978-0-12-381522-4.00005-5

RATIONALE FOR INTERVENTION

Individuals may seek more sleep than they need when idiographic sleep needs are defined by nomothetic goals. Individuals gifted with a short need for sleep may create an insomnia sleep pattern when they strive for the common goal of 7 hours and 30 minutes of sleep, even when less sleep is needed to satisfy their biologic need. By their night-time sleep pattern, this insomnia subtype resembles individuals who do fail to obtain sufficient sleep, but may be distinguished by the absence of daytime sequelae expected to follow inadequate sleep.

STEP BY STEP DESCRIPTION OF PROCEDURES

Neither research nor clinical experience has dictated a standard sleep compression protocol. What follows is how we typically do it.

Sleep compression begins by estimating total sleep time (TST) and time in bed (TIB). This is usually done by collecting a 2-week baseline sleep diary; longer or shorter baseline duration and other data sources, such as actigraphy, could be used instead. However, collecting data for much less than a week may mean that you will not get a representative sample of sleep (for example, including both weekend and weekdays). We have also found that sleep diaries have better utility for setting a sleep compression schedule, since they reflect patients' *perceptions* of their own sleep, and as a result patients are more likely to accept recommended changes than when baseline data are derived from an actigraphic device.

The baseline sleep assessment will yield mean TST and mean TIB. Atypical baseline nights producing unrepresentative TST or TIB values that might arise from factors such as illness or uncharacteristic socializing can be discounted. The therapeutic goal of sleep compression is to eliminate the TIB–TST discrepancy by cutting back TIB in incremental parts over the next several weeks. We will typically use about six sessions to shrink TIB to conform to TST. The number of treatment sessions may be adjusted according to the magnitude of the TIB–TST discrepancy that will be managed.

As an example, consider Jennifer, who averaged 6 hours of sleep a night during baseline but had 8 hours of TIB. The 2 hours of superfluous TIB will be cut by 120 minutes/six sessions, or about 20 minutes a week. As the sessions unfold, the pace of cutting TIB can be adjusted to accommodate changes in TST that may arise. If TST gradually increases, the number of minutes cut can slow, or the reverse if TST shrinks. Similarly, should the patient report waxing daytime impairment, the pace of reducing TIB should slow. We do not use a fixed formula, such as maintaining sleep efficiency within a specified range, in titrating TIB cuts. Typically, by the fourth or fifth session the therapist or patient may suggest that the rate of compression is too slow or too fast, and we will renegotiate the treatment course.

In the first session of sleep compression in this case example, prescribed TIB will be reduced to 7 hours, 40 minutes. Provider and patient will negotiate a fixed bedtime (e.g., 11:00 pm) and fixed wake time (e.g., 6:40 am).

We usually defer to the patient's preference in setting these TIB boundaries so long as they conform to the prescribed TIB duration. A week later, the second session will set a TIB of 7 hours and 20 minutes, and the bedtime (e.g., 11:10 pm) and/or wake time (e.g., 6:30 am) will be reset accordingly. Each of the next four weekly treatment sessions will reduce the TIB by 20 minutes, so that at the end of the sixth treatment session, the week following will see the TIB and the TST match at 6 hours.

Adherence

Adherence with sleep compression is generally less problematic than with traditional sleep restriction recommendations that precipitously reduce a client's time in bed. The leisurely process of cutting back in-bed times allows patients time to become accustomed to changing their bedtime and rising time, and because the overall reduction in bed time is less abrupt, there is usually less initial reactance to the plan. Unlike the common injunction "Don't go to bed unless sleepy" characteristic of the stimulus control procedure, sleep compression instructions encourage patients to stick with the prescribed bedtime and wake time each week. We want the compression of TIB to proceed in an orderly, slow fashion. Some patients want to rush the process and are tempted to cut back at a faster pace. In our experience, this may excite side effects, such as increased daytime sleepiness and irritability, and invite unstable, disruptive circadian rhythms. Patients whose life circumstance dictates an inconsistent sleep schedule, such as rotating shiftwork, may be poor candidates for sleep compression treatment. Based on correlation with treatment outcome, greater consistency of time spent in bed per night and a more consistent arising time are aspects of adherence that should receive the most attention [1].

Though many of us would relish the newfound time liberated by compressed sleep, some patients rebel at the prospect of having to find something to do late at night or early in the morning, and this may fuel lapses in adherence. Therapists should assist patients in creating a menu of low-key activities for the evening and alerting activities for the morning. Another concern with adherence arises in the case of persons whose TST improves to match in-bed time before the full 6-week protocol is complete. For example, if Jennifer comes back at the end of the third week reporting that she was in bed every night for 7 hours and asleep for an average of 6 hours and 45 minutes per night, a decision must be made. Continuing to pursue the sleep compression schedule as planned may invite resistance, since the desired goal of a high nightly sleep efficiency has been achieved. In such a case, we would typically encourage the client to "hold the course" at 7 hours per night for the next few weeks to see whether the improvement is permanent or transitory. If, the following week, Jennifer's sleep has again deteriorated, then we would recommend reducing an additional 20 minutes per night, picking up where we left off with a target goal of 6 hours per night as originally set. Although in cases where one is following a standardized research protocol this kind of variation in procedure may not be permitted, in the average clinical setting such flexibility empowers the patient and reduces the risk of the patient and therapist developing an adversarial relationship around the sleep scheduling program.

POSSIBLE MODIFICATIONS/VARIANTS

There are few published modifications of sleep compression. The protocol just described is a modification from the protocol used in the initial case study, which was conducted weekly for 2 months and then biweekly for the final 6 months [2]. Subsequent studies have all been conducted using between four and six sessions, conducted once a week [3–6]. Two of these studies demonstrated the efficacy of sleep compression as an independent intervention [3,6].

Another variation regarding the timing of individual therapy, although no supporting publications exist, would be to decrease the time in bed more rapidly, thus reaching the target total sleep time at a quicker pace. However, as was cautioned earlier, reducing time in bed too rapidly may produce side effects. An extreme modification would be akin to sleep restriction [7], in which the time in bed is immediately cut to the total sleep time. A major difference between sleep compression and sleep restriction is that sleep restriction aims to increase total sleep time after time in bed is reduced. Therefore, sleep compression is better suited for individuals with reduced sleep need, whereas sleep restriction is better suited for individuals whose sleep need falls within the normal range. (See Chapter 1 in this volume for a more detailed description of sleep restriction.)

Another modification is the use of group treatment for the presentation of sleep compression. A study utilizing treatment groups consisting of five participants yielded positive outcomes for the use of sleep compression [3]. Subsequent studies utilized groups of three to six individuals. However, these studies combined sleep compression in a treatment package, making it difficult to separate out the specific treatment effects of sleep compression from the combined effects of the multi-component treatment package [4,5,8]. The McCurry package consisted of relaxation, sleep hygiene, stimulus control, sleep compression, and education for caregivers of parents with Alzheimer's disease, and demonstrated improvements in sleep during treatment and at a 3-month follow-up compared to wait list control [5]. These findings suggest that whether independent or as part of multi-component treatment, sleep compression presented via group therapy can be effective for insomnia and provides all the usual benefits of group treatment.

PROOF OF CONCEPT/SUPPORTING DATA/EVIDENCE BASE

Sleep compression is a method of behavior modification for insomnia that includes the gradual, step-wise reduction of time in bed until the target total sleep time is reached. Sleep compression has been shown to be effective as monotherapy [2,6] and as part of a multi-component treatment package [4,5]. Recently, sleep restriction/sleep compression was recommended as one of two evidence-based psychological treatments (EBTs) for insomnia in older adults [9]. The other recommended EBT is multi-component cognitive-behavioral therapy, which could include sleep compression.

REFERENCES

[1] B.W. Riedel, K.L. Lichstein, Strategies for evaluating adherence to sleep restriction treatment for insomnia. Behav. Res. Ther. 39 (2001) 201–212.

[2] K.L. Lichstein, Sleep compression treatment of an insomnoid, Behav. Ther. 19 (1988) 625–632.

[3] B.W. Riedel, K.L. Lichstein, W.O. Dwyer, Sleep compression and sleep education for older insomniacs: Self-help versus therapist guidance, Psychol. Aging 10 (1995) 54–63.

[4] S.M. McCurry, R.G. Logsdon, L. Teri, Behavioral treatment of sleep disturbance in elderly dementia caregivers, Clin. Gerontol. 17 (2) (1996) 35–50.

[5] S.M. McCurry, R.G. Logsdon, M.V. Vitiello, L. Teri, Successful behavioral treatment for reported sleep problems in elderly caregivers of dementia patients: a controlled study, J. Gerontol.: Psychol. Sci. 53B (1998) P122–P129.

[6] K.L. Lichstein, B.W. Riedel, N.M. Wilson, K.W. Lester, R.N. Aguillard, Relaxation and sleep compression for late-life insomnia: a placebo-controlled trial, J. Consult. Clin. Psychol. 69 (2001) 227–239.

[7] A.J. Spielman, P. Saskin, M.J. Thorpy, Treatment of chronic insomnia by restriction of time in bed, Sleep 10 (1987) 45–56.

[8] N.K. Vincent, H. Hameed, Relation between adherence and outcome in the group treatment of insomnia, Behav. Sleep Med. 1 (2003) 125–139.

[9] S.M. McCurry, R.G. Logsdon, L. Teri, M.V. Vitiello, Evidence-based psychological treatments for insomnia in older adults, Psychol. Aging 22 (2007) 18–27.

RECOMMENDED READING

K.L. Lichstein, B.W. Riedel, N.M. Wilson, et al., Relaxation and sleep compression for late-life insomnia: a placebo-controlled trial, J. Consult. Clin. Psychol. 69 (2001) 227–239.

S.M. McCurry, R.G. Logsdon, M.V. Vitiello, L. Teri, Successful behavioral treatment for reported sleep problems in elderly caregivers of dementia patients: a controlled study, J. Gerontol.: Psychol. Sci. 53B (1998) P122–P129.

B.W. Riedel, K.L. Lichstein, W.O. Dwyer, Sleep compression and sleep education for older insomniacs: self-help versus therapist guidance, Psychol. Aging 10 (1995) 54–63.

Chapter 6

Paradoxical Intention Therapy

Colin A. Espie
University of Glasgow Sleep Centre, Sackler Institute of Psychobiological Research, University of Glasgow, Scotland, UK

PROTOCOL NAME

Paradoxical Intention (PI) therapy.

GROSS INDICATION

Paradoxical intention is thought to be ideal for insomnia disorder, particularly where there is intense preoccupation about sleep, sleep loss, and its consequences. The psychophysiological insomnia phenotype, as characterized in ICSD-2, couples sleep preoccupation with the notion of "striving" to sleep, and the maladaptive relationship between effort to sleep and ability to sleep [1].

SPECIFIC INDICATION

There is no evidence to suggestion that Paradoxical Intention (PI) therapy is differentially effective in the sleep onset and sleep maintenance insomnia subtypes. The rationale for PI therapy, however, seems particularly appropriate for the psychophysiological insomnia phenotype (as stated above). There are two studies that suggest that reduction of sleep-related anxiety and performance effort may be the mechanism by which PI has its effect [2,3], but there are no formal clinical trials that demonstrate greater efficacy of PI in those insomnia patients who exhibit greater sleep effort.

CONTRAINDICATIONS

Two related notes of caution when considering PI therapy. First, PI is not suitable for patients who adopt a very concrete approach [4], or who are cognitively impaired. PI instructions (such as "remain awake for as long as possible") are not literal commands to be implemented in an unthinking, mechanistic way. Rather, PI presents a cognitively challenging perspective on insomnia. It is important that patients understand that PI is a vehicle for a change in outlook as well as a change in behavior. Second, whereas aspects of

Behavioral Treatments for Sleep Disorders. DOI: 10.1016/B978-0-12-381522-4.00006-7

PI are incorporated in all elements of CBT for insomnia (see Table 6.2, later), the particular use of PI, and certainly its use as a single insomnia therapy, may require a high level of therapist skill. In these circumstances, it should be regarded as a more advanced form of sleep psychotherapy [5].

RATIONALE FOR INTERVENTION

The guiding rationale is that because sleep is essentially an involuntary physiological process, attempts to place it under voluntary control are likely to make matters worse. PI is thought to work by reducing performance anxiety (the poor sleeper's inability to produce the criterion performance for good sleep) and by reducing associated sleep worry and sleep preoccupation.

Paradoxical techniques in psychotherapy have been described for a long time – for example, 100 years ago, methods were described of treating impotence through the simultaneous prescription of intimate physical contact and the prohibition of sexual intercourse. Further work in the 1960s and 1970s developed this into a treatment program for sexual dysfunction, to good effect. Psycho-physiological relationships seem particularly relevant to PI. People have sexual responses when they try not to; people blush when they try not to blush; people stammer when they try to prevent stammering; … and people remain awake when they try to get to sleep. The paradoxical nature of early behavior therapy treatments is also worth noting – for example, "negative practice" to break undesirable habits, "massed practice" for motor tics, "flooding" for fears and phobias (see Seltzer [6] or Espie [5] for review).

The use of PI for insomnia was adapted from Viktor Frankl's (1955 onwards) work [7] by Michael Ascher and others in the late 1970s [8,9], when it was observed that people with insomnia had more success falling asleep when they tried to remain awake than they had when they tried to fall asleep. Contemporary understanding of PI fits with the Psychobiological Inhibition/Attention–Intention–Effort model [10,11], where mental and behavioral focus on the sleep process is regarded as inhibitory to sleep engagement.

STEP BY STEP DESCRIPTION OF PROCEDURES

The following elements of PI therapy should be regarded as sequential but, for the purposes of tailoring therapy for an individual patient, they may be taken out of order, and some elements may be regarded as more or less important to include.

Consider Sleep "Normalcy"

A good starting point is to consider, with your patient, "How does a good sleeper do it?" It must be a difficult thing to be a good sleeper, or so people with insomnia might think. They usually have spent months, more likely years, trying to find a solution to their problem; to find a key that will unlock their sleep. But here there is a special secret. Good sleepers are good sleepers precisely because what they do is second nature to them. They just don't really think about it, nor do they "do" anything in particular.

Consider that good sleepers may not even be the best at following good routines. Maybe some of them are neglectful of so-called "sleep hygiene". The point is that the good sleeper is different from the person with insomnia because whatever it is that they do is not done deliberately or anxiously with the purpose of influencing sleep. They are not preoccupied about sleep … and so they sleep. If they don't sleep so well, then because they are not preoccupied about that it tends to sort itself out again.

Consider the purpose of "sleep hygiene"; you might even venture the idea that most good sleepers don't deserve to sleep well because they pay so little attention to it! This introduces a helpful component of the PI approach: the use of humor, which, in skilled therapeutic hands, is a very effective, and perhaps ultimate, de-catastrophizing agent [5].

Measure Sleep Normalcy

Ask your patient to complete a sleep effort scale [12], in the manner they think that a good sleeper might complete it. There is one such scale in Figure 6.1.

The following seven statements relate to your night-time sleep pattern *in the past week*. Please indicate by circling *one* response how true each statement is for you (score 2, 1 or 0 for each statement)

1.	I put too much effort into sleeping when it should come naturally	Very much	To some extent	Not at all
2.	I feel I should be able to control my sleep	Very much	To some extent	Not at all
3.	I put off going to bed at night for fear of not being able to sleep	Very much	To some extent	Not at all
4.	I worry about not sleeping if I cannot sleep	Very much	To some extent	Not at all
5.	I am no good at sleeping	Very much	To some extent	Not at all
6.	I get anxious about sleeping before I go to bed	Very much	To some extent	Not at all
7.	I worry about the consequences of not sleeping	Very much	To some extent	Not at all

FIGURE 6.1 The Glasgow Sleep Effort Scale. *(Broomfield & Espie)*

Each item reflects a common concern or preoccupation for people with insomnia. Their task, though, is to fill out the scale from the perspective of a good sleeper. Hopefully, they will see that the good sleeper's score would be zero, or pretty close to zero.

Develop a Formulation of Insomnia as a Sleep Effort Syndrome

By the time we see the majority of people with insomnia at a clinic, they may have spent years trying and trying to find a solution. PI offers a potential exit from that vicious cycle – by giving up trying. So, the next therapeutic task is to consider whether the patient would share a collaborative formulation that sees insomnia as a psychophysiological "sleep effort syndrome" [13].

Having considered what the "sleep psychology" of the good sleeper is like, you could now ask the patient to complete the Glasgow Sleep Effort Scale from his or her own perspective. Commonly, patients will endorse putting a lot of effort into trying to sleep, wishing they could control it, the build up of fear as bedtime approaches, excessive worry and anxiety about sleep and its consequences, and an overall feeling that they are just no good at sleep. In short, they may begin to realize that they see sleep as a "doing thing", and that this is counter-productive.

It can be helpful to get people to understand that they should "draw the thin line" (Figure 6.2) [14]. Here is the challenge of this exercise. On the one side, there should be recognition that they need to put 100 percent commitment into putting good advice into practice, but on the other that it is crucial they stop trying so hard. Motivation and commitment are good; effort and preoccupation are bad. You should work alongside individuals toward a steady, calm, assured approach as the best way to go. The emphasis should be upon determination and not giving up, but if they cross the line from productive commitment to unproductive effort, then they will be focussing their efforts again too much

Being motivated	Trying too hard
Following advice	Getting more preoccupied
Sticking to the program	Forcing sleep
Returning to the program	Trying to win
Refusing to give up	Getting desperate

FIGURE 6.2 The thin line between commitment and unproductive effort. (*From Espie, 2006*)

upon trying to sleep, trying to defeat insomnia. They will lose that battle. Help patients to consider that the good sleeper is no conquering hero. They have to abandon their attempts to drive insomnia from their bedroom door, and instead to start permitting sleep to come to them in its own way and in its own time.

Draw Helpful Parallels

PI therapy requires an attitudinal shift: just as it is helpful to consider the perspective of the normal sleeper, and to contrast that with the insomnia perspective, it can be helpful to draw parallels with other problems and with other situations.

For example, a paradox sometimes occurs when people with insomnia actually sleep better when they come into a sleep lab than they do at home. This may be because they are relaxed about whether or not they sleep well; they may even want their sleep problem to be evident to others. When they have this different outlook, their sleep may actually be more normal. Another illustration that most people understand is that normal sleepers, who do occasionally have bad nights, are familiar with the experience of wakeful periods spent wishing that morning would come quickly. When finally it is close to morning, they feel relieved about it and think "well, at least I can get up now"; upon which they promptly fall asleep, being no longer concerned and no longer trying to sleep.

Moreover, in a general sense, tapping into what people already know and so what they believe to be true, can be very helpful in therapy. The laudable sporting failure is a good example(!), where the commendable desire to achieve something becomes counter-productive and impairs performance. Get people to generate their own examples. That will help them get the point – trying not to scratch something that is itchy, trying to get that tune out of your head, the audition performance that didn't go as well as it might have, thinking too hard about your golf swing, trying to thread a needle, etc. Whether these are simple motor activities, social, sporting, or interpersonal goals, the point is that too much can spoil.

Another technique you can use for this part of the therapy is the "try not to think of a white bear" experiment, commonly used in social psychology. This demonstrates that active attempts to suppress (thoughts of a white bear) actually cause an increased frequency of such thoughts returning. There are a number of thought suppression strategies and games on the Internet which people can try. They all illustrate the importance of ironic (paradoxical) control processes.

Give Up Trying to Sleep

So what advice would PI therapy specifically offer for sleep-related behavior? Table 6.1 describes two methods for implementing PI therapy in bed.

TABLE 6.1 Methods for Giving Up Trying to Sleep (from Espie, 2006)

Method 1	Method 2
• Turn the tables • Take every opportunity to be carefree about your insomnia • Relish opportunities to get out of bed whenever you can • Be prepared to accept you have insomnia • Try to imagine as many catastrophes as you can that will happen just because you are awake at night; see them as exaggerated and absurd • Think of wakefulness as an opportunity, not a disaster; use the time when you are up to do something useful or something you enjoy	• Try to stay awake • Lie comfortably in your bed with the lights off, but keep your eyes open • Give up any effort to fall asleep • Give up any concern about still being awake • When your eyelids feel like they want to close, say to yourself gently "Just stay awake for another couple of minutes, I'll fall asleep naturally when I'm ready" • Don't purposefully make yourself stay awake, but if you can shift the focus off attempting to fall asleep, you will find that sleep comes naturally

Method 1 is a "giving up trying" method (after Fogle and Dyall [2]); an extension of the attitudinal shift that you will have been working on together, and parts of it come close to the notion of acceptance and mindfulness that are reported elsewhere in this book (see Chapter 14). This method has been referred to as "turning the tables" [4]. The use of humor is powerful in helping people to take a different perspective. It helps to reduce to dust the edifices of our exaggerated conclusions and emotions. Encourage people to think "what is the worst that can happen?", BUT rather than just challenging the true likelihood of all their wild imaginings (as you would do in cognitive restructuring; see Chapter 12) try instead going with the flow, rather than against it, by posing less resistance. Consider the scripted example in Box 6.1.

Method 1 may or may not appeal to your patient, but this more lighthearted approach could help to reduce anxiety and effort around sleep. Patients using this approach often talk about developing a completely different attitude. Indeed, the idea of accepting situations, rather than fighting them all the time has its roots in a number of ancient philosophies and religions. Acceptance leads to a problem having a less dominating position and influence. Where sleep is concerned, a more mellow perspective is an adaptive outlook, and one that can lead to improved sleep.

Method 2 is more explicitly paradoxical, where patients (paradoxically) encourage the symptoms that they don't want to have, to keep going. The goal becomes that of staying awake, instead of getting to sleep. By deciding to stay awake, the patient is completely giving up trying to sleep. When that happens, there is a strong possibility that individuals will find themselves falling asleep, in spite of their efforts to remain awake. It can be enormously reassuring for

Box 6.1 The Use of Humor in Paradoxical Intention Therapy

Patient: It is pretty awful really when I think about it. I can't sleep at night, and then to make matters worse insomnia just ruins my day.
Therapist: What do you mean?
Patient: Well, I can't think straight, and I get irritable, and I don't get through as much work as I should.
Therapist: That's shocking.
Patient: What's shocking?
Therapist: Well, that you don't get through your work. I mean that's pretty bad.
Patient: Well it's not that I don't get my work done, it's more that ...
Therapist: Sorry, you are the one that said you didn't get through your work ... So what effect does that have?
Patient: Well, it might get noticed. I mean, my boss might notice it.
Therapist: Really! ... I guess he wouldn't like that!?
Patient: Em, no, he'd probably have something to say about it. It could affect my job.
Therapist: Wow, that's worrying. You're not getting through your work, your boss is maybe going to notice, and you might lose your job.
Patient: Yeah, it's possible.
Therapist: Have you thought about reducing your financial commitments?
Patient: What?
Therapist: ... like maybe giving up your golf club membership, or taking the kids out of private school?
Patient: No, no I haven't, but why ...?
Therapist: I mean, if these things are likely to happen then you are best to take responsible action.
Patient: I think this is maybe getting a bit exaggerated, I mean it is not that bad ... it is not even likely I think.
Therapist: Thank goodness for that! (takes out handkerchief and mops brow).
Patient: (smiles)
Therapist: (smiles, laughs): I thought I was going to have an anxiety attack there!
Patient: (laughs): Yeah, I'm like a dog with a bone about this sleep problem!
Therapist: I was just about to check if I had some loose change to give you!!
Patient: (laughs): ... very thoughtful of you.
Therapist: You know, I think you're just trying too hard in every department, ... to sleep ... and also during the day. Why don't you give yourself a break!?
Patient: (laughs): ... you're not the first person to have suggested that!

patients to find that they are overtaken by sleep. They often say things like "I don't know what happened last night. I was trying to stay awake just a few minutes longer, and the next thing I knew it was morning". This is when patients begin to realize that they can be normal sleepers.

In the Method 2 approach, people should go to bed at a normal time when they feel sleepy and put the lights off; however, their explicit intention is to remain awake rather than to fall asleep, and therefore they are instructed to keep their eyes open and to make no effort whatsoever to sleep. This is a passive approach rather than an active one, in the sense that they should not deliberately try to keep themselves aroused. They are not given explicit direction to think about something stimulating, to move their arms and legs, or whatever, to remain awake; rather, to resist the tendency for their eyelids to close by re-opening them and keeping them open, and encouraging themselves to remain awake until sleep comes naturally. They should follow the same instructions if they waken during the night and do not quickly return to sleep. Like the good sleeper, sleep should be allowed to come to them.

POSSIBLE MODIFICATIONS AND VARIANTS

There is essentially no difference in the treatment instruction for PI when it is used for sleep onset insomnia compared with sleep maintenance insomnia or mixed type insomnia. However, there are, as we have seen, alternative ways of presenting the PI instructions.

In addition, it is important to note that there are elements of PI incorporated into almost all the proven CBT interventions for insomnia. This is illustrated in Table 6.2. The first column refers to the CBT technique itself, the second column refers to the insomnia problem that the technique is addressing, and the third column explains why the technique might be seen as paradoxical. Table 6.2 also illustrates how some of the processes in CBT (like keeping a diary) may also seem paradoxical.

PROOF OF CONCEPT/SUPPORTING DATA/EVIDENCE BASE

Paradox has been part of psychological theory and practice for a long time. Frankl's concern that patients took control of their symptoms stemmed from an existentialist philosophy [7]. His logotherapeutic approach comprised two related techniques; paradoxical intention and de-reflection. The former was concerned with increasing the frequency of responses already occurring too often; the latter involved attempting further to inhibit already infrequent responses. It is the latter response deficit which is the core of insomnia. Paradoxical intention in this sense involves "prescribing the symptom". The work of Ascher [7,8] and Seltzer [6] has been associated with the integration of PI into behavioral therapies, and there are parallels with Wegner's theories of ironic control [15,16]. PI also resonates with contemporary psychological perspectives on insomnia [10,11,17].

Treatment outcome data provide evidence for the efficacy of PI as a single therapy. Randomized, placebo controlled trials have been available for decades, demonstrating significant reductions in the principal insomnia dimensions of sleep onset latency and wakefulness after sleep onset [18,19]. In light of such data, the Standards of Practice Committee of the American Academy

TABLE 6.2 Paradoxical Aspects of Other CBT Methods

CBT method	Patient concern	Therapeutic response
Sleep Restriction Therapy	*I have got insomnia. I feel I am not getting enough sleep.*	*What we are going to do is to reduce the time you spend in bed so you need to stay awake for longer ...*
Stimulus Control	*I keep wakening up during the night and can't get back to sleep.*	*Get up out of your bed, and get out of your bedroom, and go and read a book instead.*
Progressive Muscle Relaxation	*I feel wound up and unable to let go.*	*Tense up the muscles in your fingers and your hands to make a fist, keep the tension going at a steady rate, ...*
Cognitive Therapy	*I feel that if I don't sleep soon, then I am going to be completely useless tomorrow.*	*So what's the worst that could happen if you don't sleep? You could try that as an experiment.*
Keeping a Sleep Diary	*I just can't stop thinking about my sleep. How I sleep and how I feel the next day is constantly on my mind.*	*I would like you to start keeping a detailed and careful note of your sleep pattern and sleep quality in a diary. Now every day you need to fill this in accurately...*

of Sleep Medicine regards PI as an evidence-based treatment for insomnia [20,21]. Moreover, PI is often included as an element of multi-component CBT, which, like PI alone, is an effective treatment for insomnia disorder [22,23].

REFERENCES

[1] American Academy of Sleep Medicine, International Classification of Sleep Disorders. Diagnostic and Coding Manual, second ed., American Academy of Sleep Medicine, Westchester, IL, 2005.

[2] D.O. Fogle, J.A. Dyall, Paradoxical giving up and the reduction of sleep performance anxiety in chronic insomniacs, Psychother. Theory Res. Pract. 20 (1983) 21–30.

[3] N. Broomfield, C.A. Espie, Initial insomnia and paradoxical intention: An experimental investigation of putative mechanisms using subjective and actigraphic measurement of sleep, Behav. Cogn. Psychother. 31 (2003) 313–324.

[4] C.A. Espie, W.R. Lindsay, Paradoxical intention in the treatment of chronic insomnia; Six case studies illustrating variability in therapeutic response, Behav. Res. Ther. 23 (1985) 703–709.

[5] C.A. Espie, The Psychological Treatment of Insomnia, J. Wiley & Sons Ltd, Chichester, 1991.

[6] L.F. Seltzer, Paradoxical Strategies in Psychotherapy: A Comprehensive Overview and Guidebook, J. Wiley & Sons, Chichester, 1986. (Wiley Series on Personality Processes).

[7] V.E. Frank, The Doctor and the Soul: From Psychotherapy to Logotherapy, Knopf, New York, NY, 1955.

[8] L.M. Ascher, J.S. Efran, The use of paradoxical intention in a behavioural program for sleep-onset insomnia, J. Consult. Clin. Psychol. 8 (1978) 547–550.

[9] L.M. Ascher, R.M. Turner, Paradoxical intention and insomnia: An experimental investigation, Behav. Res. Ther. 17 (1979) 408–411.

[10] C.A. Espie, Insomnia: Conceptual issues in the development, persistence and treatment of sleep disorder in adults, Annu. Rev. Psychol. 53 (2002) 215–243.

[11] C.A. Espie, N.M. Broomfield, K.M.A. MacMahon, et al., The attention-intention-effort pathway in the development of Psychophysiologic Insomnia: A theoretical review, Sleep Med. Rev. 10 (2006) 215–224.

[12] N.M. Broomfield, C.A. Espie, Toward a reliable, valid measure of sleep effort, J. Sleep Res. 14 (2005) 401–407.

[13] C.M Morin, C.A. Espie, Insomnia: A Clinical Guide to Assessment and Treatment, Kluwer Academic/Plenum Publishers, New York, NY, 2003.

[14] C.A. Espie, Overcoming Insomnia and Sleep Problems: A Self-Help Guide Using Cognitive Behavioral Techniques, Constable & Robinson Ltd, London, 2006.

[15] D.M. Wegner, Ironic processes of mental control, Psychol. Rev. 101 (1994) 34–52.

[16] M.E. Ansfield, D.M. Wegner, R. Bowser, Ironic effects of sleep urgency, Behav. Res. Ther. 34 (1996) 523–531.

[17] A.G. Harvey, A cognitive model of insomnia, Behav. Res. Ther. 40 (2002) 869–893.

[18] R.M. Turner, L.M. Ascher, Controlled comparison of progressive relaxation, stimulus control, and paradoxical intention therapies for insomnia, J. Consult. Clin. Psychol. 47 (1979) 500–508.

[19] C.A. Espie, W.R. Lindsay, D.N. Brooks, et al., A controlled comparative investigation of psychological treatments for chronic sleep-onset insomnia, Behav. Res. Ther. 27 (1989) 79–88.

[20] A.L. Chesson, W.M. Anderson, M. Littner, et al., Practice parameters for the nonpharmacologic treatment of chronic insomnia, Sleep 22 (1989) 1128–1133.

[21] T. Morgenthaler, M. Kramer, C. Alessi, et al., Practice parameters for the psychological and behavioral treatment of insomnia: an update. An American Academy of Sleep Medicine Report, Sleep 29 (2006) 1415–1419.

[22] C.M. Morin, P. Hauri, C.A. Espie, et al., Nonpharmacologic treatment of chronic insomnia: An American Academy of Sleep Medicine Review, Sleep 22 (1999) 1134–1156.

[23] C.M. Morin, R.R. Bootzin, D.J. Buysse, et al., Psychological and behavioural treatment of insomnia. Update of the recent evidence (1998–2004) prepared by a Task Force of the American Academy of Sleep Medicine, Sleep 29 (2006) 1398–1414.

Chapter 7

Behavioral Experiments

Allison G. Harvey, Lisa S. Talbot
Golden Bear Sleep and Mood Research Clinic, Psychology Department, University of California, Berkeley, CA

PROTOCOL NAME

Behavioral experiments.

GROSS INDICATION

Behavioral experiments provide:

- an approach to challenging unhelpful beliefs about sleep and developing/testing new (and helpful) beliefs about sleep;
- an approach to facilitating awareness of perpetuating cognitive and behavioral processes and bringing about change in/reversal of these processes.

SPECIFIC INDICATION

There is no evidence that this form of therapy is differentially effective for subtypes of insomnia.

CONTRAINDICATIONS

Based on clinical experience, this treatment modality may be difficult to utilize when the context only allows for short therapy sessions (i.e., therapy sessions less than 50 minutes) because most behavioral experiments need time to set up and then, in a subsequent session, debrief.

Specific behavioral experiments have contraindications (see Chapters 8–10 in this volume for examples).

RATIONALE FOR INTERVENTION

Because verbal techniques like directly questioning the logical basis of thoughts and beliefs, Socratic questioning, and guided discovery are typically not enough on their own to bring about profound change, behavioral experiments are used. Behavioral experiments are "planned experiential activities, based

Behavioral Treatments for Sleep Disorders. DOI: 10.1016/B978-0-12-381522-4.00007-9

on experimentation or observation, which are undertaken by patients in or between ... therapy sessions. Their design is derived directly from a ... formulation of the problem, and their primary purpose is to obtain new information which ... [includes] ... contributing to the development and verification of the ... formulation" [1]. Behavioral experiments encourage patients to become scientists (i.e., to make judgments in their lives based on data they collect, rather than based solely on their subjective feelings).

STEP BY STEP DESCRIPTION OF PROCEDURES

There are essentially six steps to completing a behavioral experiment [1]:

1. Precisely identify the belief/thought/process the experiment will target.
2. Collaborate with your patient to brainstorm ideas for an experiment; be as specific as you can.
3. Write predictions about the outcome and devise a method to record the outcome.
4. Anticipate problems and brainstorm solutions.
5. Conduct the experiment.
6. Review the experiment and draw conclusions.

Finally, identify follow-up experiments if needed.

Before explaining each of these steps in more detail, it is important to note that conducting behavioral experiments requires an openness to any outcome. The purpose of the experiment is to facilitate your patient to have new experiences and to discover new possibilities (even if they are not the experiences/outcomes you expected). Very often, the experience of a behavioral experiment brings about profound disconfirmation of unhelpful beliefs or stunning demonstrations that certain behaviors or thoughts are important contributors to the insomnia. They can also provide deep experiential learning that new thoughts/beliefs/behaviors can reduce distress/anxiety and improve sleep.

If you are going to make use of behavioral experiments, introduce the idea in Session 1. Explain to the patient that:

A big part of this treatment is that you and I will be thinking together creatively to devise ways of working out which of the things that you are currently doing are helpful or unhelpful. We'll do this by setting up and completing behavioral experiments. Behavioral experiments are just like experiments that scientists do. They enable us to collect data on important issues in our lives and they are also a means of generalizing what we're working on in session to your day-to-day life so that the changes really "stick". We'll also use behavioral experiments to figure out what works best for you. Everyone is different, so it is important that you are willing to experiment to find out what works for you. That is, we'll be trying new things or stopping doing some familiar things. And I'll be asking you to tell me honestly how these changes work out for you. Based on your experience, we will learn what helps and what makes things worse. The more experiments you do, the faster we can figure out what will help you.

Then ask, “Are you willing to do some experiments and then report what you notice?”

Also, when possible, it may be better to do behavioral experiments within the therapy hour rather than across 2 or more days, as it creates a more controlled environment (i.e., fewer potential confounding variables). However, as will become clear in this chapter and in Chapters 8–10 in this volume, many behavioral experiments for insomnia need to be conducted *between* therapy sessions. For these experiments, particular care is needed to ensure maximally efficient and effective learning. Be very specific when planning the experiment. Operationalize exactly what the experiment involves, define the outcomes and – this is very important – when possible, *practice* the skills needed for the conduct of the experiment within the therapy session *before* the patient goes home to try the experiment. When possible, we also suggest that experiments conducted during the daytime be conducted within 1 day. If conducted over 2 days, the results can be attributed to sleeping better on one of the nights or to differences inherent to the days (e.g., the work I was doing wasn’t so hard that day) [2].

We’ve found that therapy outcome is better when we really move the treatment along. That is, if an opportunity arises to do a behavioral experiment, go for it. The therapist should try to accumulate as much evidence as possible (against unhelpful beliefs, etc.) as quickly as possible. Aim to complete at least one behavioral experiment per session.

Now to return to the step-by-step process of setting up a behavioral experiment.

Step 1: Precisely Identify the Belief/Thought/Behavior/Process the Experiment will Target

Be clear about the reason for doing the experiment. Define the target. Write it down as the “aim” of the experiment. Sometimes the aim is to challenge a currently held unhelpful belief, a style of thinking, or an unhelpful behavior. Sometimes the aim of the experiment is to test a new (more helpful) belief, style of thinking, or behavior. Sometimes an experiment compares these two. Other times the experiment is “observational” [1]. The survey experiment described in Chapter 8, on unhelpful beliefs, is an example of this. This involves gathering evidence regarding specific beliefs and behaviors related to sleep. In the example we will discuss in this chapter (patient John), frequent worrying in bed was identified as an unhelpful behavioral process to target through a behavioral experiment (see Table 7.1).

Step 2: Collaborate with your Patient to Brainstorm Ideas for an Experiment

Be as specific as you can. Define a time and a place for the experiment. Identify people and resources needed to complete the experiment [1]. Be creative, and try

TABLE 7.1 Behavioral Experiment Record Sheet for John

Aim and prediction	Experiment	Outcome	What I learned
What do I want to find out? What do I think will happen?	How will I test my prediction?	What actually happened? Was the prediction correct?	
Aim: Determine whether savoring is a process that will reduce my worrying in bed and improve my sleep. *Prediction*: Savoring will make lying awake more pleasant, but will not help my sleep quality.	On 3 nights, when lying awake in bed, try the process of *savoring* (recall, appreciate, and enhance positive experiences of the day; focus on each experience in an in-depth way by remembering feelings, words, scents, and other details associated with the experience)	*Night 1:* Sleep quality rating (1–10): 5 Pleasantness rating (1–10): 6 (Time spent savoring: 15 min) *Night 2:* Sleep quality rating (1–10): 8 Pleasantness rating (1–10): 7 (Time spent savoring: 25 min) *Night 3:* Sleep quality rating (1–10): 6 Pleasantness rating (1–10): 8 (Time spent savoring: 20 min)	Savoring made me feel calmer and it was much more pleasant than worrying. I felt less anxious. Savoring seemed moderately helpful for my sleep quality. It might become even more helpful if the process is more "natural" for me. I plan to practice it during the day so that savoring becomes easier for me.

to arouse a patient's curiosity and interest. If your patient comes up with an idea for an experiment that tests beliefs or behaviors, go with it. This may increase interest in this approach and motivation to complete the experiment. Write down all of the decisions made. In the example of John (see Table 7.1) he believed that worrying in bed was likely to be unhelpful, but he could not think of alternative cognitive strategies that could occupy his mind. The therapist suggested the concept of savoring – a process that involves recalling, appreciating, and enhancing positive experiences of the day. John expressed interest in this idea, particularly given that he was working on developing a more positive approach to his life in general. John and the therapist decided to test the effectiveness of savoring by having John try it, instead of worrying, while lying awake in bed on 3 nights.

Step 3: Write Down Predictions about the Outcome and Devise a Method to Record the Outcome

This should be done as soon as possible after the experiment is completed. This is critically important. If a patient waits until the next therapy session, a number of days later, to report the outcome, the memories may be vague and inaccurate. In such a case, the learning would be greatly reduced. In John's experiment, he predicted that savoring would not help him fall asleep faster but would make the experience of lying awake in bed more pleasant. The outcome variables of "sleep quality" and "pleasantness", with 1–10 scales, were listed for John to rate each morning after completing savoring during the previous night. In addition, John estimated how long he tried savoring during the night (see Table 7.1).

Step 4: Anticipate Problems and Brainstorm Solutions

Ask, "What things might prevent you from doing this?" Collaborate with your patient to identify possible obstacles, and think together about how to prevent these from becoming impediments to the conduct of the experiment. We emphasize again that it is really important to *practice* the skills needed for the conduct of the experiment within the therapy session *before* your patient goes home to try the experiment. In the case of John, he expressed a genuine interest in trying savoring, but also discussed his concern that he was naturally a "more negative guy". The therapist reassured him that the two of them would practice savoring in session. After reviewing the guidelines of the savoring process, the therapist and the client each closed their eyes for 2 minutes and tried savoring. The therapist then asked John about his experience. He expressed that he had experienced a few moments where he felt he was attending to the "positives" of the day, but that he also felt frustrated that his mind jumped between experiences. The therapist and John brainstormed ways he could enhance his connection with savoring, such as through focusing on each experience in a more in-depth way by remembering the feelings, words, scents, and other details associated with the experience. John wrote down these ideas associated with savoring to review at home. At the end of the session, he felt more confident in his ability to use savoring as an in-bed process.

Step 5: Conduct the Experiment

In John's case, he attempted savoring while in bed on 3 nights during the week between therapy sessions, and each time completed the ratings in the morning (see Table 7.1).

Step 6: Review the Experiment and Draw Conclusions

Ask the patient to summarize the session/main point learned. Help the patient by filling in the gaps. Write down the conclusions; make a copy for the patient to take home and keep a copy for the files.

In our example, John returned to the next therapy session with his behavioral experiment form completed. It indicated that on all 3 nights John found the experience of savoring pleasant (scores of 6, 7, and 8 consecutively on a 1–10 scale). Interestingly, on each successive night the experience became more pleasant. He believed this upward trend was a result of the process becoming easier with more practice. To John's surprise he also found that his sleep quality generally improved following savoring, though there was some variation (ratings of 5, 8, and 6, see Table 7.1). He concluded that savoring increased his sense of calm and pleasure when lying awake in bed, while decreasing his anxiety. He found it moderately helpful for his sleep quality.

Keep a look out for, and a list of, the conclusions drawn for each experiment. In subsequent sessions, keep reminding the patient about these. The goal is to promote deep encoding of the new material. Repetition of the core conclusion helps with this.

Sometimes an experiment will not generate the outcome you or your patient were expecting. When this happens, walk patients through the experiment step-by-step. Start with an understanding of the context (What was their mood? Where were they? Had anything significant happened just prior to starting the experiment?). Then cycle through questions like, "What happened next?", "What did you do then?", "What did you think?", and, again, "What happened next?", until you have a hypothesis about what happened. Typically, via careful questioning, learning can be derived from an experiment regardless of the outcome. In John's case, the therapist and patient discussed that his sleep had improved, albeit not dramatically, on the savoring nights. After some questioning regarding his experience of the savoring, John hypothesized that his sleep quality might improve if savoring became more "second nature" for him. He suggested that he practice savoring during the day three times in the next week, in addition to continuing to implement it during the night.

Step 7: Identify Follow-up Experiments if Needed

If the experiment wasn't completed fully, or if the outcome was ambiguous and raised another question, return to Step 1 and devise a further experiment.

POSSIBLE MODIFICATIONS/VARIANTS

While a stock of behavioral experiments useful for patients with insomnia is beginning to accrue (see, for example, Ree and Harvey [2]), behavioral experiments should be personalized for each patient. As such, there is an infinite range of possibilities (see Chapters 8–10 in this volume for examples). The use of behavioral experiments in therapy creates opportunities to collaborate with your patient, being highly creative together, while making substantial progress in the treatment.

PROOF OF CONCEPT/SUPPORTING DATA/EVIDENCE BASE

There is preliminary evidence that conducting a behavioral experiment, relative to traditional verbal/educational approaches, is more helpful in the context of insomnia [3]. There is no evidence for this specific approach as a monotherapy. However, there is evidence from an open trial that behavioral experiments used as part of a multi-component approach to insomnia are effective [4]. We emphasize, though, that testing within a randomized controlled trial is required.

REFERENCES

[1] J. Bennett-Levy, G. Butler, M.J.V. Fennell, et al., The Oxford Handbook of Behavioural Experiments, Oxford University Press, Oxford, 2004.

[2] M. Ree, A.G. Harvey, Insomnia, in: J. Bennett-Levy, G. Butler, M. Fennell, et al., (Eds.), Oxford Guide to Behavioural Experiments in Cognitive Therapy, Oxford University Press, Oxford, 2004, pp. 287–305.

[3] N.K. Tang, A.G. Harvey, Altering misperception of sleep in insomnia: Behavioral experiment versus verbal feedback, J. Consult. Clin. Psychol. 74 (4) (2006) 767–776.

[4] A.G. Harvey, A. Sharpley, M.J. Ree, et al., An open trial of cognitive therapy for chronic insomnia, Behav. Res. Therapy 45 (2007) 2491–2501.

RECOMMENDED READING

J. Bennett-Levy, G. Butler, M.J.V. Fennell, et al., The Oxford Handbook of Behavioural Experiments, Oxford University Press, Oxford, 2004.

M. Ree, A.G. Harvey, Insomnia, in: J. Bennett-Levy, G. Butler, M. Fennell, et al., (Eds.), Oxford Guide to Behavioural Experiments in Cognitive Therapy, Oxford University Press, Oxford, 2004, pp. 287–305.

Chapter 8

Intervention to Reduce Unhelpful Beliefs about Sleep

Allison G. Harvey, Polina Eidelman
Golden Bear Sleep and Mood Research Clinic, Psychology Department, University of California, Berkeley, CA

PROTOCOL NAME

Intervention to reduce unhelpful beliefs about sleep.

GROSS INDICATION

This intervention is an approach to challenging unhelpful beliefs about sleep and developing/testing new (and helpful) beliefs about sleep.

SPECIFIC INDICATION

There is no evidence that this form of therapy is differentially effective for subtypes of insomnia.

CONTRAINDICATIONS

The Fear of Poor Sleep experiment may involve some short-term sleep deprivation. As such, this experiment should not be attempted with patients who will need to drive, operate a machine/industrial tool, or engage in other activities the day following the experiment if these activities, attempted under conditions of sleep deprivation, would compromise the safety of the patient or other people entrusted to the patient.

RATIONALE FOR INTERVENTION

Unhelpful beliefs about sleep held by patients with insomnia relate to the amount of sleep required (e.g., "I must get 8 hours of sleep most nights", "If I have to get up to go to the bathroom my night's sleep is wrecked"), fear of the short- and long-term consequences of insomnia (e.g., "After a poor night's sleep, I know that I'll find it impossible to cope at work the next day", "This is having

Behavioral Treatments for Sleep Disorders. DOI: 10.1016/B978-0-12-381522-4.00008-0

serious effects on my physical health"), and the belief that it is possible to lose control over one's ability to sleep (e.g., "When I have trouble getting to sleep, I should stay in bed and try harder", "I'll go to bed early to ensure I get at least some sleep", "I must actively control my sleep"). The Dysfunctional Beliefs about Sleep Scale (DBAS) [1] is a useful aid for identifying unhelpful beliefs about sleep. The approach to challenging unhelpful beliefs described here makes use of behavioral experiments (for the rationale for this approach, see Chapter 7).

STEP BY STEP DESCRIPTION OF PROCEDURES

There is an enormous variety of unhelpful beliefs about sleep held by patients with insomnia. Hence, while some of the most commonly used behavioral experiments for tackling beliefs are described below, it is emphasized that these experiments should be individualized for each patient, and new experiments should be devised for other beliefs held by your patients. Several of these experiments have also been described elsewhere [2].

Each experiment is described in terms of seven "set up" steps (see Chapter 7 for the steps involved in devising each experiment).

Example 1: Daytime Fatigue

1. *Precisely identify the belief/thought/process the experiment will target.*
   A common belief held by patients with insomnia is that "I have a fixed pot of energy that I must conserve. It progressively drains away throughout the day. The only way I can top up my energy is via sleep."
   You may introduce this experiment and help patients identify this belief by asking them what they typically do and avoid doing during a day that follows a night of insomnia. Approaches to conserving energy commonly used by patients with insomnia include engaging in mundane activities such as paperwork and data entry, and avoiding meetings and socializing. Note that while these coping strategies may initially make a lot of sense, they can actually lead to feeling more tired, and contribute to the day being unpleasant, boring, and unproductive. Furthermore, it probably contributes to increased stress (because important activities in the day were avoided) and worry (there will be fewer distractions from worry), which may further impede sleep, hence contributing to a vicious cycle.
2. *Collaborate with your patient to brainstorm ideas for an experiment. Be as specific as you can.*
   The key to this experiment is for the patient to compare and contrast conserving and using energy. There are many variants on this experiment, but one that seems to work particularly well is to conduct the experiment over 2 days. On the first day, the patient spends one 3-hour block conserving energy, and then a 3-hour block using energy. The following day they do this again, but in the reverse order. Prior to the experiment,

through careful questioning, try to understand exactly what conserving energy means for your patient. Also, spend time brainstorming strategies for using energy. These might include going for a 10-minute walk, returning all phone calls, arranging to have a coffee with a colleague, getting on top of paperwork, going to the water cooler to get a drink, and walking to a local shop to buy a magazine or snack.

3. *Write down predictions about the outcome and devise a method to record the outcome.*

   Typically, the prediction made by patients with insomnia will be that "after a poor night's sleep, I will cope better and feel less fatigued and moody if I conserve my energy".

   Measurement method: After each 3-hour block, the patient rates their fatigue, mood, and coping on a 0 ("not at all") to 10 ("very much") scale. In addition to measuring specific aspects of functioning or mood, encourage your patient to note what they have learned from the experiment.

4. *Anticipate problems and brainstorm solutions.*

   The patient may not know or only have a vague idea how to engage in using energy – so very clearly define and discuss. Get super specific. To increase the chance that your patient will do the experiment over the coming week, it may be useful to plan the specific time when it will be done. To increase the chance that your patient will do the experiment over the coming week, it may be useful to plan the specific time when it will be done and to practice specific skills for using/generating energy in the session.

5. *Conduct the experiment.*
6. *Review the experiment and draw conclusions. Write down the conclusions.*

   Typically, a patient with insomnia will discover that there may be other factors than sleep that influence energy levels, and that mood and energy are improved by "using" energy. In other words, "using" energy becomes synonymous with "generating" energy.

   We often then develop a new metaphor with that patient – that energy levels are like elastic; they can be stretched quite easily. This is in contrast to their original view that energy levels progressively deplete throughout the day (like a leaky battery). To conclude the experiment, it is often useful to generate a list of ways to decrease the adverse effects of poor sleep through energy generation. Patients may benefit from preparing a list that works in the different contexts of their life (workplace energy generating, weekend energy generating, working from home, etc.).

Example 2: Poor Sleep is Dangerous

A belief commonly held by patients with insomnia is that poor sleep is dangerous. This belief needs to be pulled out by the roots. It is only then that fewer episodes of tiredness will be noticed. Patients will always feel somewhat tired unless we deal with the belief, because they'll always be monitoring for/watching out for tiredness and then, of course, they'll notice it more. Accordingly, a behavioral experiment can be conducted to show that poor sleep is not dangerous. This is also an opportunity to practice new skills for managing the consequences of not sleeping. This experiment works best toward the latter part of treatment, when the patient has learned and practiced a number of effective coping strategies for the day. Additionally, for patients who have experienced a significant improvement in their sleep, this experiment may be conceptualized as a sort of celebration and a way to prove to themselves that they do not need to be fearful of a night of poor sleep.

It's often helpful to explain the fact they have done the experiment by accident on several occasions. The reason for doing it more formally is that these accidental experiments are often easily forgotten, or can be attributed to flukes or the particular circumstances in which they occurred.

It is very important that patients feel you are with them and right behind them, so it can be helpful to phone them to review the experiment the evening before – this can be brief and focused. It will be hard *not* to do the experiment if you are going out of your way in this manner. You could also call them in the morning to remind them how to cope with a poor night of sleep.

1. *Precisely identify the belief/thought/process the experiment will target.*

   A belief commonly held by patients with insomnia is that "to function well the next day, I must get at least 8 hours of sleep a night. Less than 8 hours of sleep will have serious consequences for my health. If I don't get 8 hours sleep per night, I won't be able to cope with anything."
2. *Collaborate with your patient to brainstorm ideas for an experiment. Be as specific as you can.*

   The experiment usually works well when sleep is kept to about 1–1.5 hours less on the night of the experiment compared to a usual night of sleep. It is fine to be flexible with this amount. However, be mindful of the patient's anxiety in response to the suggested sleep restriction – this anxiety is a manifestation of the exact belief targeted by the experiment, and is a useful point to which you should draw the patient's attention. Collaboratively, you might decide to sleep just 6.5 hours one night. Specify whether this will involve going to bed later than usual or waking up earlier in the morning. Discuss how to stay awake later or how to wake up earlier in the morning. Try to select activities that will ensure that the experiment is enjoyable and memorable (for example, watching a movie with family, walking the dog, playing a musical instrument, getting up early to go for a swim, etc.).
3. *Write down predictions about the outcome and devise a method to record the outcome.*

   The predictions often include some version of the following: "I won't cope, I'll feel awful, low, sick, tired, and I won't want to do anything or see anyone. If I aim to sleep for only 6.5 hours I'll end up sleeping much less. If I have 1 night of poor sleep this will trigger others."

In order to assess the predictions, develop a form to help patients monitor the effect of the experiment on their ability to cope, tiredness, productivity, and mood. Also, patients should continue to complete the sleep diary each morning immediately on waking.

4. *Anticipate problems and brainstorm solutions.*

If patients are anxious about trying this experiment, capitalize on their past experiences – for example, ask "Have there been times when you have slept less than 8 hours and gotten on with the day OK?", "Have there even been times when you have had a poor night's sleep and actually had a good day?", "What did you make of these times?". Often the patient will discount these experiences. This is then an opportunity to say, "OK, so you've noticed that you can get away with X hours sleep and feel OK but this may have been due to X, Y, and Z, so the only way you can really know what this means is if you actively choose to have less than 8 hours sleep". In other words, it can be helpful to begin by recruiting a past experience that doesn't fit with their belief (if I sleep poorly it's a disaster, I find it so hard to cope) and is consistent with an alternative belief (if I sleep poorly I might feel rotten but cope OK). This helps sow the seeds of doubt that the belief is correct.

You should also generate a list of effective daytime coping strategies collaboratively with your patient. This can serve as a reminder during the day following the night of "poor sleep". Additionally, it may be useful to remind patients that the hour they will be cutting from their night can be used as a time for pleasurable activities that they might otherwise not have time to do.

5. *Conduct the experiment.*

6. *Review the experiment and draw conclusions. Write down the conclusions.*

Patients are typically surprised by how well they cope with 6.5 hours sleep, and they get to discover that restricted sleep does not necessarily trigger poor sleep on subsequent nights. When reviewing the experiment, it is important to spell out the take away message – poor sleep might be unpleasant, but it is not dangerous and it is definitely something with which the patient can cope. Remind patients that this experience is an important one to remember. This is a night where they chose to sleep "poorly" and still made it through the day, coping well. This is a helpful experiment for reducing the fear of poor sleep.

Table 8.1 depicts an example of a behavioral experiment that was completed with a patient who conducted the Fear of Poor Sleep experiment. This patient wanted to reduce his sleep to 5.5 or 6 hours. He concluded that one night of reduced sleep did mean he felt more tired but he coped. For this patient the Fear of Poor Sleep experiment was a celebration of his new-found confidence in his ability to sleep (as opposed to the significant fear of poor sleep he had felt previously).

TABLE 8.1 Fear of Poor Sleep Experiment
Record Sheet for Behavioral Experiments

Aim	The experiment (i.e., what you plan to do)	What do you predict will happen?	What actually happened?	Outcome
To purposefully have a shorter night's sleep	Either stay up later – watch stars, moonlit walk (1 am to bed) OR get up earlier and go for a run in the countryside. Aim for 5.5–6 hours of sleep (in bed for around 6.5 hours)	Might even sleep better? I'll feel fine in the morning. It'll be interesting to see	Went out to see friends. Back midnight. Watched film until 1:30 am Bed 1:45–7:45 Slept 2 am to 7 am (5 hours) one or two awakenings	Did feel tired on waking and at times during the day but functioned fine and coped okay – paperwork at desk, gardening odd jobs, saw friends. Can do it! Can survive okay on 5 hours!

Example 3: Control of Sleep

1. *Precisely identify the belief/thought/process the experiment will target.*
   A common belief held by patients with insomnia is, "I am terrified of losing control over my ability to sleep. I have to try really hard to sleep and try to get control back over it."
2. *Collaborate with your patient to brainstorm ideas for an experiment. Be as specific as you can.*
   One example that has worked well is that on the first night the patient does everything he or she can to control sleep. On the second night, the patient drops all attempts to sleep.
3. *Write down predictions about the outcome and devise a method to record the outcome.*
   A typical prediction is that "unless I try very hard to get to sleep and be perfectly still, I will have a night of insomnia".
   The sleep diary kept by the patient will indicate the amount of time it took to get to sleep and how long he or she was awake over the course of the night – these are useful outcome measures for this experiment. Additional outcome measures can be collaboratively developed with the patient.
4. *Anticipate problems and brainstorm solutions.*
   Brainstorming the specifics of what a patient will do when trying to control sleep, and how he or she might drop these attempts at

controlling sleep, is a useful way to prevent obstacles. These will likely vary person to person, and it is important to outline them in some detail before the experiment is attempted.

5. *Conduct the experiment.*
6. *Review the experiment and draw conclusions. Write down the conclusions.* Patients typically conclude that the more they try to control their sleep, the more out of control it is. So actively trying to control sleep makes it worse. This experiment is also a good basis for having a discussion about sleep being an automatic biological process that does not need to be controlled.

Example 4: Survey

The goal of this experiment is to broaden the patient's thinking about what constitutes "normal sleep". By administering a survey to a set of individuals who are close to the patient's age, the patient can gather data about the variety of sleep obtained by self-described good sleepers. Additionally, he or she may survey peers to gather ideas for coping strategies for the daytime and can begin to see that individuals without sleep difficulty often see their daytime mood and energy levels as being affected by many factors other than sleep.

Pre-session preparation: We suggest administering the DBAS [1] before this experiment is attempted. For all items rated as higher than halfway on the rating scale, prepare survey questions designed to help your patient to obtain corrective/helpful information. For example, if your patient believes that he or she must sleep 8 hours every night in order to cope the next day, you could include the following questions: "Do you regard yourself as a normal sleeper or someone with insomnia?" or "Each week, what is the typical number of hours of sleep that you get per night?" Also, go through your notes for the past few sessions to identify other unhelpful beliefs the patient holds. Prior to the session, prepare drafts of survey questions designed to tackle these.

1. *Precisely identify the belief/thought/process the experiment will target.* Introduce this experiment by discussing with patients how they developed their ideas about sleep. Do they have some ideas about how good sleepers sleep? Do they have some curiosity about these ideas? Many individuals with insomnia are eager to learn more about the way other people sleep, and to approach this in a scientific manner. The key beliefs targeted by the survey will vary person to person, and will be based on the highly endorsed DBAS items. Some common unhelpful beliefs include:
   - It's not normal to have difficulty with sleep.
   - Most people sleep about 8 hours a night and wake up feeling bright and alert.
   - It's not normal to feel tired and experience some lapses in memory and concentration at times during the day.

2. *Collaborate with your patient to brainstorm ideas for an experiment. Be as specific as you can.*

   Design a survey collaboratively with your patient to address different beliefs and attitudes about sleep. Surveys are a great reminder as to how well good sleepers really sleep (i.e., the reality is that good sleepers have poor nights of sleep now and then, and they feel tired during the day at times). Often patients with insomnia have forgotten the realistic picture of what being a good sleeper is. You can also include questions asking about strategies that others use to increase their energy when they feel tired. In one recent experiment, we included questions about how other people coped with daytime tiredness. Many, many strategies were suggested, and only a small proportion of them involved resting or sleeping. In fact, most strategies suggested things like a change in environment, getting fresh air, going for a walk, drinking cold water, having a snack. The patient realized that energy can be increased by other things than rest and sleep, and that boredom was the biggest trigger to feeling tired. The above experiment can also be very helpful for eliciting reasons for daytime tiredness that are not sleep-related. Answers might include that work is boring, and that everyone gets tired in the afternoon.

   Questions might include:
   - How long, on average, does it take you to fall asleep?
   - What would be the maximum time it takes you to fall asleep?
   - How many hours of sleep do you think you need?
   - How many hours of sleep do you actually get?
   - Most people wake up in the night; how many times do you wake up, even if for a few seconds?
   - Do you ever find it difficult to get back to sleep (after waking up)?
   - Do you ever feel tired/lethargic when you wake up in the morning? Can you describe how you feel?
   - Do you ever feel tired during the day? Can you describe this? What are some reasons why you might feel this way?

   Typically, the patient will try to collect 10–20 responses and the therapist will try to collect some responses too. We always try to target people within 5 years of age either side of the patient's age (given sleep-related changes with age).

3. *Write down predictions about the outcome and devise a method to record the outcome.*

   Ask your patient his or her predictions about what the responses will be. Before the next session, devise a form for collating the data from the survey experiment. In the session, show the patient the form for collating the data. Work together to collate the data for a couple of the completed questionnaires. Set the rest of the collation for homework. If there are only a small number of respondents, feel free to complete the collation in session. An example of a collated survey, along with the associated conclusions (in bold), is included as Figure 8.1.

Sleep survey – results

1. How long, on average, does it take you to fall asleep (in minutes)?

0–10	11–20	21–30	31–40	41–50	51–60	61+
12	5	7		1	1	

Many people take a long time to fall asleep.

2. What would be the maximum time it takes you to fall asleep?

11–20	21–30	31–40	41–50	51–60	61–70	71–80	81+
5	3	1	2	6			7

3. How many hours of sleep do you think you need?

4	5	6	7	8	9	10
		4	8	7	4	1

4. How many hours of sleep do you actually get?

4	5	6	7	8	9	10
	1	2	11	5	1	

Average sleep was less than 8 hours.

5. If you got less than your ideal amount of sleep, how many hours could you get by with per night for two nights in a row?

3	4	5	6	7	8	9
2	4	8	10			

Average hours to get by with was 5 hours.

6. Do you think about sleep during the day?

Yes	No
5	14

7. Most people wake up at night. How many times do you wake up, even if for a few seconds?

0	1–2	2–3	3–4	4–5	5–6	7+
2	10	6	2	2	1	

Most people wake up during the night between one and three times.

8. Do you ever find it difficult to get back to sleep after waking up?

Yes	No
5	8

9. Do you ever have times in the day when you feel lethargic/tired?

Yes	No
23	3

How often does this happen?

Almost every day	*Most days*	*After lunch*	*In the mornings*	*Occasionally*
2 times/week	*1 time/week*	*Early afternoon*	*Lunchtime*	*2 times/day*

10. If you feel tired during the day, what strategies do you use to help you feel less tired?

Try to reinvigorate	Work	Keep busy	Motivate self	Walk
Sports	Keep going	Eat more	Drink tea, coffee, water	Power nap
Fresh air	Focus on work	Be active	Snack	

11. What things, other than lack of sleep, lead to feelings of tiredness for you?

Certain foods	Meal	Lack of food	Exercise	Low blood pressure
Worry	Work, stress, pressure	Dark, cold	Sitting in one place	Children
Driving	Problem solving	Heat	Junk food	Difficult work

FIGURE 8.1 An example of a collated survey.

4. *Anticipate problems and brainstorm solutions.*
   Include a discussion about survey design more generally, covering things like the fact that your results will be more valid if the sample size is reasonable (the larger the sample, the less likely your results will be skewed by unusual responders), the importance of the age group of respondents (given that age influences sleep), and other sources of potential bias. This discussion not only educates the patient about how to collect valid data to make their mind up about important issues in their lives, but also sets up a basis for discussing the results (e.g., if there are a small number of respondents then you can remind the patient in the next session about the potential for bias). Be mindful of patients who have some anxiety about administering the survey to peers. To trouble-shoot this, you might problem-solve the reasons for this anxiety. For instance, if the patient does not want to ask friends to complete the survey in person, he or she might choose to set up an online survey, the link for which can be emailed to others. Alternately, the therapist may administer the bulk of the surveys to collect the data without triggering the patient's anxiety.
5. *Conduct the experiment.*
6. *Review the experiment and draw conclusions. Write down the conclusions.*
   The survey is likely to reveal that the majority of people get less than 8 hours of sleep; have some trouble with sleep when feeling stress; and feel tired when they wake up, and again after lunch. Most people have trouble sleeping at least some of the time. It is not realistic to expect 8 hours sleep every night. The patient's expectations of sleep and daytime tiredness are adjusted, and anxiety about attaining "perfect" sleep is reduced. Strategies for coping with poor sleep are generated.

PROOF OF CONCEPT/SUPPORTING DATA/EVIDENCE BASE

There is preliminary evidence that conducting a behavioral experiment, relative to a verbal approach, is more helpful in the context of insomnia [3]. There is no evidence on this specific approach as a monotherapy. Although there is no evidence on this specific approach as a monotherapy, evidence from an open trial suggests that behavioral experiments used as part of a multicomponent approach to insomnia are effective [4]. However, we emphasize that testing within a randomized controlled trial is required.

REFERENCES

[1] C. Morin, Insomnia: Psychological Assessment and Management, The Guilford Press, New York, 1993.

[2] M. Ree, A.G. Harvey, Insomnia, in: J. Bennett-Levy, G. Butler, M. Fennell, et al., (Eds.), Oxford Guide to Behavioural Experiments in Cognitive Therapy, Oxford University Press, Oxford, 2004, pp. 287–305.

[3] N.K. Tang, A.G. Harvey, Altering misperception of sleep in insomnia: behavioral experiment versus verbal feedback, J. Consult. Clin. Psychol. 74 (4) (2006) 767–776.

[4] A.G. Harvey, A. Sharpley, M.J. Ree, et al., An open trial of cognitive therapy for chronic insomnia, Behav. Res. Ther. 45 (2007) 2491–2501.

RECOMMENDED READING

J. Bennett-Levy, G. Butler, M.J.V. Fennell, et al., The Oxford Handbook of Behavioural Experiments, Oxford University Press, Oxford, 2004.

M. Ree, A.G. Harvey, Insomnia, in: J. Bennett-Levy, G. Butler, M. Fennell, et al., (Eds.), Oxford Guide to Behavioural Experiments in Cognitive Therapy, Oxford University Press, Oxford, 2004, pp. 287–305.

Chapter 9

Intervention to Reduce Misperception

Allison G. Harvey, Lisa S. Talbot
Golden Bear Sleep and Mood Research Clinic, Psychology Department, University of California, Berkeley, CA

PROTOCOL NAME

Intervention to reduce misperception.

GROSS INDICATION

This intervention is an approach to reversing misperception of sleep and misperception of daytime functioning.

SPECIFIC INDICATION

There is no evidence that this form of therapy is differentially effective for subtypes of insomnia.

CONTRAINDICATIONS

Be mindful that there is a significant subgroup of patients who accurately perceive their sleep and daytime dysfunction. Tread gently with the approaches suggested here in case your patient falls into this group; these interventions then cease to be relevant.

RATIONALE FOR INTERVENTION

There is a significant subgroup of people with insomnia who display a tendency toward misperceiving their sleep. Specifically, they perceive that they have slept significantly less than they have actually slept. Also, people often assume that they can accurately gauge the quality of their sleep by how they feel on waking. Using feelings on waking to judge sleep quality is likely to lead to erroneous conclusions, as these feelings may be influenced by many

Behavioral Treatments for Sleep Disorders. DOI: 10.1016/B978-0-12-381522-4.00009-2

factors. For example, patients often notice that if the day ahead involves challenges at the office, they feel worse on waking relative to if the day ahead involves a relaxing and fun outing with good friends. Moreover, for 3–20 minutes immediately on waking there is a period, known as sleep inertia, which is a transitional state between sleep and waking. During this time most people feel very tired, and experience body sensations such as a sore, heavy head and tired, heavy eyes. Monitoring at this time can lead to misinterpretations of normal feelings of tiredness on waking (e.g., "I had a rotten night's sleep last night"). The approach to reducing misperception of sleep and daytime functioning described here makes use of natural opportunities and behavioral experiments (for rationale, see Chapter 7).

STEP BY STEP DESCRIPTION OF PROCEDURES (SEE CHAPTER 7 FOR THE STEPS INVOLVED IN DEVISING EACH EXPERIMENT)

Step by Step Description of Procedures for Misperception of Sleep

In all sessions, first watch for natural opportunities to explore the possibility your patient is misperceiving, and cover the content at the end of this section when such opportunities arise. However, if a natural opportunity does not arise and/or if the misperception is hard to alter, then use a behavioral experiment such as the ones described below.

An example of a natural opportunity that might arise is that patients will often come in to a session and report a possible misperception experience. Here is an example:

Something weird happened last night. I honestly thought I'd hardly slept at all but when I told my wife over breakfast this morning she laughed and said that I was fast asleep, and breathing heavily, all night – she knew because she wasn't feeling well so she was awake a lot. You know, I believe her, because she's very supportive of me and wouldn't say I was asleep if I wasn't.

If this happens, seize the opportunity to ask, "What sense do you make of that?". If your patient doesn't raise it, ask, "One other possibility that comes to my mind is …" [and cover the content that seems most relevant below listed as points 1 to 8].

Often it does not work to try *verbally* to convince patients that sleep is hard to estimate. However, it can be incredibly powerful to set up, and draw attention to, the patient's own experience of difficulty perceiving sleep. The latter is done through the use of behavioral experiments. One of the first behavioral experiments we do in the treatment aims to reduce misperception of sleep. This involves demonstrating the discrepancy between an objective estimate of sleep (measured via actigraphy or polysomnography) and the patient's own subjective estimate (measured via the sleep diary) (see Tang and Harvey [1] for a full description). Patients are taught to download the watch (actigraph) and compare their sleep recorded on the watch with the sleep in the diary in order to calculate how accurately they perceive their sleep. Typically, patients learn that they get more sleep than they think they are getting (and note that it is easily possible to be misperceiving sleep AND still be sleep deprived; for example, patients who think they aren't sleeping at all often discover they are getting 2–4 hours of sleep per night). In addition, and particularly if an objective measure of sleep is not available, we use a number of other methods to demonstrate misperception of sleep. For instance, we give patients a handheld counter (e.g., a golf counter) to place under their pillow to test beliefs like "I wake up more than 30 times each night". When they wake in the morning, patients may find that in fact the handheld counter was only pressed three times. When conducting this experiment, it is important that patients *first* record how many times they thought they woke during the night and *then* look at the counter for the objective information.

In working with misperception of sleep, we make sure to cover the following points, in any order (this will depend on the patient):

1. Emphasize that sleep is incredibly difficult to perceive reliably, because sleep onset is defined by the absence of memories.
2. This provides an opportunity to draw a distinction between how much sleep you FEEL you get and how much you ACTUALLY get, and that it is easy to feel you get less sleep than you actually do.
3. We tend to give two examples of the difficulties perceiving sleep:

   Example A. I have often had the experience of meaning to nap, on a Sunday afternoon, for just 10–20 minutes, but then waking up 2 hours later unable to believe how much time has passed.

   Example B: Particularly vivid to me is sitting on a plane going to Europe from the US, falling asleep, thinking I was asleep for 2–3 hours and then waking up to find I had only slept for 20 minutes!
4. Discuss the influences on our perception of time. Ask, "Have you noticed situations in which time flies and situations in which time crawls?" Using Socratic questioning, try to draw out the point that time seems to go slowly when we're upset, unhappy, worried, or bored, but seems to go fast when we're having fun.
5. Discuss the difficulties associated with accurately estimating time of falling asleep using the clock, because sleep is defined by the absence of memories. Also, the following examples may help make this point:

   Example A. Have you ever been on a jogging machine and decided you were going to be really good that day and jog for a whole 20 minutes? If so, and if you kept a close track of every second that passed, it may have seemed like forever. On the other hand, if you became involved in your thoughts, watching the TV or listening to music, the time may have gone by in a flash.

Example B. When you were a child at school, do you remember sitting in class, knowing that there were 5 minutes until the bell signaling "home-time" sounded? You may have watched the second-hand tick, second-by-second – it seemed to take forever.

These are examples of time distortion due to clock monitoring.

6. Make sure you let the patient give their own examples too.
7. The bottom-line message is that it is very difficult to determine whether you have fallen asleep and, if so, how long you have been asleep.
8. Make sure you introduce the notion of sleep inertia here by saying something like:

   "On waking, most of us, most mornings have a period of between 3 minutes and 20 minutes when we feel dazed, sleepy, and 'out of it'. This is a normal transitional state called *sleep inertia.* Sleep inertia is a term that simply refers to the transition between a state of sleep and a state of wakefulness. It is not a pleasant feeling, especially if you have to rush around and get ready for work or get your children off to school, but it is a normal transitional state and doesn't necessarily mean that you had a poor night of sleep."

Step by Step Description of Procedures for Misperception of Daytime Functioning

If you hypothesize that your patient is suffering from misperception during the daytime, devise one or more behavioral experiments to explore this. Common daytime misperceptions are that the sleep problem is ruining my ability to concentrate or remember, or is causing me to age prematurely.

Example Experiment: Does Tiredness Noticeably Affect My Appearance?

When you have a patient who is very concerned that the effects of tiredness are very noticeable to others, try this behavioral experiment (or a variant of it). First, identify the associated beliefs, which tend to be along the lines of: "I look terrible in the morning. Everyone can tell how tired I am by looking at me. I can't be as confident when I'm tired because I look terrible." Then ask the patient to take his or her own photo every day for 1 week (using the "date" camera function so that the date is saved on each photo). The photo should be taken at the same time of the day (just before leaving for work), and under the same conditions (e.g., not wearing make-up in any of the photos). Ask the patient to also keep a sleep diary, recording estimated time slept and how he or she felt at the time of the photograph (e.g., tired, lethargic, headache, lively, etc.). Then in the next session look at the photos and ask the patient to pick the photo in which he or she looks most tired. Typically, most people either cannot choose a photo because they all look similar, or they choose a photo that does not correspond with the morning when he or she felt most tired.

Example Experiment: Does Tiredness Ruin My Ability to Concentrate?

When you have a patient who believes that daytime concentration difficulties are directly connected to sleep, try this experiment. First, identify the associated beliefs, which are usually along the lines of "I can't concentrate because of my poor sleep". Then set up an experiment in which the patient rates his or her concentration on a 1–5 scale three times per day. Operationalize exactly when the recordings will be taken, such as daily upon arrival at work, post-lunch, and before dinner, for 1 week. The recordings should be kept on a log separate from the sleep diary. Then, in the next session, look at the ratings with the patient and relate them to the information in the sleep diary for each of the days. Typically, there is not a direct correlation between sleep and concentration ratings. This helps the patient to see that other factors besides sleep must contribute to concentration fluctuations.

POSSIBLE MODIFICATIONS/VARIANTS

While a stock of behavioral experiments useful for patients with insomnia is beginning to accrue (see, for example, Ree and Harvey [2]), behavioral experiments should be personalized for each patient. As such, there is an infinite range of possibilities.

PROOF OF CONCEPT/SUPPORTING DATA/EVIDENCE BASE

There is preliminary evidence that conducting the behavioral experiment described above that compares the sleep diary to actigraphy is more effective, relative to verbal instruction, for reducing the anxiety associated with misperception of sleep [1].

REFERENCES

[1] N.K. Tang, A.G. Harvey, Altering misperception of sleep in insomnia: behavioral experiment versus verbal feedback, J. Consult. Clin. Psychol. 74 (4) (2006) 767–776.

[2] M. Ree, A.G. Harvey, Insomnia, in: J. Bennett-Levy, G. Butler, M. Fennell, et al. (Eds.), Oxford Guide to Behavioural Experiments in Cognitive Therapy, Oxford University Press, Oxford, 2004, pp. 287–305.

RECOMMENDED READING

J. Bennett-Levy, G. Butler, M.J.V. Fennell, et al., The Oxford Handbook of Behavioural Experiments, Oxford University Press, Oxford, 2004.

M. Ree, A.G. Harvey, Insomnia, in: J. Bennett-Levy, G. Butler, M. Fennell, et al., (Eds.), Oxford Guide to Behavioural Experiments in Cognitive Therapy, Oxford University Press, Oxford, 2004, pp. 287–305.

Chapter 10

Intervention to Reduce Use of Safety Behaviors

Allison G. Harvey, Polina Eidelman
Golden Bear Sleep and Mood Research Clinic, Psychology Department, University of California, Berkeley, CA

PROTOCOL NAME

Intervention to reduce use of safety behaviors.

GROSS INDICATION

This intervention is an approach to reducing the use of safety behaviors. Safety behaviors include overt and subtle attempts to cope with inadequate sleep and to increase control over sleep. Safety behaviors are problematic because they increase the symptoms of the disorder and/or prevent disconfirmation of unhelpful beliefs about sleep.

SPECIFIC INDICATION

There is no evidence that this form of therapy is differentially effective for subtypes of insomnia.

CONTRAINDICATIONS

There is currently no evidence relating to contraindications. However, based on clinical experience, this treatment modality may be difficult to utilize when the context requires therapy sessions that are shorter than 50 minutes (because most behavioral experiments need time to set up and then, in a subsequent session, to debrief).

RATIONALE FOR INTERVENTION

Safety behaviors include overt and subtle attempts to cope with inadequate sleep and to increase control over sleep [1]. A key point to note is that safety

Behavioral Treatments for Sleep Disorders. DOI: 10.1016/B978-0-12-381522-4.00010-9

behaviors arise from beliefs/worries about sleep such as "I can't cope without 8 hours sleep", or "If I don't get to sleep I have to make up for it by napping or conserving my energy". Unfortunately, safety behaviors serve to prevent disconfirmation of these beliefs, and many safety behaviors have the effect of increasing the likelihood of the feared outcome [2,3]. For example, safety behaviors can impact [4]:

- the regularity of the sleep cycle (e.g., sleeping late in the morning, napping during the day, going to bed early);
- getting to sleep (e.g., thinking through plans for the next day, drinking coffee); some trigger a paradoxical fueling of thoughts (e.g., tell myself to stop worrying, try to stop thinking about my problems, tell myself I must go to sleep now);
- feelings of daytime sleepiness (e.g., taking the day easy, canceling all appointments);
- the day being unpleasant or boring (e.g., avoiding other people, slowing down the pace of the day, reducing self-expectations);
- preoccupation with sleep (e.g., making plans based on how much sleep is obtained, keeping a calculation of the sleep obtained, formulating plans for catching up on sleep).

STEP BY STEP DESCRIPTION OF PROCEDURES (SEE CHAPTER 7 FOR THE STEPS INVOLVED IN DEVISING EACH EXPERIMENT)

Measures have been developed to assist in assessing for the use of safety behaviors in insomnia and monitoring for sleep-related threats. The former is known as the Sleep-Related Behaviors Questionnaire (SRBQ) [5]; the latter is known as the Sleep Associated Monitoring Index (SAMI) [6]. Below we describe some of the most common experiments we have used to reduce the use of safety behaviors and monitoring.

Example 1: Symptom Monitoring (If You Look for Trouble, You Find Trouble)

1. *Precisely identify the belief/thought/process/behavior the experiment will target.*

   Many patients with insomnia focus a great deal of their attention during the day on monitoring their mood, energy, and performance as a way of gauging their tiredness, whether they got enough sleep the night before, and whether they are coping. This internal focus typically amplifies feelings of tiredness, and contributes to concern about and preoccupation with sleep.

   It can be helpful to design an experiment that targets thoughts like: "monitoring helps me to keep a check on how I am doing and helps me to adjust my daytime activities accordingly", and "monitoring my tiredness is automatic and I can't control it".

2. *Collaborate with your patient to brainstorm ideas for an experiment. Be as specific as you can.*

   Work with your patient to identify when monitoring is occurring for them. For instance, some patients tend to be quite vigilant for noises or time passing when awake in the middle of the night, while others may be more likely to attend to their energy level in the middle of the day. By pinpointing the specific difficulties with monitoring pertaining to your patient, you will be better able to target their beliefs through the experiment. Discuss specific ways to monitor and not to monitor for sleep-related symptoms, and practice both within the session.

   Taking the daytime as an example, it is often helpful to discuss monitoring versus not monitoring as putting attention outward versus inward. When attention is focused out, patients are not monitoring because they are directing their attention to the external environment by concentrating on sights, sounds, and smells around them. In contrast, when patients are monitoring, they are focusing inward toward bodily sensations, cognitive processes, and mood. For the experiment, consider asking the patient to monitor sleep-related symptoms for 2 hours during the day and then spend the next 2 hours *not* monitoring the sleep-related symptoms. Then ask the patient to repeat this pattern three times over the week. At the end of each period, the patient records how much he or she managed to be sleep-focused (i.e., monitor) and not sleep focused (i.e., attend to the external environment), and rate mood, performance, and fatigue. A concentrated and effective version of this experiment can be done when the patient is exercising or taking a walk outside (concentrating on the sunshine and trees versus concentrating on sore muscles or achy feet). It's really important that you clearly operationalize and practice monitoring and not monitoring in the session.

3. *Write down predictions about the outcome and devise a method to record the outcome.*

   A common prediction is that "I won't be able to stop monitoring throughout the day. A focus on my mood, energy, and performance throughout the day helps me feel in control because I can check out what's happening. Focusing on external things will not make any difference."

   We ask the patient to keep a diary of his or her mood, energy, and performance three times a day throughout the experiment.

4. *Anticipate problems and brainstorm solutions.*
5. *Conduct the experiment.*
6. *Review the experiment and draw conclusions. Write down the conclusions.*

   Patients will typically feel better when they do not monitor sleep-related symptoms. Monitoring actually makes us more likely to notice natural (and harmless) changes in mood, energy, and performance, and makes us more likely to worry. Patients also learn that they can choose not to monitor (and instead to smell the flowers). Many patients report an uplifting mood and energy effect that comes from not monitoring.

Example 2: Clock-watching

1. *Precisely identify the belief/thought/process/behavior the experiment will target.*

   Many patients with insomnia monitor the clock in order to see how long it takes to fall asleep and, if awake at night, how many hours of sleep remain. On waking, many patients also calculate the number of hours they slept. This clock-watching behavior typically serves to fuel anxiety, as the patient very rarely gets good news by checking the clock. As anxiety and frustration increase, patients are likely to have even greater difficulty sleeping.
2. *Collaborate with your patient to brainstorm ideas for an experiment. Be as specific as you can.*

   Make sure that the rationale for the experiment is clear to the patient. Then ask the patient to act as usual for 2 nights (i.e., monitor the clock) and then, for the next 2 nights, put the clock under the bed before turning out the light.
3. *Write down predictions about the outcome and devise a method to record the outcome.*

   Predictions made by patients include: "I won't be able to resist the urge to look at the clock, it will be really hard. It's a habit that I cannot break, I'll still find some way to calculate my sleep (e.g., by what was on the TV in the next room before falling asleep). Calculating how much sleep I get reduces my anxiety by letting me be prepared. I will be too anxious to sleep if I can't tell what time it is during the night."

   Add questions to the morning sleep diary to assess anxiety during the night and difficulty not looking at the clock (for the third and fourth nights).
4. *Anticipate problems and brainstorm solutions.*

   These will differ from patient to patient. However, one common concern is worry about oversleeping. This can be easily addressed by having the patient set an alarm before putting the clock under the bed.
5. *Conduct the experiment.*
6. *Review the experiment and draw conclusions. Write down the conclusions.*

   Watching the clock typically makes the patient worry more, which, in turn, interferes with getting to sleep. Removing the clock typically helps reduce anxiety about sleep. Dropping clock-monitoring helps

TABLE 10.1 A Behavioral Experiment for Clock-watching
Record Sheet for Behavioral Experiments

Aim	The experiment (i.e., what you plan to do)	What do you predict will happen?	What actually happened?	Outcome
To see if looking at the time is helpful or not.	3 nights without the watch/clock (put clock under the bed). 3 nights with the watch.	It might make me more stressed to know what time it is. It might be helpful not to see the time – less pressure on sleep.	I didn't worry as much about what the time was; therefore, less pressure to sleep.	I was able to not think about the time, and therefore leave that out of the equation. This meant one less stimulus to keep my brain active in my sleep. Whether I could maintain the strategy during a bad night is debatable.

people sleep more soundly. It may be helpful to encourage patients who have engaged in clock-monitoring for a long period of time to continue the experiment for a week or longer before drawing conclusions, with the rationale that it may be necessary to take a longer amount of time to break long-standing habits.

An example of a clock-monitoring experiment is included as Table 10.1.

Example 3: Napping during the day

1. *Precisely identify the belief/thought/process/behavior the experiment will target.*

   Sometimes patients with insomnia learn to cope with their daytime tiredness by taking naps (e.g., in front of the television in the evening). The beliefs that are typically associated with napping are "I can't cope without my naps; I must nap in order to catch up on lost sleep".

2. *Collaborate with your patient to brainstorm ideas for an experiment. Be as specific as you can.*

   In introducing the experiment, it is often helpful to discuss the effects napping has on the sleep homeostat (e.g., "By taking an afternoon nap, you are relieving the pressure building for sleep, so when you try to go to sleep at night the decreased pressure for sleep might contribute to your difficulty falling asleep."). Further, it may be useful to increase patients' interest in trying the experiment by pointing out the time they will gain by not napping during the day. In the first week, we tend not to make any changes. In the second week, the patient attempts to abstain from dozing, regardless of the amount of sleep obtained on the previous night. Pleasant and engaging activities are scheduled for the times the patient would ordinarily doze. Unless a pleasant alternative is planned, patients will typically find it difficult to stop napping. Patients keep a diary to record the frequency of naps, their tiredness, and how well they felt they were coping.

3. *Write down predictions about the outcome and devise a method to record the outcome.*

   A typical prediction would be: Dozing reduces tiredness because it helps me catch up on lost sleep. Not dozing will be associated with an increase in tiredness and poorer coping.

4. *Anticipate problems and brainstorm solutions.*

   It is important to conduct this experiment over at least 2 weeks – a minimum of 1 week of napping and 1 week of not (or limited) napping. Looking at 1 day of not napping, for example, would not give the sleep cycle sufficient time to adjust to the new routine.

   In the short term, this experiment can result in patients feeling more tired. It is important to warn them of this potential short-term effect and encourage them to continue with the experiment. In these instances, it is particularly important to spend time problem-solving given the specific life circumstances of the patient. Think carefully with them about the sorts of activities they might engage in as an alternative to napping. Conceptualizing this time as an "active rest" may help them to maintain dedication to the experiment as they conceptualize the time when they used to nap as a time to revitalize themselves by doing something else.

   For older adults, a nap of less than 1 hour, before 3 pm, may help overcome the natural tendency, with ageing, to sleep less at night [7].

5. *Conduct the experiment.*

6. *Review the experiment and draw conclusions. Write down the conclusions.*

   During this experiment, patients typically learn that if they do not nap during the day they will be able to cope, and improve their night-time sleep. An added benefit is that patients typically end up with more time in the week and thus feel less stressed and more able to cope. The additional time also often presents an opportunity for patients to engage in rewarding and interesting activities for which they might otherwise not have made time during the day.

Example 4: Drinking coffee

1. *Precisely identify the belief/thought/process/behavior the experiment will target.*

   Do this experiment (or a variant of it) if your patient believes that drinking lots of coffee is the only way he or she can get through the day.
2. *Collaborate with your patient to brainstorm ideas for an experiment. Be as specific as you can.*

   It is helpful to begin with a discussion of how caffeine affects sleep, and the manner in which constantly drinking coffee could contribute to insomnia. Peak your patient's interest in generating other strategies to cope during the day. A good set-up for this experiment is to contrast several days of regular coffee-drinking with several days when the patient limits coffee to two medium-strength cups before 4 pm and then tries other energy-increasing strategies after 4 pm (see Example 1 in Chapter 7 regarding unhelpful beliefs).
3. *Write down predictions about the outcome and devise a method to record the outcome.*

   Typical predictions might include: "I won't be able to function without coffee; caffeine is the only thing that will help me have enough energy to make it through the day; it will be too hard/not worth the trouble to stop drinking coffee in the afternoon."

   In addition to collecting the sleep data that are always recorded by the patient in their sleep diary, it is helpful for patients also to rate their energy level during the days when they drink coffee as usual and the days when they switch to other energy-generating behaviors at 4 pm.
4. *Anticipate problems and brainstorm solutions.*
5. *Conduct the experiment.*
6. *Review the experiment and draw conclusions. Write down the conclusions.*

   Other strategies are typically as effective as coffee at increasing energy. Furthermore, the patient will typically feel sleepier at bedtime, and may also take less time to fall asleep at night.

Example 5: Drinking alcohol to sleep

1. *Precisely identify the belief/thought/process/behavior the experiment will target.*

   Do this experiment (or a variant of it) if your patient believes that drinking alcohol helps him or her to sleep.
2. *Collaborate with your patient to brainstorm ideas for an experiment. Be as specific as you can.*

   It is helpful to begin with a discussion of how alcohol impacts sleep and sleep architecture. Psychoeducation about the effects of alcohol and the manner in which it has been empirically shown to disrupt sleep may be an effective way to introduce the experiment. A good set-up for this experiment is to contrast several days when the patient does nothing to change his or her drinking habits with several days of no more than two standard drinks per day and no drinking within (at least) an hour of bedtime.

3. *Write down predictions about the outcome and devise a method to record the outcome.*
   Typical predictions might include: "I won't be able to fall asleep without a nightcap; this habit will be too difficult to break."
   In addition to collecting the sleep data that are always recorded by patients in their sleep diary, it is helpful for patients to also rate their mood before bed, and their anxiety about not drinking.
4. *Anticipate problems and brainstorm solutions.*
   Warn patients that it may take a few nights for their sleep to readjust to not drinking alcohol before sleep.
5. *Conduct the experiment.*
6. *Review the experiment and draw conclusions. Write down the conclusions.*
   Typically, patients find that alcohol is more disruptive to their sleep over the course of the night than is not drinking. Thus, conclusions often include something like: "When I didn't drink alcohol to help me get to sleep, it took slightly longer to fall asleep at the beginning of the night, but I woke in the middle of the night less frequently. Perhaps alcohol helps me get to sleep, but it worsens my sleep quality and means I wake up early. No need to rely on alcohol to sleep."

POSSIBLE MODIFICATIONS/VARIANTS

While a stock of behavioral experiments useful for patients with insomnia is beginning to accrue (see, for example, Ree and Harvey [5]), behavioral experiments should be personalized for each patient. As such, there is an infinite range of possibilities, particularly because there is an infinite range of safety behaviors that patients can use.

PROOF OF CONCEPT/SUPPORTING DATA/EVIDENCE BASE

For information about the use of behavioral experiments to treatment insomnia, see Chapter 7. There is research showing that patients with insomnia use more sleep-related safety behaviors [5] and engage in more sleep-related monitoring [6] than normal sleepers, and there is evidence that clock-monitoring increases anxiety about sleep and contributes to sleeplessness [8]. However, there have been no specific evaluations of the use of the behavioral experiments described above.

REFERENCES

[1] P.M. Salkovskis, The importance of behaviour in the maintenance of anxiety and panic: a cognitive account, Behav. Psychother. 19 (1991) 6–19.

[2] D.M. Clark, Anxiety disorders: why they persist and how to treat them, Behav. Res. Ther. 37 (Suppl. 1) (1999) S5–27.

[3] P.M. Salkovskis, Cognitive-behavioural factors and the persistence of intrusive thoughts in obsessional problems, Behav. Res. Ther. 27 (1989) 677–682.

[4] A.G. Harvey, A cognitive model of insomnia, Behav. Res. Ther. 40 (2002) 869–894.

[5] M. Ree, A.G. Harvey, Investigating safety behaviours in insomnia: the development of the sleep-related behaviours questionnaire (SRBQ), Behav. Change 21 (2004) 26–36.

[6] C. Neitzert Semler, A.G. Harvey, Monitoring for sleep-related threat: a pilot study of the sleep associated monitoring index (SAMI), Psychosom. Med. 66 (2004) 242–250.

[7] C.M. Morin, C. Colecchi, J. Stone, et al., Behavioral and pharmacological therapies for late-life insomnia, J. Am. Med. Assoc. 281 (1999) 991–999.

[8] N.K.Y. Tang, D.E. Schmidt, A.G. Harvey, Sleeping with the enemy: clock monitoring in the maintenance of insomnia, J. Behav. Ther. Exper. Psych. 48 (2007) 40–55.

RECOMMENDED READING

J. Bennett-Levy, G. Butler, M.J.V. Fennell, et al., The Oxford Handbook of Behavioural Experiments, Oxford University Press, Oxford, 2004.

M. Ree, A.G. Harvey, Insomnia, in: J. Bennett-Levy, G. Butler, M. Fennell, et al., (Eds.), Oxford Guide to Behavioural Experiments in Cognitive Therapy, Oxford University Press, Oxford, 2004, pp. 287–305.

P.M. Salkovskis, The importance of behaviour in the maintenance of anxiety and panic: a cognitive account, Behav. Psychother. 19 (1991) 6–19.

Chapter 11

Cognitive Therapy for Dysfunctional Beliefs about Sleep and Insomnia

Charles M. Morin, Lynda Bélanger
Université Laval, Québec City, Canada

PROTOCOL NAME

Cognitive therapy for dysfunctional beliefs about sleep and insomnia.

GROSS INDICATION

This intervention is indicated for primary and comorbid insomnia, acute or chronic duration.

SPECIFIC INDICATION

This therapeutic approach is indicated specifically for individuals with evidence of dysfunctional sleep cognitions and, particularly, faulty sleep-related beliefs. There is no evidence that it is more or less effective for specific subtypes of insomnia (initial, middle, mixed) or diagnostic subgroups (primary or comorbid insomnia). Clinically, cognitive therapy is likely to be more helpful for patients with psychophysiological or paradoxical insomnia, relative to idiopathic insomnia, as the former patients tend to endorse more unhelpful beliefs which may perpetuate their sleep difficulties.

CONTRAINDICATIONS

There is no absolute contraindication for using cognitive therapy for insomnia. As for most psychotherapy, however, this therapeutic approach requires some psychological mindedness and a minimum capacity of introspection in order to explore the validity of beliefs and thoughts that are likely to contribute to insomnia. It may also be necessary to adapt or simplify the level of cognitive therapy with some patients.

Behavioral Treatments for Sleep Disorders. DOI: 10.1016/B978-0-12-381522-4.00011-0

RATIONALE FOR INTERVENTION

Cognitive therapy seeks to alter sleep-related cognitions (e.g., beliefs, attitudes, expectations, and attributions) that are presumed to contribute to the maintenance or exacerbation of insomnia. The basic premise of this approach is that appraisal of a given situation (sleeplessness) can trigger negative emotions (fear, anxiety) that are incompatible with sleep. For example, when a person is unable to sleep at night and begins dwelling on the possible consequences of sleep loss on the next day's performance, this can set off a spiral reaction and feed into the vicious cycle of insomnia, emotional distress, and more sleep disturbances (see Figure 11.1).

Within this conceptual framework, cognitive therapy is designed to guide patients in identifying some unhelpful sleep-related cognitions and beliefs and in reframing them with more adaptive substitutes in order to short-circuit the self-fulfilling nature of this vicious cycle [1,2]. Specific treatment targets include (but are not limited to):

- unrealistic expectations about sleep requirements ("I must get my 8 hours of sleep every night");
- faulty attributions about the causes of insomnia ("My insomnia is entirely due to a biochemical imbalance");

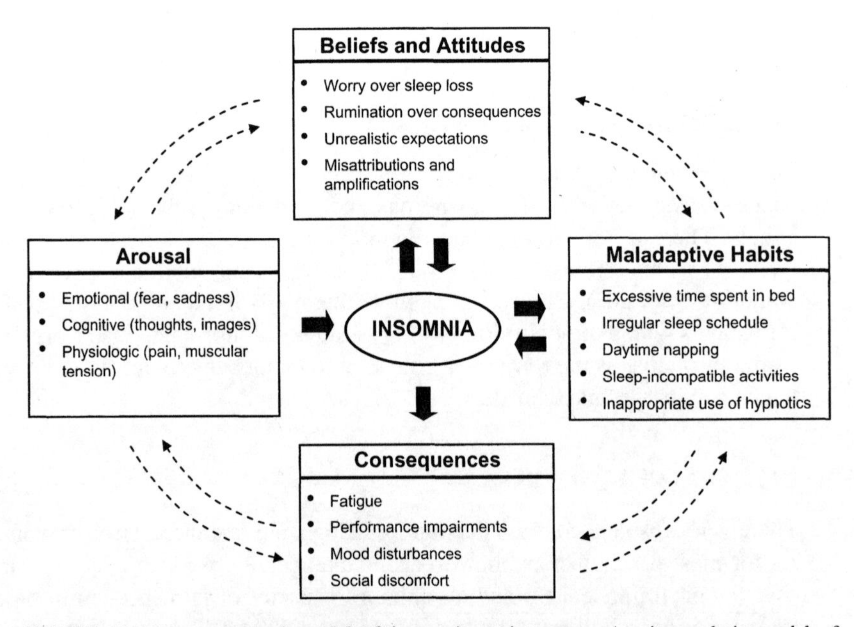

FIGURE 11.1 A conceptual model of insomnia maintenance. A microanalytic model of chronic insomnia showing how maladaptive beliefs and sleep habits can contribute to perpetuate insomnia. Reproduced with permission from Morin (1993).

- excessive worry about sleep loss and amplification of its consequences ("Insomnia will have serious consequences on my health");
- misconceptions about healthy sleep practices ("If I only try harder, I'll eventually return to sleep").

STEP BY STEP DESCRIPTION OF PROCEDURES

Cognitive therapy for unhelpful sleep-related beliefs relies on the same clinical procedures (e.g., reappraisal, reattribution, decatastrophizing, attention shifting, hypothesis testing) used in the cognitive management of other disorders such as anxiety and depression. Through cognitive techniques such as Socratic questioning, collaborative empiricism, and guided discovery [3,4], the therapist aims at helping patients to (1) identify their negative automatic thoughts about sleep and insomnia which are hypothesized to maintain the target problem; (2) recognize the connections between cognitions, emotions, and behaviors; (3) examine the evidence for and against their sleep-related distorted automatic thoughts; (4) substitute more realistic interpretations for these biased cognitions; and (5) learn to identify and modify their core beliefs which predispose to distorted perceptions of the problem [5].

As a preliminary step to implementing these procedures, it is particularly important to provide patients with a conceptual framework of insomnia – that is, an explanation of the role of cognitive processes in regulating emotions, physiological arousal, and behavior (i.e., cognitive theory of emotions) (Figure 11.2). This process is facilitated by starting off with examples unrelated to insomnia that can trigger various negative emotions (e.g., being late for an appointment and stuck in traffic; not being selected for a job; a friend

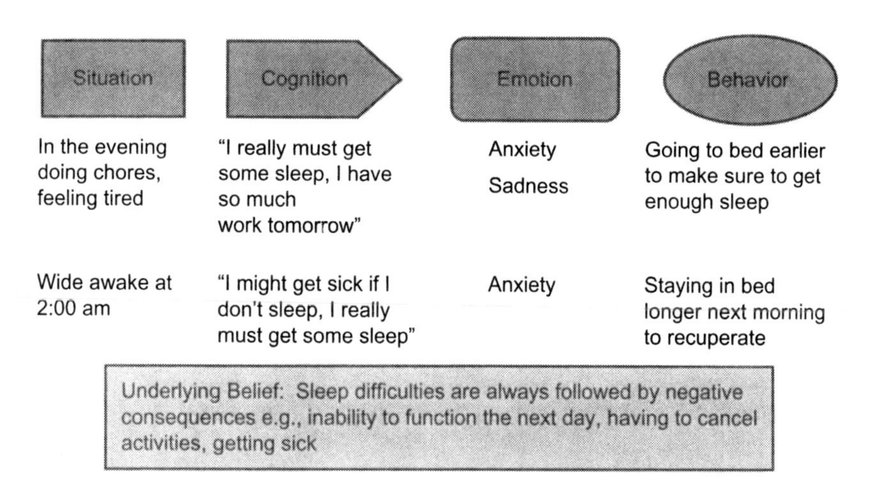

FIGURE 11.2 Basic Premise of the Cognitive Model. Relationship between cognitions (beliefs), emotions and behaviors.

being late for an appointment). It is important that the patient understands how a person's interpretation of a given situation may modulate the types of emotional reaction to that situation. Collaboratively, therapist and patient can elicit several examples to illustrate the relationship between thoughts, emotions, and behaviors, and then move on to more specific examples related to insomnia.

Once the cognitive model is understood and the importance of targeting beliefs and attitudes about sleep is integrated, the next step is to identify patient-specific dysfunctional sleep cognitions in order to eventually question their validity and replace them with more rational substitutes. Self-monitoring is usually a very effective strategy to identify automatic thoughts. It can be achieved in the office through the use of Socratic verbal questioning and imagery recollection. Starting from a recent example when the patient had trouble sleeping, the therapist guides the patient to identify his or her automatic thoughts and associated emotions. The therapist can ask questions such as, "What was running through your mind when you were unable to sleep last night?", "How did you feel at that time?", "What did you think then?".

Home practice is highly important in cognitive therapy. The automatic thoughts record form [3,4] is a very useful assessment tool to monitor a wider variety of dysfunctional thoughts than those reported during treatment sessions and is a practical tool to help patients continue monitoring their sleep-related negative automatic thoughts between sessions. Table 11.1 presents an example of this record form, with the standard three-column format. Patients are asked to identify: (1) the situation or event which led to the unpleasant emotion, (2) the automatic thoughts and/or images that went through their mind at that time, and (3) the emotional reactions (e.g., helplessness, anxiety, anger) and their intensity. The emotion's intensity is rated on a scale from 0 to 100. Patients should pay particular attention to their automatic thoughts when they

TABLE 11.1 Example of a Standard Three-column Automatic Thoughts Record Form

Situation (Specify Date and Time)	Automatic Thoughts (What was Going Through Your Mind?)	Emotions (Rate Each Emotion's Intensity on a Scale of 1–100%)
09/28 Watching TV in the evening	"I must sleep well tonight, I have so much work tomorrow"	Anxious (50%)
09/29 Lying in bed awake at 2 am	"This has to stop! I can't go on living like this. This is going to make me ill" "I have to get some sleep!"	Anxious (75%) Discouraged/sad (60%)

have trouble sleeping at night or have trouble functioning during the day, or when they worry about sleep.

Self-report questionnaires can also be useful to help identify and select relevant treatment targets to be addressed in therapy. In our clinical practice and research, we use the Dysfunctional Beliefs and Attitudes about Sleep Scale (DBAS) [1]. This self-report scale was designed to assess a variety of sleep-related beliefs and identify those that are more strongly engrained and emotionally laden. A 30-item and a 16-item version are available (see Appendix 11.1 for the 16-item version). Patients indicate the extent to which they agree or disagree with each statement on a scale ranging from 0 (strongly disagree) to 100 (strongly agree). The content of the items reflects several themes (listed above) related to expectations about sleep requirements, explanations of the causes of insomnia, perception of its consequences, and beliefs about sleep-promoting practices. Higher scores in one or more of these domains have been linked to more severe sleep disturbances and higher distress associated with insomnia [6–8].

Once patient-specific sleep cognitions have been identified and patients are comfortable with thought-monitoring, the next step is to encourage patients in viewing their thoughts as only one of many possible interpretations. The next step of therapy thus consists of finding alternatives to the dysfunctional sleep cognitions by using cognitive restructuring techniques in order to weaken the association between sleeplessness and the negative thoughts that are hypothesized to maintain the aroused state. To guide patients in evaluating the validity and usefulness of their cognitions, the therapist can ask probing questions such as:

- What is the evidence for this idea?
- What is the evidence against?
- What makes you think this will happen?
- What are the chances that this will happen?
- What is the worst that could happen?
- Could you live through it?
- Are there any alternative ways of seeing this situation?
- What is the most realistic outcome?

Here are some examples.

In the following example, clinician and patient work collaboratively to reduce the degree of attention given to insomnia consequences on daytime functioning and to examine if some other factors might also explain some daytime impairments.

Therapist: During the evaluation you mentioned that you are quite worried about the possible consequences of insomnia on your ability to function, that you often feel that you won't be able to function at all during the day after a poor night's sleep. Did I understand this correctly?

Patient: Yes, that looks like it.

Therapist: Let's look at this concern more closely … Have there been times recently when this has happened?

Patient: Yes there have been a few.

Therapist: Would you say that every time you have had a poor night's sleep lately you were unable to function the next day?

Patient: Well … probably not every time, maybe 50 percent of the time.

Therapist: Can you remember times recently when you were able to function fairly well during the day despite having slept poorly the preceding night?

Patient: This has happened a couple of times and each time I find myself wondering about how I managed …

Therapist: Let's look at the opposite situation: have there been times when you had difficulties functioning or had no energy during the day even though you had slept well the night before?

Patient: Yes, that has happened several times as well.

Therapist: Are there other situations or activities you do either at work or at home that could also explain how you feel during the day?

Patient: Well … I had never looked at this from this angle before … I guess that when I'm under a lot of pressure at work or out of a big meeting; chances are that I'll feel tired at the end of the day, even if I have slept well the night before … Perhaps because I feel a lot of stress during some of those meetings …

Therapist: If we take another look at this belief that you're always unable to function after a poor night sleep, how do you see this now?

Patient: Well, I think that the point we are getting at is that probably sleeping poorly is not the only cause of how I may feel or function during the day …

Patient: hmm … and although I may feel more tired during the day after a poor night's sleep, most of the time I can still function fairly well, at least I can get most things done.

Therapist: That's really interesting! It seems that the more a person worries about those daytime impairments, the greater the chance that it will take longer to fall back to sleep; this is because of the negative emotions they are feeling and worry during the day about this may even affect their sleep the following night. This is like a self-fulfilling prophecy …

Patient: I guess that really makes a lot of sense … I have often thought that everything seems worse in the middle of the night … I should wait before judging and definitively avoid panicking.

Self-monitoring is still extremely useful at this stage in order to help the patient modify his or her thinking about sleep and realize how much the emotional reaction changes depending on the nature of the thoughts entertained. For that purpose, two columns are added to the three-column automatic thoughts form: a fourth column where patients are asked to identify possible alternative ways of seeing things (i.e. more rational and realistic thoughts) – for example, finding evidence for and against the thought/belief, listing the impact that the thought has on his or her emotions, or estimating the probability that the feared outcome will take place; and a fifth column where the associated emotions are reassessed as a function of this alternative thinking. Table 11.2 presents an example of a standard five-column automatic thoughts record form [4].

TABLE 11.2 Example of a Standard Five-column Automatic Thoughts Record Form

Situation (Specify Date and Time)	Automatic Thoughts (What was Going Through Your Mind?)	Emotions (Rate each Emotion's Intensity on a Scale of 1–100%)	Alternative Thoughts (How Can I See This Situation Differently?)*	Emotions (Rate Each Emotion's Intensity on a Scale of 1–100%)
10/08 Wide awake in the middle of the night	"Oh no, not again! What type of day will I have tomorrow? I definitely won't be able to function at work"	Anxious (90%)	"There is really no point in worrying about this right now … I can't force sleep anyway …" "I can usually still get some work done after a poor night's sleep, worrying will only make things worse and keep me awake even longer." Even if feeling tired is unpleasant I can find ways to cope. I always end up okay in the end …"	Anxious (15%)

*You can use the following questions to help you revise each negative automatic thought: "What are the evidences for and against this thought?", " What are the chances that this will happen?", "How does thinking this way make me feel?"

POSSIBLE MODIFICATIONS/VARIANTS

Cognitive therapy uses a variety of procedures to change cognitions; some of these strategies are more verbal in nature and others may be more performance-based (i.e., behavioral experiments) [4]. The level of cognitive therapy that is necessary (e.g., addressing core beliefs) varies across patients, and has to be adapted to the severity of their problem and their capacity to identify and question their own thoughts and emotions. The dosage (intensity) of cognitive interventions for unhelpful beliefs about sleep as well as treatment response can thus vary greatly across patients. Although most people will be able to grasp the main concepts in cognitive therapy, questioning one's way of thinking may be more difficult for some individuals (e.g., patients with cognitive impairment, some patients with lower education or reduced introspection capacity). The main implication for treatment may be to remain very concrete and use many practical examples. The amount of time devoted to cognitive interventions, both within a given session and in relation to the multifaceted therapy for insomnia, may also need to be adapted to each patient's capacity and acceptance. It is better to change one unhelpful belief at a time, making sure that the point is well understood, rather than risk losing the patient with too much information.

On the other hand, some patients may not be receptive to this type of intervention, or may be reluctant to question and monitor their beliefs and attitudes. It is important to verify whether such reluctance is due to a resistance to consider psychological factors as potential contributing factors to insomnia, or to a lack of insight into one's problem. Once the nature of the difficulty has been identified, it is important to work it through with the patient. Sometimes it may be necessary to take a step back and re-examine the conceptual model of insomnia. It may also be useful to revise the possible causes of insomnia, with an emphasis on the role of unhelpful thoughts and beliefs in the etiology of maladaptive behaviors and negative emotions which serve to maintain insomnia. Many patients are convinced that their insomnia problem is the result of a physical disorder such as a chemical imbalance. The idea is not to try to convince patients that there is no biological cause to their sleep difficulty, but rather to help them understand that there are usually several causes to insomnia and that they can have an active role in controlling some of them – namely, the psychological factors. In addition to verbal interventions, planning behavioral experiments to directly test the validity of some unhelpful beliefs may be quite effective. Such experiments can be presented as a "test" for patients to conduct by themselves in order to discover how some of their thoughts are directly related to their sleep difficulty [9].

Formal cognitive therapy may not always be necessary, as didactic teaching about good sleep practices, sleep requirements, and the impact of insomnia may be sufficient to correct erroneous beliefs. For instance, presenting the negative effects of excessive daytime napping, or of spending too much time in bed on the circadian system, may be sufficient to change the patients' perceptions regarding the usefulness of these strategies, and consequently encourage them to change these maladaptive behaviors. When working with older adults, topics that should be carefully addressed, and perhaps considered as a standard theme, are the age-related changes in sleep architecture and their consequences on the experience of sleep. This educational intervention may sometimes be sufficient to modify beliefs about unrealistic sleep standards based on younger years' sleep and individual differences in sleep duration requirements.

PROOF OF CONCEPT/SUPPORTING DATA

There is increasing evidence that some sleep-related beliefs may be instrumental in perpetuating or exacerbating insomnia. Not surprisingly, cognitive therapy has become a standard therapeutic component in most multi-component approaches to treating insomnia [10]. Cognitive therapy is considered a critical therapy component for successful insomnia treatment outcomes [10,11] and for long-term maintenance of sleep improvements following therapy [12,13]. Although there has been no direct evaluation of the unique contribution of cognitive therapy to overall treatment efficacy, one open clinical trial has evaluated the contribution of a different version of cognitive therapy relative to that described in the present chapter [14]. The results of that study have been very promising, although they need replication due to the small sample size and uncontrolled study design. There is currently one large multi-center randomized clinical trial examining the unique contribution of cognitive therapy relative to its behavioral counterpart and the full cognitive behavior therapy (Morin and Harvey, in progress).

REFERENCES

[1] C.M. Morin, Insomnia: Psychological Assessment and Management, Guilford Press, New York, NY, 1993.

[2] C.M. Morin, C.A. Espie, Insomnia: A Clinical Guide to Assessment and Treatment, Kluwer Academic/Plenum Publishers, New York, NY, 2003.

[3] A.T. Beck, J.A. Rush, B.F. Shaw, G. Emery, Cognitive Therapy of Depression, Guilford Press, New York, NY, 1979.

[4] J.S. Beck, Cognitive Therapy: Basics and Beyond, Guilford Press, New York, NY, 1995.

[5] L. Bélanger, J. Savard, C.M. Morin, Clinical management of insomnia using cognitive therapy, Behav. Sleep Med. 4 (2006) 179–202.

[6] C.E. Carney, J.D. Edinger, R. Manber, et al., Beliefs about sleep in disorders characterized by sleep and mood disturbance, J. Psychosom. Res. 62 (2007) 179–188.

[7] C.E. Carney, J.D. Edinger, Identifying critical beliefs about sleep in primary insomnia, Sleep 29 (2006) 444–453.

[8] C.M. Morin, A. Vallières, H. Ivers, Dysfunctional beliefs and attitudes about sleep (DBAS): validation of a brief version (DBAS-16), Sleep 30 (2007) 1547–1554.

[9] M. Ree, A. Harvey, Insomnia, in: J. Bennett-Levy, J. Butler, M. Fennell, et al., (Eds.), Oxford Guide to Behavioural Experiments in Cognitive Therapy, Oxford University Press, New York, NY, 2004.

[10] C.M. Morin, R.R. Bootzin, D.J. Buysse, et al., Psychological and behavioral treatment of insomnia: update of the recent evidence (1998–2004), Sleep 29 (2006) 1398–1414.

[11] J.D. Edinger, C.E. Carney, W.K. Wohlgemuth, Pretherapy cognitive dispositions and treatment outcome in cognitive behavior therapy for insomnia, Behav. Ther. 39 (2008) 406–416.

[12] J.D. Edinger, W.K. Wohlgemuth, R.A. Radtke, et al., Does CBT alter dysfunctional beliefs about sleep? Sleep 24 (2001) 591–599.

[13] C.M. Morin, F. Blais, J. Savard, Are changes in beliefs and attitudes about sleep related to sleep improvements in the treatment of insomnia? Behav. Res. Ther. 40 (2002) 741–752.

[14] A.G. Harvey, A.L. Sharpley, M.J. Ree, et al., An open trial of cognitive therapy for chronic insomnia, Behav. Res. Ther. 45 (2007) 2491–2501.

RECOMMENDED READING

J.S. Beck, Cognitive Therapy: Basics and Beyond, Guilford Press, New York, NY, 1995.

L. Bélanger, J. Savard, C.M. Morin, Clinical management of insomnia using cognitive therapy, Behav. Sleep Med. 4 (2006) 179–202.

C.M. Morin, Insomnia: Psychological Assessment and Management, Guilford Press, New York, NY, 1993.

C.M. Morin, C.A. Espie, Insomnia: A Clinical Guide to Assessment and Treatment, Kluwer Academic/Plenum Publishers, New York, NY, 2003.

APPENDIX 11.1

The Dysfunctional Beliefs and Attitudes about Sleep Scale

Dysfunctional Beliefs and Attitudes about Sleep

Instructions. Several statements reflecting people's beliefs and attitudes about sleep are listed below. Please indicate to what extent you personally agree or disagree with each statement. There is no right or wrong answer. For each statement, circle the number that corresponds to your own **personal belief**. Please respond to all items even though some may not apply directly to your own situation.

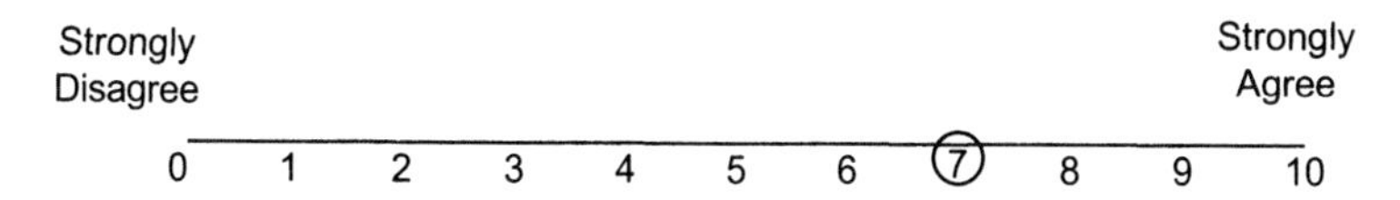

1. I need 8 hours of sleep to feel refreshed and function well during the day.

0 1 2 3 4 5 6 7 8 9 10

2. When I don't get proper amount of sleep on a given night, I need to catch up on the next day by napping or on the next night by sleeping longer.

0 1 2 3 4 5 6 7 8 9 10

3. I am concerned that chronic insomnia may have serious consequences on my physical health.

0 1 2 3 4 5 6 7 8 9 10

4. I am worried that I may lose control over my abilities to sleep.

0 1 2 3 4 5 6 7 8 9 10

5. After a poor night's sleep, I know that it will interfere with my daily activities on the next day.

0 1 2 3 4 5 6 7 8 9 10

6. In order to be alert and function well during the day, I believe I would be better off taking a sleeping pill rather than having a poor night's sleep.

0 1 2 3 4 5 6 7 8 9 10

7. When I feel irritable, depressed, or anxious during the day, it is mostly because I did not sleep well the night before.

0 1 2 3 4 5 6 7 8 9 10

8. When I sleep poorly on one night, I know it will disturb my sleep schedule for the whole week.

0 1 2 3 4 5 6 7 8 9 10

9. Without an adequate night's sleep, I can hardly function the next day.

0 1 2 3 4 5 6 7 8 9 10

10. I can't ever predict whether I'll have a good or poor night's sleep.

0 1 2 3 4 5 6 7 8 9 10

11. I have little ability to manage the negative consequences of disturbed sleep.

0 1 2 3 4 5 6 7 8 9 10

12. When I feel tired, have no energy, or just seem not to function well during the day, it is generally because I did not sleep well the night before.

0 1 2 3 4 5 6 7 8 9 10

13. I believe insomnia is essentially the result of a chemical imbalance.

0 1 2 3 4 5 6 7 8 9 10

14. I feel insomnia is ruining my ability to enjoy life and prevents me from doing what I want.

0 1 2 3 4 5 6 7 8 9 10

15. Medication is probably the only solution to sleeplessness.

0 1 2 3 4 5 6 7 8 9 10

16. I avoid or cancel obligations (social, family) after a poor night's sleep.

0 1 2 3 4 5 6 7 8 9 10

Chapter 12

Cognitive Restructuring: Cognitive Therapy for Catastrophic Sleep Beliefs

Michael L. Perlis

Department of Psychiatry, University of Pennsylvania Center for Sleep and Respiratory Neurobiology, University of Pennsylvania; School of Nursing, University of Pennsylvania, Philadelphia, PA

Philip R. Gehrman

Department of Psychiatry, University of Pennsylvania Center for Sleep and Respiratory Neurobiology, University of Pennsylvania, Philadelphia, PA

PROTOCOL NAME

Cognitive restructuring: cognitive therapy for catastrophic sleep beliefs.

GROSS INDICATION

- Excessive focus on thoughts/beliefs pertaining to the potential catastrophic consequences of sleep continuity disturbance and/or sleep loss;
- Obvious and large probability overestimates regarding the potential catastrophic consequences of sleep continuity disturbance and/or sleep loss.

SPECIFIC INDICATION

To date, there is no evidence to suggest that this form of therapy is differentially effective for one or another type of insomnia (psychophysiologic vs idiopathic vs paradoxical insomnia) or for any of the phenotypes/subtypes of insomnia (initial vs middle vs late insomnia).

CONTRAINDICATIONS

While there is no evidence to show "where and when" this form of therapy is contraindicated, it stands to reason that this treatment modality may not be

Behavioral Treatments for Sleep Disorders. DOI: 10.1016/B978-0-12-381522-4.00012-2

useful, or may be complicated, in the following cases:

- Patients who do not exhibit an excessive focus on thoughts/beliefs pertaining to the potential catastrophic consequences of sleep continuity disturbance and/or sleep loss (**NOTE**: It may not be evident that a patient has such thoughts/beliefs until one engages in the exercise that lies at the heart of this protocol)
- Patients who have experienced severe life experiences that they attribute to their insomnia (e.g., an accident that involved severe injury or loss of life)
- Patients with cognitive impairment due to brain injury, dementia, or other illnesses that may interfere with their ability to engage in a cognitive intervention.

RATIONALE FOR INTERVENTION

There is no doubt that theorists and therapists differ about the role of cognition as a precipitating and/or perpetuating factor for chronic insomnia. Some suggest that cognitive factors are critical (e.g., serve to trigger abnormal attentional processes or counterproductive effort behaviors). Others argue that such factors serve to exacerbate insomnia, but are not primary (e.g., patients with chronic insomnia are not awake because they are worrying, but instead are worrying because they are awake). Still others may take the position that cognitive factors are simply epiphenomenon (e.g., insomnia occurs in association with behavioral factors and conditioning, period). If one subscribes to the first or second of the above positions, then attention to cognitive factors is warranted, and all that is required is a determination regarding whether this particular form of Cognitive Therapy (CT) is useful. As noted above, this form of therapy is likely to be useful with patients who exhibit an "excessive focus on thoughts/beliefs pertaining to the potential catastrophic consequences of sleep continuity disturbance and/or sleep loss".

STEP BY STEP DESCRIPTION OF PROCEDURES

There are essentially eight steps to the process:

1. Introduce the exercise
2. Calculate how long the patient has had their insomnia (in days)
3. Identify and record 3–10 catastrophic thoughts
4. Assess and record the patient's probability estimates
5. Determine the actual frequency of occurrence of the anticipated "catastrophes"
6. Calculate the frequency rate that corresponds to the certainty estimate
7. Discuss with the patient how it is that one is prone to such overestimates
8. Set a countering "mantra".

Each of these stages is explicated below.

Introduce the Exercise

How the exercise is introduced is, in part, dependent upon the centrality placed upon CT. In the treatment regimen laid out by our group [1], this component is delivered during the second half of treatment and is explained as an exploration of a factor that is thought to be "wind to the flame" (i.e., how one thinks about insomnia may make it worse). Regardless of when the procedure is introduced, when undertaking this exercise with a patient it needs to be introduced in a considerate way – one that avoids any hint that the therapist is being pedantic or patronizing. This caveat is proffered based on the concern that it is easy to slip into a haughty role when one knows the answer to a question … or, perhaps more aptly, when one is accustomed to probabilistic thinking and making judgments on the basis of sampled evidence. One possible way to introduce the exercise is as follows.

Therapist: As you may have noticed, the work we've done to date doesn't much address the role of worry in insomnia. I know that some folks think that being a worrier is what causes insomnia … and this may be so early on … But once the insomnia is chronic, our sense is that the disorder continues not so much because of worry, but rather because of the other factors that we have talked about. That is, the mismatch between sleep ability and sleep opportunity that comes from extending sleep opportunity (going to bed early, sleeping in, and napping during the day). And it seems that we have made some real distance by focusing our efforts on these issues. [This is a good time to pull out the graphs and review them with the patient.] But the fact is, worry is not irrelevant. In the context of chronic insomnia, it can be "gas to the fire" or "wind to the flame". In the case of both of these analogies … they make the point that neither wind nor gas started the fire, but they sure can make things worse. So today I want to spend the session focused on this issue and have you play a game with me. It's a bit of a silly game, but I think when we're done, the point of the game won't be lost on you.

Calculate How Long the Patient has had Their Insomnia (in Days)

This first step only requires asking patients to estimate how long they have had their insomnia. While this information is likely to have been acquired during the initial evaluation, if it wasn't then this step may be complicated by a patient's unwillingness to give a "hard number". Often when asked, the patient will simply say that he or she has had insomnia "forever". In this instance, it may be useful to do a brief biographical assessment. That is, "tell me of a vivid memory when your were 4, 10, in Elementary School, in Junior High, in High School, in College, during your first job as a _______, when you first got married, when you had your first child, etc.". Once a life event anchor is had for each time period, the therapist can then query, per event, "when you ________ did you have trouble sleeping then?" Once a date is established, all that is required is that duration of the insomnia be calculated in terms of days and recorded (ideally on a whiteboard or on a sheet of paper that can be viewed by both the therapist and the patient). Calculating the number of days can, and should be, done conservatively. If the patient has had insomnia for 10 years, this translates to 3650 days. This assumes, however, that insomnia occurs on a nightly basis. This is unlikely, and this represents an ideal time to query the patient about frequency of insomnia per week. Data from the sleep diaries may also be used to address the point. Regardless of how it is decided, the final number should reflect that insomnia does not occur nightly. If it is decided, for example, that 5 days per week is more accurate, then the final assessment will be closer to 2600 days.

Identify and Record 3–10 Catastrophic Thoughts

There are two parts to this component of the exercise: first, eliciting material (thoughts) from the patient; and second, if necessary, helping the patient to unmask the underlying catastrophic thought. Eliciting thoughts can be done as follows:

Therapist: Settle back in your chair a bit. Maybe close your eyes and imagine you're in bed. Think back to a time before you sought out treatment. You've been lying in bed for 30 minutes – maybe more. What thoughts pop into your head when you're thinking "If I don't fall asleep, tomorrow I'll ______________? Fill in the blank … "If I don't fall asleep, tomorrow I'll ______________…"

Unmasking the underlying catastrophic thought is required when the patient provides a thought that is not only relatively benign but is also a high probability event ("tomorrow I'll feel tired"). The task then is for the therapist to get the patient to associate from the given thought to the related/derivative catastrophic thought. One way to do this is to set up a "T" chart on a whiteboard where the therapist lists the initial-antecedent thought (I'll be tired) on the left side of the board and encourages the patient to "continue with that line of thought" towards other potential consequences ("I'll be so tired that I'll *wreck my car*"). Table 12.1 provides some typical "antecedent" and "consequent" type statements.

Assess and Record the Patient's Probability Estimates

Assessing patients' sense of certainty requires that they tell you how certain they are in terms of percentages (0 percent certain to 100 percent) regarding each catastrophic event. For example:

Therapist: Your first example was "If I don't fall asleep, tomorrow I'll wreck my car". At the time you thought this … lying awake

TABLE 12.1 Common Worries and Catastrophic Thoughts

If I Don't Get Enough Sleep Tonight Then ...

Worry	Associated Catastrophic Thought
I'll be irritable and short with my wife	My wife will leave or divorce me
I'll be irritable and short with my kids	My kids will hate me – never speak to me again
I won't socialize well	I'll lose my friends
I'll do poorly at work	I'll be fired
I'll make a mistake at work	I'll kill someone
I'll make a mistake at work	I'll be sued
I'll be fired	I'll be ruined financially
I'll feel poorly	I'll get sick
I'll get sick	I'll die
I'll lose my mind	I'll go crazy – have a nervous breakdown
I won't fall asleep	I'll be awake all night
I'll fall asleep behind the wheel (or space out)	I'll total my car
I'll have an accident	I'll wreck my car and kill myself or someone else
I'll look old and unattractive	People will turn away from me in disgust

in the middle of the night ... and you heard in your head "If I don't fall asleep tomorrow I'll wreck my car" ... At that moment, how certain were you that this would happen?

Often the patient will provide very high certainties (100 percent, 99 percent, etc.). While these high estimates may accurately represent the patient's feeling at the time, the exercise works better if the therapist uses more conservative estimates *and makes it clear to the patient that he or she is "rounding down"*. Rounding down will leave the patient with the impression that the probability estimates revealed during the exercise, high as they may be, are still lower than those that occur when experiencing insomnia.

Therapist: So in the middle of the night you are 95 percent certain that if you don't fall asleep, you'll wreck your car. That's very certain! Let's round this to 90 percent ...

Determine the Actual Frequency of Occurrence of the Anticipated "Catastrophes"

Determining the frequency of occurrence requires that the therapist queries, by each item, the number of times each of the catastrophic events occurred. This can be tricky to the extent that the therapist is unaware that a catastrophic event may indeed have occurred (e.g., a school bus driver had an accident ascribed to fatigue/sleepiness where there was a loss of life). Ideally, such information should be discovered during the initial interview and a judgment about whether to deploy this form of cognitive therapy made *before* the exercise is begun. This said, for the purposes of this summary (and in keeping with the running example), let's say the patient reports having one car accident in 10 years, though they're not entirely sure it was related to fatigue or sleepiness.

Calculate the Frequency Rate that Corresponds to the Certainty Estimate

This step requires that the therapist calculates (or, better yet, has the patient calculate) the number of instances each event should have occurred, given the number of opportunities (days of insomnia) and the patient's certainty estimates (Table 12.2 provides an example). This step is the "A-ha!" step, and should be delivered with care. For example:

Therapist: Here comes the game aspect to this exercise. One way of thinking about and judging the reasonableness of one's certainties is to see how well they match "the facts". To do this we need to compare the actual occurrences of the events we've listed here with how often they should have happened, given your level of certainty and the number of opportunities you have had for the events to have occurred.

TABLE 12.2 Cognitive Restructuring
Number of Days with Insomnia 1500

1	2	3	4
Event	Certainty When Lying Awake and Unable to Sleep	No. of Event Occurrences	No. of Event Occurrences Given Certainty
Stay awake all night	85%	1	1200
Wreck the car	80%	2	1200
Be fired	90%	0	1300

Let's start with *wrecking your car*. If you've had insomnia for 2600 nights and your certainty about the possibility of wrecking your car was reasonable, you'd have experienced it on 90 percent of the occasions when you've had insomnia … so that would be 0.90 × 2600, or 2340 times. Hmmm – let's call it 2300 times. So … how many times have you wrecked your car? Once. Not 2300 times. Not 500 times. Once. And even in this instance, you're not completely ready to say it happened because of the insomnia.

So here's the interesting bit – somehow when you're lying in bed it seems reasonable to think, and to be very certain of the factualness of it, that its likely "that you'll wreck your car" when your experience tells you otherwise. Your experience tells you that this is actually a "low probability event" – in fact, an unbelievably low probability event.

As part of the exercise, it would be useful to calculate (or have the patient calculate) the actual probability. In the present example, given the number of occurrences to date (1) and the number of opportunities (2600), the probability is closer to 0.04 percent.

Discuss with the Patient How it is that One is Prone to Such Overestimates

At this juncture, the patient should be oriented, and in as many ways as possible, to the paradox that at night things may seem certain, but that in the clear light of day such certainties seem improbable, if not downright foolish. This can lead to a discussion of the effects of sleep loss and circadian phase on brain function and/or logical thought, and how we're all vulnerable to irrational thinking in the middle of the night … or, as we tend to say in therapy, *"it's a bad thing to be awake when reason sleeps"*.

Set a Countering "Mantra"

The final step is to provide patients with a tool (a mnemonic) so that they might recall this session when prone to worry at night. To accomplish this, we recommend setting a countering mantra. For example:

Therapist: Bottom line – when you are having trouble falling asleep and you start thinking the "If I don't fall asleep I may … ", it helps to remember in that moment when you think, "I may…" to counter with "I may not … in fact it's downright unlikely that I may …" In fact, just thinking *"not likely"* when you have catastrophic worries is helpful. We like to refer to this as a countering "mantra" – a thing that you can say in your head that will remind you of this exercise.

POSSIBLE MODIFICATIONS/VARIANTS

To date, no modifications or variants for this kind of cognitive restructuring have been developed for use with patients with chronic insomnia.

PROOF OF CONCEPT/SUPPORTING DATA/EVIDENCE BASE

Cognitive restructuring is a core form of therapy for CBT for depression and anxiety and panic disorders. Some years ago we recommended that this form of therapy could be applied to the treatment of sleep-related worry [1]. While there are no efficacy or effectiveness studies on this specific approach as a monotherapy, there are effectiveness data related to its use as part of multi-component therapy. Moreover, its effectiveness in the related disorders and its clear clinical utility in the treatment of insomnia suggest that this is an important component to include in CBT-I.

REFERENCE

[1] M. Perlis, C. Jungquist, M. Smith, D. Posner, Cognitive Behavioral Therapy for Insomnia: A Session by Session Guide, Springer Press, New York, NY, 2005, pp. 89–96.

RECOMMENDED READING

D.H. Barlow, Cognitive-behavioral approaches to panic disorder and social phobia, Bull. Menninger Clin. 52 (1992) A14–A28.

D.H. Barlow, M.G. Craske, J.A. Cerny, J.S. Klosko, Behavioral treatment of panic disorder, Behav. Ther. 20 (1989) 261–282.

N.M. Broomfield, A. Gumley, C.A. Espie, Candidate cognitive processes in insomnia, J. Cogn. Psychother. 19 (2005) 3–15.

C.A. Espie, Insomnia: conceptual issues in the development, persistence and treatment of sleep disorder in adults, Annu. Rev. Psychol. 53 (2002) 215–243.

Chapter 13

Intensive Sleep Retraining: Conditioning Treatment for Primary Insomnia

Jodie Harris
Adelaide Institute for Sleep Health, Repatriation General Hospital, Adelaide, South Australia

Leon Lack
Department of Psychology, Flinders University, Adelaide, South Australia

PROTOCOL NAME

Intensive Sleep Retraining (ISR): conditioning treatment for primary insomnia.

GROSS INDICATION

This is indicated for chronic primary (psychophysiologic) insomnia, with evidence of conditioning (learned insomnia) and/or behavioral contributors or maintaining factors.

SPECIFIC INDICATION

Initial data indicate that this treatment is effective for those with sleep onset, or sleep onset and maintenance insomnia. However, there is some support for a greater treatment effect with sleep onset difficulties.

CONTRAINDICATIONS

Specific contraindications include patients with a particular susceptibility to sleep deprivation (e.g., epilepsy or seizure disorders, bipolar disorder).

ISR treatment has to date only been applied to a carefully selected subsection of insomnia sufferers, with no evaluation of effectiveness for early morning awakening insomnia, circadian rhythm disturbances, or so-called "secondary" insomnia. However, if we assume that these co-morbid disorders may involve some conditioning factors in the sleep disturbance, ISR may prove to be applicable to a wider range of insomnia presentations.

Behavioral Treatments for Sleep Disorders. DOI: 10.1016/B978-0-12-381522-4.00013-4

RATIONALE FOR INTERVENTION

Conditioning factors are proposed to be involved in the precipitation and perpetuation of chronic insomnia. Learning theory suggests that insomnia may be a "learned" arousal or wakefulness response, or alternatively may be a "learned" absence of de-arousal associated with internal and external cues for sleep [1]. As such, the cues to produce a sleep-conducive state, and to aid the subsequent sleep experience, may then be less effective or absent.

Traditional behavioral therapies for insomnia often involve a gradual build-up of sleep debt in early weeks of treatment application, a heightened homeostatic drive that gradually enables more and more experiences of shorter sleep onsets at night. Rapid sleep onsets, occurring at increasing frequency with time, are thought to condition sleep-conducive cues in the bedroom environment.

ISR is proposed to act by using an acutely increased homeostatic drive to facilitate rapid sleep onsets in a series of sleep opportunities in a single treatment session. Thereby, conditioning treatment, as might occur with traditional behavioral therapies such as Stimulus Control Therapy (SCT [2]) and Sleep Restriction Therapy (SRT [3]), is applied in a shorter time frame.

STEP BY STEP DESCRIPTION OF PROCEDURES

The following procedures are a description of the ISR treatment that has been used in the research to date.

1. *Treatment preparation.* A pre-treatment night of sleep restriction allows an initial build-up of sleep pressure. This is set at a period of 5 hours time in bed, independent of sleep time, using an alarm to awaken. In addition, naps and caffeine are avoided in the 24 hours prior to treatment start.
2. *Treatment.*
   a. Treatment occurs in the sleep laboratory in order to enable EEG sleep onset monitoring. Arrival in the laboratory is followed by the application of relevant EEG (C3-A2, C4-A1, O1-A2), EOG and EMG electrodes as per a standard 10–20 system.
   b. Treatment "sleep trials" begin at 10:30 pm on night 1 of treatment.
   c. A "sleep trial" involves the treatment recipient getting into bed in order to attempt to initiate sleep in a laboratory bedroom-simulation environment. (It may be advantageous to mimic the home environment as closely as possible, including bringing personal pillows, bedding, pyjamas, etc.).
   d. Once settled in bed, just prior to a sleep trial start, an assessment of subjective sleepiness (Stanford Sleepiness Scale; SSS [4]) is completed.
   e. The half-hourly sleep trials start with lights out, and an instruction to "get comfortable, lie still and allow yourself to fall asleep", after which time the bedroom lights are extinguished.

f. EEG monitoring in the adjacent sleep laboratory area allows measurement of sleep onset latency (SOL), and restriction of the amount of sleep obtained in any nap opportunity. Participants are awoken following 3 consecutive minutes of (any stage of) sleep, if obtained within each 20-minute nap opportunity.
g. Following each sleep trial, participants are asked whether they experienced and recognized sleep within the sleep trial. Feedback is then provided as to whether sleep was obtained according to the EEG, in order to facilitate some sleep–wake discrimination training. This is consistent with research data suggesting that individuals with insomnia are prone to report prior wakefulness following an awakening from sleep, and that feedback about sleep state may improve sleep in insomnia sufferers [5].
h. Following the end of each sleep trial treatment, recipients get out of bed and maintain quiet wakeful activities (i.e. reading, watching DVDs). Wakefulness is corroborated by on-line EEG. The laboratory remains a "time-free" environment throughout treatment.
i. Half-hourly trials are held throughout a 25-hour treatment period, resulting in a total of 50 opportunities to initiate sleep under sleep deprivation conditions.

3. *Post-treatment.*
   a. A post-treatment recovery sleep is limited to a period of 8 hours in bed in order to maintain circadian rhythmicity, and encourage the maintenance of some homeostatic sleep drive to encourage ongoing treatment response.
   b. Daily sleep diaries are completed throughout the 2 weeks prior to treatment, and for at least 6 weeks immediately following ISR.

POSSIBLE MODIFICATIONS/VARIANTS

1. Research indicates that ISR, although rapidly efficacious on its own, tends to be more consistently effective when combined with follow-up Stimulus Control Therapy (SCT). This treatment may then alter some of the previously maintaining factors in patients' insomnia – for instance, spending excessive amounts of time in bed. SCT has been implemented on the first post-ISR treatment day, with a series of five weekly sessions with a clinical psychologist.
2. One case series pilot study attempted to implement this conditioning treatment for a period of 36 hours, starting at 10:30 am [6]. However, sleep onsets were less likely to be obtained within the first treatment day, and the routine was therefore altered in future trials. To date, there is little evidence regarding the number of sleep trials or sleep onsets required for effective treatment.
3. Future research will attempt to examine the "type" of insomnia, and the sleep and psychological profiles of participants most likely to benefit from ISR treatment. For instance, there has been a trend for a greater treatment

effect with sleep onset disturbance over sleep maintenance difficulties. However, larger-scale investigations will need to be completed before these trends can be confirmed.

PROOF OF CONCEPT/SUPPORTING DATA/EVIDENCE BASE

The largest study to date of ISR was a randomized controlled trial involving 79 participants with chronic sleep onset insomnia (with or without sleep maintenance insomnia) [7]. Treatment groups were ISR, SCT, ISR plus SCT, and a sleep hygiene control (concurrently administered in other treatment groups). ISR was administered in a weekend treatment period, followed up with five weekly treatment sessions. Figure 13.1 illustrates the average heightened sleepiness levels and decreased sleep onset latencies across the 25-hour treatment period.

Figure 13.2 illustrates the effect of ISR on immediate mean post-treatment (daily) sleep variables of total sleep time and sleep onset latency in a pilot study. There is evidence of rapid and significant changes in these variables.

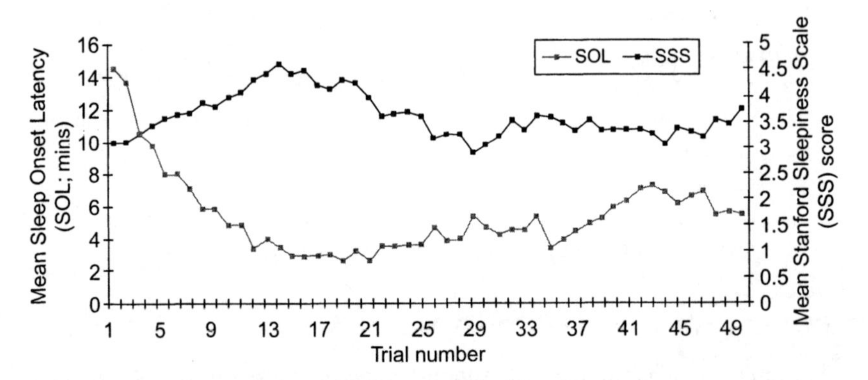

FIGURE 13.1 Mean Sleep Onset Latency (SOL) and Stanford Sleepiness Scale (SSS) scores at each sleep trial time throughout the ISR treatment procedure (n = 39).

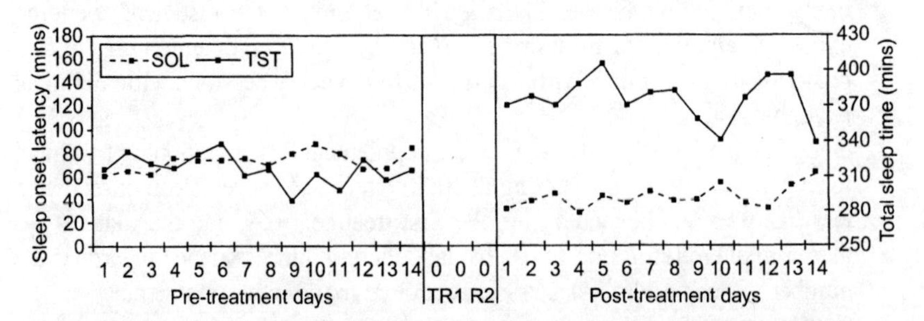

FIGURE 13.2 Mean daily Sleep Onset Latency (SOL) and Total Sleep Time (TST) immediately prior to, and following ISR T (treatment), R1 (recovery night 1) and R2 (recovery night 2). N = 17, ISR administered in isolation [8].

In the most recent larger RCT study, the active treatment groups (ISR, SCT, ISR + SCT) all resulted in significant improvements in sleep diary sleep onset latency and sleep efficiency, with moderate to large effect sizes, from pre-treatment to post-treatment. Wake time after sleep onset decreased significantly in the SCT and ISR + SCT groups. Total sleep time increased significantly in the ISR and ISR + SCT treatment groups. There were few statistically significant differences between active treatment groups, indicating a comparable treatment response.

In this largest trial, ISR was implemented with follow-up sleep hygiene recommendations addressing caffeine and other stimulants, exercise, alcohol, the bedroom environment, and a "wind-down" time prior to sleep. These instructions, also applied as a control treatment, showed little independent treatment effect. However, it has been suggested that the effectiveness of CBT treatments may be threatened if these factors are not concurrently addressed.

Trends indicated that the combination ISR+SCT group demonstrated the largest effect sizes for both sleep and daytime functioning variables, and resulted in a greater proportion of treatment responders, with 61 percent reaching "good sleeper" status (vs 38 percent with SCT, and 47 percent with ISR alone). Subjective (sleep diary) treatment gains achieved by post-treatment in the active treatment groups were largely maintained throughout follow up periods, up to 6 months.

In conclusion, Intensive Sleep Retraining is a brief, laboratory-based, conditioning treatment for chronic sleep onset insomnia, which results in very rapid improvements in sleep variables. The ISR treatment response seems to be comparable to other traditional behavioral therapies, and when used in combination may speed up and enhance the response to these therapies.

REFERENCES

[1] J.A. Robertson, N.M. Broomfield, C.A. Espie, Prospective comparison of subjective arousal during the pre-sleep period in primary sleep-onset insomnia and normal sleepers, J. Sleep Res. 16 (2) (2007) 230–238.

[2] R.R. Bootzin, Stimulus control treatment for insomnia, Proc. Am. Psychol. Assoc. 7 (1972) 395–396.

[3] A.J. Spielman, P. Saskin, M.J. Thorpy, Treatment of chronic insomnia by restriction of time in bed, Sleep 10 (1) (1987) 45–56.

[4] E. Hoddes, V.P. Zarcone, H. Smythe, et al., Quantification of sleepiness: a new approach, Psychophysiology 10 (1973) 431–436.

[5] J. Mercer, L. Lack, R. Bootzin, Feedback of sleep/wake state improves subjective and objective sleep of insomniacs, Sleep 28 (2005) 242.

[6] L.C. Lack, M. Baraniec, Intensive sleep onset training for sleep onset insomnia, Sleep 25 (2002) A478.

[7] J. Harris, L. Lack, K. Kemp, et al., A randomised controlled trial of Intensive Sleep Retraining (ISR); A brief conditioning treatment for chronic insomnia, Sleep (2010) (submitted).

[8] J. Harris, L. Lack, H. Wright, et al., Intensive sleep retraining (ISR) treatment for chronic primary insomnia: a preliminary investigation, J. Sleep Res. 16 (2007) 276–284.

Chapter 14

Mindfulness-Based Therapy for Insomnia

Jason C. Ong

Department of Behavioral Sciences, Rush University Medical Center, Chicago, IL

Rachel Manber

Department of Psychiatry and Behavioral Sciences, Stanford University, CA

PROTOCOL NAME

Mindfulness-Based Therapy for Insomnia (MBTI): applying the principles of acceptance and letting go.

GROSS INDICATION

MBTI may be particularly useful in treating the distress and emotional reactivity associated with chronic insomnia.

SPECIFIC INDICATION

MBTI is indicated for primary insomnia and for psychophysiological insomnia.

CONTRAINDICATIONS

There are no specific contraindications for this technique. However, there are contraindications for the MBTI program. Individuals with a current psychiatric diagnosis of major depressive disorder, bipolar disorder, psychotic disorder, post-traumatic stress disorder, and substance abuse or dependence are not appropriate candidates for MBTI because these conditions are likely to interfere with the practice of meditation or participation in the group, or the underlying psychiatric condition could be exacerbated by engaging in meditation.

RATIONALE FOR INTERVENTION

A disorder of insomnia is defined by the presence of disturbed sleep and associated distress or impairment of function [1,2]. Current pharmacological and psychological treatments for insomnia are generally aimed at improving sleep,

Behavioral Treatments for Sleep Disorders. DOI: 10.1016/B978-0-12-381522-4.00014-6

with relatively little direct attention given to the waking symptoms associated with poor sleep. MBTI is a group program that integrates mindfulness principles with behavior therapy for insomnia using experiential and didactic techniques. It is designed to treat the full range of nocturnal and daytime insomnia symptoms by integrating empirically supported behavioral treatments of insomnia (stimulus control, sleep restriction, sleep hygiene) that target sleep disturbance with mindfulness-based techniques that target the emotional distress that is characteristic of the waking symptoms. The mindfulness principles are cultivated through meditation practices and mindfulness exercises, based on the Mindfulness-Based Stress Reduction Program (MBSR) [3,4] and the Mindfulness-Based Cognitive Therapy (MBCT) for depression program [5]. The behavioral components of MBTI include stimulus control [6], sleep restriction [7], and sleep hygiene [8], delivered within a mindfulness-based framework. The overall goal of the MBTI program is to reduce unwanted wakefulness at night and manage negative emotional reactions to disturbed sleep. The MBTI program is delivered in groups of six to eight participants and consists of eight weekly 2-hour sessions plus one all-day retreat.

The step-by-step procedures below demonstrate how two specific mindfulness principles, acceptance and letting go, can be utilized to help patients work with negative emotional reactions in response to disturbed sleep. These principles, which are practiced during formal meditations, help guide the individual to recognize his or her attachment to rigid beliefs and expectations about sleep and daytime functioning, and then develop a flexible approach to the process of sleep. Adopting an accepting stance is hypothesized to reduce sleep-related arousal and distress.

STEP BY STEP DESCRIPTION OF PROCEDURES

In the MBTI program, each session begins with a period of formal mindfulness meditation, followed by a period of didactics and group dialogue, which is used to teach the principles of mindfulness (see Table 14.1), discuss the meditation practice, and explain the connection between mindfulness and insomnia. A patient-centered approach is used, allowing group participants to discover thoughts and feelings that arise during the implementation of the behavioral components (e.g., stimulus control) and the meditation practice. A point of emphasis in MBTI is using the principles of acceptance and letting go to work with negative emotional reactions to disturbed sleep. Below are sample dialogues demonstrating how these two principles are discussed and applied to sleep disturbance in the MBTI program.

There are three key points to emphasize in these discussions:

1. Not getting ideal sleep does not have to be a burden or another task on the list of things to fix.
2. Acceptance and letting go are not passive; rather, they involve actively choosing to take a non-reactive stance.

TABLE 14.1 Applying Mindfulness Principles to Sleep

In the spirit of cultivating mindfulness, this program will help guide your personal inquiry into your own sleep needs and the optimal state of mind for initiation of sleep (at the beginning or middle of the night). In doing so, bring attention to changing your *relationship* to sleep rather than to the amount of sleep you get each night. As you begin to change this relationship, you might notice an improvement in the quality of your sleep. Later, you will likely see an increase in the amount of sleep you get. This approach requires discipline and consistency but follows the principles of mindfulness discussed in this program.

Beginner's Mind: Remember that each night is a new night. Be open and try something different! What you have been doing to this point is probably not working well.
Non-striving: Sleep is a process that cannot be forced, but instead should be allowed to unfold. Putting more effort into sleeping longer or better is counterproductive.
Letting go: Attachment to sleep or your ideal sleep needs usually leads to worry about the consequences of sleeplessness. This is counterproductive and inconsistent with the natural process of letting go of the day to allow sleep to come.
Non-judging: It is easy to automatically judge the state of being awake as negative and aversive, especially if you do not sleep well for several nights. However, this negative energy can interfere with the process of sleep. One's relationship to sleep can be a fruitful subject of meditation.
Acceptance: Recognizing and accepting your current state is an important first step in choosing how to respond. If you can accept that you are not in a state of sleepiness and sleep is not likely to come soon, why not get out of bed? Many people who have trouble sleeping avoid getting out of bed. Unfortunately, spending long periods of time awake in bed might condition you to being awake in bed.
Trust: Trust your sleep system and let it work for you! Trust that your mind and body can self regulate and self correct for sleep loss. Knowing that short consolidated sleep often feels more satisfying than longer fragmented sleep can help you develop trust in your sleep system. Also, sleep debt can promote good sleep as long as it is not associated with increased effort to sleep.
Patience: Be patient! It is unlikely that both the quality and quantity of your sleep will be optimal right away.

These are just some ways that the mindfulness principles are related to sleep. You might discover other connections between these principles and the process of going to sleep or falling back asleep. We encourage you to explore this for yourself and share your experience throughout this program.

3. The principles of mindfulness, along with the meditation practice, promote a more flexible way to look at sleep and work with sleep disturbance.

Letting Go

Therapist: Many people have expectations about how much sleep they need. However, when we become attached to the idea that we need to be asleep at a specific time or that we need a certain amount of sleep every night, we can become inflexible and anxious about how we sleep. This is counterproductive, and can maintain the cycle of insomnia.

Patient: I have been practicing my meditation and sometimes it helps me to relax, but what should I do when meditation does not help me sleep better at night?

Therapist: Mindfulness meditation is not another form of relaxation. It is the practice of paying attention without engaging. When you find yourself awake at night, allow yourself to let go of the notion that you need to do something about it. Remember that sleep naturally unfolds when we allow ourselves to let go of conscious activities, including deliberate efforts to make it happen. We have been practicing letting go in the formal meditations throughout the program. For example, during the body scan meditation we bring attention to each area of the body and then let go of that area, shifting our attention to the next body area. We allow our attention to move to another area without judging or becoming engaged in problem-solving of how to relieve tension in the previous area. Another example is how we have been paying attention to the breath. With each exhalation, we let go of that breath and move to the next.

Patient: I have tried to push away my thoughts at night and clear my mind, but they keep coming back. Letting go doesn't seem to be working for me.

Therapist: Remember, letting go is different than clearing your mind or forcing thoughts to go away. How many of you have tried pushing your thoughts away, only to find that the thoughts keep coming back? Instead, letting go is a way to allow thoughts to be as they are and to allow them to run their course. You might find that if you let these thoughts come in and out of your conscious awareness without getting engaged in them, they will eventually subside. It's a very different and counterintuitive way to approach thoughts that you wished you did not have!

Acceptance

Therapist: Accepting that sleep may not happen exactly when we want or for as long as we would like is another key to breaking the cycle of insomnia. It might seem reasonable to expect that we will meet our ideal sleep needs each night. Yet in modern society we often fall short of this ideal. As you have likely noticed, our brain is quite a resilient organ and it works even under less than optimal conditions, including when we have been sleeping very little. Accepting that sleep cannot be forced means that it is futile to put much mental effort into sleeping. Instead, when we cannot sleep at a given moment at night we can view it as a sign that our minds or bodies are not yet ready for sleep at this moment. Accepting that struggling with sleep is counterproductive means we might just as well get out of bed. Has anyone found that continuing to struggle with sleep makes the time you spend awake in bed rather unpleasant? Have you considered the possibility that this struggle and frustration could make it even more difficult to sleep?

Patient: But how can acceptance of a problem be helpful?

Therapist: By cultivating acceptance, we can step out of our automatic reactions and increase the range of responses to the problem. For example, acceptance is helpful for people who experience chronic anxiety and worry. Researchers have found that non-acceptance, putting things off, and avoidance of the problem tends to "fuel" anxiety rather than relieve it. It seems that worry serves the purpose of "giving the mind something to do" so it does not have to face the real problem. A worried response to a stressful challenge tends to make people more rigid in their reactions to stress. In fact, one of the most effective strategies for helping people with phobias and serious anxiety issues is exposure to the feared stimulus. For example, an individual with a phobia of bridges can benefit from gradual exposure to being on a bridge (e.g., starting with a picture of bridge, then going on a small bridge, then on a larger bridge), whereas avoiding bridges generally reinforces the anxious response. Perhaps when you accept that you may or may not fall asleep easily on a given night, you will be approaching bedtime with less apprehension. As your apprehension about sleep creates tension that is likely to interfere with sleep, decreasing this apprehension will likely result in shorter time to fall asleep.

Has anyone ever thought about what people with insomnia avoid? People with insomnia usually try very hard to avoid sleep deprivation or being in a state of fatigue. However, trying to avoid this by going to bed is not likely to help you sleep better. You might learn that you do not have to be afraid of sleep deprivation, and that acceptance of a little bit of sleep deprivation can even help you sleep better!

Patient: But isn't acceptance or letting go kind of like giving up hope or being passive?

Therapist: It is actually quite the opposite! Rather than giving up, you are making a conscious decision to accept or embrace what is happening. You are choosing to actively respond by allowing or letting the feeling or experience be, rather than automatically avoiding, fixing, or changing the unpleasant feeling or experience. By doing so, you might even find that the experience changes – that the negative emotions really were not as bad as you thought. Or, you might find that an alternative solution is possible when previously you thought there was no way out. The key point is that it is not always helpful to try to fix or solve things. Acceptance provides another way to relate to the problem. It often leads to a deeper understanding of the problem and allows creative solutions to emerge.

Patient: So just accepting that I am not getting the sleep I need right now is going to help me sleep better in the future?

Therapist: Remember, letting go and acceptance are only two of the principles of mindfulness. Other principles, such as non-judging and beginner's mind, are also important. See what happens if you are able to accept that sleep at this moment is not happening without judging what might happen to you tomorrow or the next night. Perhaps you will still be able to function the following day. See if you are able to approach each night with a beginner's mind (i.e., "this is a new night and it doesn't matter what happened the night before and it won't help to worry about what I have to do tomorrow"). Over time, this shift in attitude might give your brain and body a chance to self-regulate. Rather than using acceptance and letting go as techniques intended to help you sleep better, why not pay attention to what is going on for you at this moment and see what your mind and body are telling you?

Overall Discussion

Following a discussion of these two principles, it is helpful to reinforce how taking a mindfulness approach allows us to examine whether or not we always have to move away from negative experience. The therapist might discuss any observations from patients about acceptance or the ability to let go. Questions that might be raised for discussion include:

1. Is being awake when we don't want to always a bad thing?
2. Are there ways to be more flexible in responding to wakefulness?
3. In what other situations might it be helpful to use acceptance and letting go?
4. Can you practice these principles in your own meditation practice?

POSSIBLE MODIFICATIONS/VARIANTS

In addition to the principles of acceptance and letting go, other principles of mindfulness (see Table 14.1) can be used to work with the emotional reactivity that arises during the course of chronic insomnia. For example, the principle of beginner's mind can be used to teach participants how to approach each night as an independent event, avoiding the temptation of making changes to their sleep-related behavior based upon contingencies from the day or previous night (such as, "Last night was bad so I need to make sure I am going to get more sleep tonight"). More broadly, meditations can be used to bring awareness to the mental and physical sensations that differentiate sleepiness and fatigue. Upon learning how to identify the sensations associated with the state of sleepiness, participants can be instructed on how to use sleepiness as a guide for when to go to bed when following instructions for stimulus control or sleep restriction.

PROOF OF CONCEPT/SUPPORTING DATA/EVIDENCE BASE

There is general support for the efficacy of mindfulness-based programs as applied to psychiatric illness and coping with chronic medical illness. The MBSR program has been used in the treatment of a variety of disorders, including chronic pain, generalized anxiety disorder, fibromyalgia, psoriasis, cancer, and depression. Significant reductions in self-reported cognitive and somatic anxiety have been found following MBSR, with one study [9] reporting a medium effect size ($d = 0.50$) for pre- to post-treatment effects on mental health variables (e.g., anxiety, depression severity). In a randomized controlled trial, the MBCT program significantly reduced the risk of relapse/recurrence for patients with three or more previous episodes compared to treatment-as-usual over a 60-week period [10].

Given the effects of MBSR on anxiety and mood-regulation and the potential long-term benefits for preventing relapse as seen in MBCT, a mindfulness-based approach may be successfully applied to the management of chronic insomnia. The principles of mindfulness are theoretically congruent with the Spielman model of chronic insomnia [11], and appear to complement the behavioral therapies for insomnia. Also, the patient-centered approach and use of meditations as experiential learning tools might be more appealing to patients than the didactic approaches used in other behavioral interventions for insomnia.

To date, only a limited number of studies have been conducted on using mindfulness meditation for patients with insomnia. Preliminary work on an early version of MBTI has yielded promising results supporting the use of this intervention for primary insomnia. An open-label pilot study [12] evaluated a 6-week version of the MBTI program on a sample of 30 participants with psychophysiological insomnia. The intervention was found to be feasible to deliver and credible to insomnia patients. Significant pre- to post-treatment effects with moderate to large effect sizes were found on several nocturnal symptoms, including decreased total wake time ($d = -1.17$), fewer awakenings ($d = -0.61$), higher sleep efficiency ($d = 1.13$), and lower scores on the Insomnia Severity Index ($d = -1.32$). Half of the participants experienced a 50 percent or greater reduction in total wake time (TWT), and all but two participants scored below the cut-off for clinically significant insomnia on the ISI. In addition, the program resulted in significant reductions in pre-sleep arousal ($d = -1.00$), sleep effort ($d = -0.96$), and dysfunctional sleep-related cognitions ($d = -1.05$). Follow-up data revealed that the acute treatment gains achieved at the end of treatment were maintained at 6 and 12 months post-treatment, and 61 percent of participants had no relapse of insomnia during the 12 months following treatment [13].

Although these studies were not able to specify the efficacy of the mindfulness meditation component, preliminary data suggest a relationship between mindfulness meditation and insomnia symptoms. A significant negative correlation was found between total number of meditation sessions during the MBTI program and change in trait hyperarousal, suggesting that more meditation practice is related to greater decrease in arousal [12]. Also, a significant negative correlation was found between scores on a measure of mindfulness skills and daytime sleepiness, raising the possibility that mindfulness skills might improve daytime functioning [13]. Studies have also examined the impact of MBSR on sleep in cancer patients. Carlson and colleagues [14] reported pre- to post-treatment improvements in sleep quality and total sleep time in a sample of cancer patients. Shapiro and colleagues [15] investigated the impact of MBSR on sleep among women with breast cancer and found no differences between the MBSR and the control group on sleep quality and sleep efficiency, but did report a positive relationship between the practice of mindfulness and feeling refreshed after sleep.

REFERENCES

[1] J.D. Edinger, M.H. Bonnet, RR. Bootzin, et al., Derivation of research diagnostic criteria for insomnia: report of an American Academy of Sleep Medicine Work Group, Sleep 27 (8) (2004) 1567–1596.

[2] American Psychiatric Association, The Diagnostic and Statistical Manual of Mental Disorders, fourth ed., APA, Washington, DC, 2000.

[3] J. Kabat-Zinn, Full Catastrophe Living: Using the Wisdom of your Body and Mind to Face Stress, Pain, and Illness, Delacorte Press, New York, NY, 1990.

[4] S. Santoreli, J. Kabat-Zinn, Mindfulness-based Stress Reduction Progressional Training Resource Manual, Center for Mindfulness in Medicine, Health Care, and Society, Worcester, MA, 2004.

[5] Z.V. Segal, J.M.G. Williams, J.D. Teasdale, Mindfulness-based Cognitive Therapy for Depression: A New Approach to Preventing Relapse, Guilford Press, New York, NY, 2002.

[6] R.R. Bootzin, D. Epstein, J.M. Wood, Stimulus control instructions, in: P.J. Hauri, (Ed.), Case Studies in Insomnia, Plenum Press, New York, NY, 1991, pp. 19–28.

[7] A.J. Spielman, P. Saskin, M.J. Thorpy, Treatment of chronic insomnia by restriction of time in bed, Sleep 10 (1) (1987) 45–56.
[8] P.J. Hauri, Current Concepts: The Sleep Disorders, The Upjohn Company, Kalamazoo, MI, 1977.
[9] P. Grossman, L. Niemann, S. Schmidt, et al., Mindfulness-based stress reduction and health benefits. A meta-analysis, J. Psychosom. Res. 57 (1) (2004) 35–43.
[10] J.D. Teasdale, Z.V. Segal, J.M. Williams, et al., Prevention of relapse/recurrence in major depression by mindfulness-based cognitive therapy, J. Consult. Clin. Psychol. 68 (4) (2000) 615–623.
[11] A.J. Spielman, L.S. Caruso, P.B. Glovinsky, A behavioral perspective on insomnia treatment, Psychiatr. Clin. North Am. 10 (4) (1987) 541–553.
[12] J.C. Ong, S.L. Shapiro, R. Manber, Combining mindfulness meditation with cognitive-behavior therapy for insomnia: a treatment-development study, Behav. Ther. 39 (2) (2008) 171–182.
[13] J.C. Ong, S.L. Shapiro, R. Manber, Mindfulness meditation and cognitive behavioral therapy for insomnia: a naturalistic 12-month follow-up, Explore (NY) 5 (1) (2009) 30–36.
[14] L.E. Carlson, S.N. Garland, Impact of mindfulness-based stress reduction (MBSR) on sleep, mood, stress and fatigue symptoms in cancer outpatients, Intl. J. Behav. Med. 12 (4) (2005) 278–285.
[15] S.L. Shapiro, R.R. Bootzin, A.J. Figueredo, et al., The efficacy of mindfulness-based stress reduction in the treatment of sleep disturbance in women with breast cancer: an exploratory study, J. Psychosom. Res. (54) (2003) 85–91.

RECOMMENDED READING

J. Kabat-Zinn, Full Catastrophe Living: Using the Wisdom of your Body and Mind to Face Stress, Pain, and Illness, Delacorte Press, New York, NY, 1990.
J.C. Ong, S.L. Shapiro, R. Manber, Combining mindfulness meditation with cognitive-behavior therapy for insomnia: a treatment-development study, Behav. Ther. 39 (2) (2008) 171–182.
J.C. Ong, S.L. Shapiro, R. Manber, Mindfulness meditation and cognitive behavioral therapy for insomnia: a naturalistic 12-month follow-up, Explore (NY) 5 (1) (2009) 30–36.
Z.V. Segal, J.M.G. Williams, J.D. Teasdale, Mindfulness-based Cognitive Therapy for Depression: A New Approach to Preventing Relapse, Guilford Press, New York, NY, 2002.

Chapter 15

Brief Behavioral Treatment of Insomnia

Anne Germain, Daniel J. Buysse
Department of Psychiatry, University of Pittsburgh School of Medicine, Pittsburgh, PA

PROTOCOL NAME

Brief Behavioral Treatment of Insomnia (BBTI).

GROSS INDICATION

BBTI is indicated for the treatment of insomnia, defined as difficulty falling or staying asleep, early morning awakenings, or complaints of non-restorative sleep, occurring on more days than not over more than a month, and associated with significant distress or functional impairments [1].

SPECIFIC INDICATION

BBTI is indicated for the treatment of primary insomnia, or insomnia comorbid with other psychiatric, medical, or sleep disorders.

CONTRAINDICATIONS

Caution should be exercised in using BBTI with patients with a diagnosis of bipolar disorder or psychotic disorder, as the transient, mild sleep restriction induced by BBTI may exacerbate these conditions. The prescription for time in bed during BBTI with older adults should generally not be less than 6 hours to reduce the risk of falls. Because of the transient sleepiness associated with sleep restriction, caution should also be exercised for patients who operate heavy machinery or drive a car regularly.

RATIONALE FOR INTERVENTION

BBTI is similar to standard cognitive behavioral treatment of insomnia (CBT-I) in combining and emphasizing the early implementation of stimulus control and sleep restriction principles and procedures. These methods have

Behavioral Treatments for Sleep Disorders. DOI: 10.1016/B978-0-12-381522-4.00015-8

been shown to increase sleep consolidation and improve sleep quality [2–5]. Education about healthy sleep practices and behaviors that affect sleep quality and consolidation is also provided to patients in BBTI in a way that is comparable to CBT-I. However, BBTI differs from standard CBT-I in important ways. BBTI uses a reduced number of in-person visits, and a shorter length of the intervention in BBTI (two in-person visits over 4 weeks) compared to CBT-I (six to eight in-person visits over 8 weeks). In addition, BBTI does not systematically address or restructure erroneous beliefs and attitudes about sleep, insomnia, and the potential consequences of poor sleep.

BBTI was developed to address common barriers encountered in the dissemination of evidence-based CBT-I. The first barrier relates to difficulties in implementing CBT-I in the clinical settings where the majority of patients with insomnia complaints seek care (e.g., primary care clinics). CBT-I requires weekly visits over a period of 8 weeks. BBTI, with two in-person visits over a period of 4 weeks, offers a potentially more feasible format in this setting. A second barrier relates to the provider offering CBT-I. CBT-I is typically delivered by a PhD-level clinician, with extensive training in behavioral sleep medicine. Sleep specialists are rarely available in primary care settings, where the majority of patients seek care, and there is evidence that Master's-level clinicians (nurses, social workers) can effectively deliver a primary intervention for insomnia in these settings. For instance, primary care clinic nurses can effectively deliver behavioral interventions for insomnia with minimal supervision in a small-group format [2]. BBTI may offer a first-line intervention for a majority of patients seen in primary care settings, whereas CBT-I may be best for patients who require a higher "dose" of treatment, delivered in a specialty care clinic.

The general rationale for BBTI is that modifying waking behaviors can directly impact the two major physiological mechanisms that regulate sleep: the homeostatic and circadian drives (Figure 15.1). The homeostatic sleep drive refers to the increased propensity for sleep with increasing duration of wakefulness (Figure 15.1a). The circadian drive refers to the variations in brain and body biological processes that are regulated by the central pacemaker, also known as the biological clock. The circadian drive promotes or inhibits the propensity to remain alert and/or fall and stay asleep throughout the 24-hour cycle. In humans, sleep is promoted during darkness and is coincident with the peak of melatonin release from the pineal gland, and the nadir of core body temperature and cortisol secretion (Figure 15.1b). When individuals sleep at a suboptimal circadian time, as is the case with delayed sleep phase syndrome or shift work, sleep is perceived to be of poorer quality, lighter, and more disrupted. The goal of BBTI is to modify waking behaviors that increase and regulate the duration of wakefulness (homeostatic drive), and identify an individualized prescription for sleep and wake time that is consistent with the circadian process. Aligning the homeostatic and circadian drives (as indicated by the gray arrows in Figure 15.1) by changing waking behaviors, then,

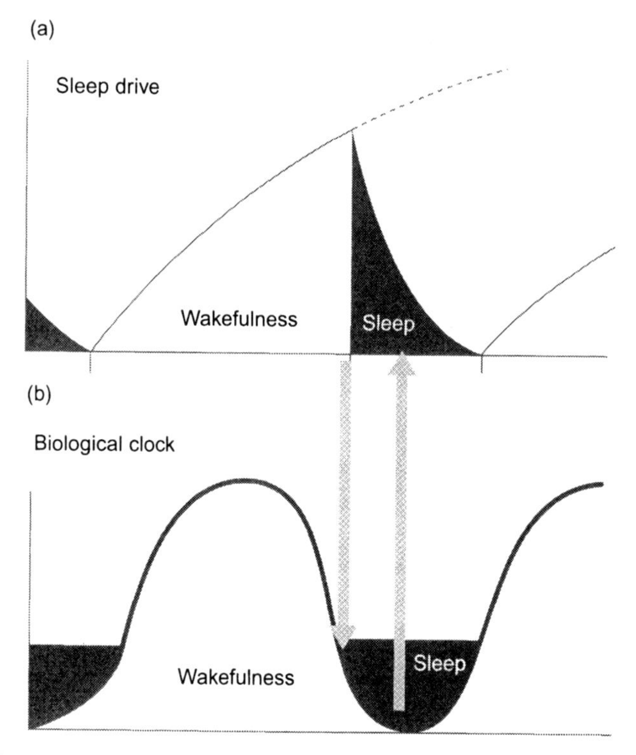

FIGURE 15.1 The two-process model of sleep regulation.

facilitates sleep onset, enhances sleep consolidation, and promotes restorative sleep and daytime alertness.

The core components of BBTI are principles of stimulus control [6] and sleep restriction [3]. Stimulus control aims at limiting the use of the sleep environment (bed, bedroom) to sleep. Sleep restriction involves the implementation of a regular sleep–wake schedule, which limits time spent in bed in order to promote sleep consolidation. Together, stimulus control and sleep restriction enhance the two major physiological processes that control sleep, thereby aligning the timing and duration of sleep. Several meta-analyses have demonstrated the efficacy and durability of these behavioral interventions for primary insomnia and comorbid insomnia (see, for example, Morin et al. [4] and Smith et al. [5]). Specifically, stimulus control and sleep restriction are associated with significant improvements in sleep latency, sleep duration, and sleep efficiency (ratio of time spent asleep/time spent in bed while awake or asleep), as well as with improvements in daytime symptoms and functioning. Thus, BBTI combines these two evidence-based techniques to reduce insomnia.

STEP BY STEP DESCRIPTION OF PROCEDURES

BBTI is a manualized intervention delivered over four consecutive weeks, which includes two individual in-person visits on Weeks 1 and 3, and telephone appointments on Weeks 2 and 4. The duration of the first treatment visit is 45 minutes, and the follow-up visit on Week 3 generally lasts no more than 30 minutes. Brief (<20 minutes) telephone sessions are conducted on Weeks 2 and 4 to address any questions or difficulties that may have arisen in the previous weeks, to encourage adherence to the prescribed sleep schedule, or to modify the prescribed sleep schedule if necessary.

The first session aims at providing accurate and concise background information about mechanisms of sleep regulation (i.e., homeostatic and circadian drives), and general information about behaviors that promote or interfere with sleep. This component provides the rationale for both stimulus control and sleep restriction. To reduce sleep-related insomnia symptoms (i.e., difficulty falling and staying asleep), stimulus control instructions and sleep restriction are then implemented. Stimulus control instructions involve limiting the bed and the sleep environment to sleep (and sexual activity). The rationale is that the timing of sleep is a learned behavior contingent upon the environment. Activities other than sleep and sexual activity, such as watching television, reading, and worrying, are prohibited in the bed and bedroom, and must be performed in other rooms. Access to the bed and the bedroom are allowed only when the person feels sleepy. When the patient awakens during the night and cannot return to sleep, the patient is instructed to leave the bed, and to perform pre-determined activities involving minimal stimulation and minimal light levels to foster sleepiness. Strict adherence to the prescribed rise time is strongly reinforced during this session. Light exposure in the morning has an important role in triggering wake signals for the biological clock.

Sleep restriction aims at limiting the number of hours in bed to match the actual number of hours spent asleep, plus 30 minutes to allow for normal time to fall asleep and nocturnal awakenings. Sleep restriction improves sleep efficiency, or the ratio of total number of hours of sleep to number of hours spent in bed. Sleep restriction is usually associated with mild sleep deprivation, which favors increased homeostatic drive, and sleep consolidation. Ideally, the prescribed sleep–wake schedule is derived from sleep diary data collected over the previous 7–14 days. In the absence of a sleep diary, retrospective estimates of recent sleep–wake patterns can be used. First selecting the rise time with the patient and then working backwards to establish bedtime is helpful. The prescribed sleep–wake schedule, as well as the list of activities identified for occupying evening, middle of the night, and morning wakefulness should also be realistic, and accommodate the patient's living conditions and responsibilities.

The first session also includes a focus on identifying activities to be performed in the morning to enhance the patient's ability to get out of bed, and adhere to the prescribed sleep–wake schedule. The temporary nature of the prescribed sleep schedule is also highlighted. Time allowed in bed can be increased over time, when sleep latency and wake time after sleep onset are less than 30 minutes per night, on most nights.

At the end of the first session, the patient receives the prescribed sleep–wake goals, and the list of selected activities to be performed out of bed when awake. Patients should also receive a sleep diary to monitor improvements in sleep, as well as to monitor adherence to the prescribed schedule.

As mentioned above, a brief follow-up telephone call is completed on Week 2 to address any questions or difficulties that may have arisen in the previous weeks, to encourage adherence to the prescribed sleep schedule, or to modify the prescribed sleep schedule if necessary.

Week 3 is an in-person visit, and serves three main purposes: (1) to address possible difficulties regarding the application of the techniques encountered during the previous week; (2) to continue close monitoring of and reinforce adherence to treatment recommendations; and (3) to provide education on how to expand time allowed in bed. Specifically, increasing time spent in bed is allowed if sleep latency and wake time after sleep onset are less than 30 minutes on most nights, based on prospective information collected with sleep diaries. The number of hours allowed in bed can then be increased by 15 minutes (by advancing bedtime or delaying rise time), and the patient is instructed to maintain the new time in bed for 1 week. If sleep latency and wake time after sleep onset (WASO) both remain below 30 minutes on most nights, then the patient is allowed to add another additional 15 minutes in bed for a week. On the other hand, if sleep latency and WASO exceed 30 minutes, then the patient is instructed to decrease time in bed by 15 minutes. In BBTI, modification to the time allowed in bed is thus determined by maintaining sleep latency and wake time after sleep onset below the clinical thresholds of 30 minutes, rather than based on sleep efficiency ≥85 percent.

On Week 4, another follow-up phone call is conducted to address any difficulties, monitor adherence, and further increase time in bed if sleep remains consolidated, but daytime sleepiness is present. A final, brief in-person visit is then scheduled after 1 or 2 weeks to review progress, to review the rationale of BBTI and the instructions for stimulus control and sleep restriction, and to review the instructions for lengthening or shortening time spent in bed.

POSSIBLE MODIFICATIONS/VARIANTS

Variants of BBTI include in-person visits rather than telephone contacts on weeks 2 and 4, and providing audiocassettes containing sleep education [7] at the end of treatment sessions. Alternative modes of BBTI delivery, such as self help, instructions delivered by mail, web-based or telephone-based delivery methods, have not yet been tested. BBTI can be used concomitantly with sleep medications if the use of hypnotics is not associated with full remission of sleep-related insomnia symptoms.

PROOF OF CONCEPT/SUPPORTING DATA/EVIDENCE BASE

There is growing evidence that BBTI and related brief therapies are associated with rapid (<4 weeks) improvements in sleep latency, wake time after sleep onset (WASO), sleep efficiency, and overall sleep quality, including reduced severity of insomnia and remission of insomnia. One trial assessed the effects of a brief behavioral intervention combining education, stimulus control, and sleep restrictions, and delivered over two 25-minute sessions delivered 2 weeks apart by a junior-level clinical psychologist, compared to a sleep hygiene education intervention equated for time spent with the therapist and on homework assignments [7]. Post-treatment assessments were conducted 2 weeks and 3 months after the end of treatment, using sleep logs and self-report questionnaires. Improvements in sleep log measures of sleep latency, WASO, and sleep efficiency were greater in the intervention group than in the control group. Furthermore, the magnitude of the improvements observed in the intervention group was similar to the improvement previously observed in the randomized clinical trial with CBT-I.

A preliminary report on an ongoing clinical trial conducted by an independent group corroborated clinically meaningful improvements in self-report and sleep log measures in older adults (age <60 years old) who received BBTI, compared to an information control (IC) condition. Post-treatment, participants who received BBTI showed clinically meaningful improvements in global self-report and sleep diary measures of sleep latency, WASO, and sleep efficiency, as well as improvements in daytime symptoms of depression and anxiety, compared to participants assigned to an information control (IC) condition. In the BBTI group, effect sizes for sleep latency (d = 0.80), WASO (d = 0.67), and sleep efficiency (d = 0.64) were comparable to those reported in CBT-I trials. Seventy-one percent of the BBTI participants and 39 percent of the IC participants met criteria for treatment response, as defined by a reduction of ≥3 points on the Pittsburgh Sleep Quality Index (PSQI; [8]), or an increase in sleep efficiency of ≥10 percent. Remission was defined as meeting response criteria, and having a PSQI score of 5 or less or sleep efficiency greater than 85 percent after treatment. Remission was observed in 53 percent of the BBTI criteria, and 17 percent of the IC participants. Preliminary analyses of follow-up data suggest that these improvements are maintained over 6 months [9]. A final report on this clinical trial, with a total of 79 older adults, is in preparation.

Another study investigated the optimal number of treatment sessions in adults with primary sleep maintenance insomnia, by randomizing participants to one, two, four, or eight individual sessions that were delivered over the course of 8 weeks, or to a wait-list control condition. All active treatment conditions involved a first session where education and specific instructions on stimulus control and sleep restriction were delivered. For groups involving more than treatment session, additional sessions consisted of review of the material provided in the first session, adherence reinforcement, and guidance on how to adjust time allowed in bed. Results indicated that one and four individual sessions delivered over the 8-week period showed significant improvements in diary and actigraphic measures of sleep efficiency, WASO, total wake time (WASO + sleep latency), and a greater rate of treatment response than the other conditions. Objective improvements in wake time and sleep efficiency were maintained in the four-session group. The authors suggested that the four-session intervention delivered biweekly may optimize the balance between patients' engagement in treatment and therapist's guidance.

PROOF OF CONCEPT/SUPPORTING DATA/EVIDENCE BASE

There is growing evidence supporting the efficacy of brief behavioral treatments, including BBTI, for primary and comorbid insomnia. A transient increase in daytime sleepiness is the main side effect reported and expected, given the mild sleep deprivation associated with sleep restriction. Improvements in sleep latency, WASO, sleep efficiency, and overall sleep quality are also associated with reductions in daytime symptoms of depression and anxiety.

REFERENCES

[1] American Academy of Sleep Medicine, P.J. Hauri, M.J. Sateia, The International Classification of Sleep Disorders, Second Edition (ICSD-2): Diagnostic and Coding Manual, American Academy of Sleep Medicine, Westchester, IL, 2005.

[2] C.A. Espie, K.M.A. MacMahon, H.L. Kelly, et al., Randomized clinical effectiveness trial of nurse-administered small-group cognitive behavior therapy for persistent insomnia in general practice, Sleep 30 (5) (2007) 574–584.

[3] A.J. Spielman, P. Saskin, M.J. Thorpy, Treatment of chronic insomnia by restriction of time in bed, Sleep 10 (1) (1987) 45–56.

[4] C.M. Morin, J.P. Culbert, S.M. Schwartz, Nonpharmacological interventions for insomnia: a meta-analysis of treatment efficacy, Am. J. Psychiatry 151 (8) (1994) 1172–1180.

[5] M.T. Smith, M.L. Perlis, A. Park, Comparative meta-analysis of pharmacotherapy and behavior therapy for persistent insomnia, Am. J. Psychiatry 159 (1) (2002) 5–11.

[6] R.R. Bootzin, P.M. Nicassio, Behavioral treatments of insomnia, in: M. Hersen, R.E. Eisler, P.M. Miller, (Eds.), Progress in Behavior Modification, Academic Press, New York, NY, 1978, pp. 1–45.

[7] J.D. Edinger, W.S. Sampson, A primary care "friendly" cognitive behavioral insomnia therapy, Sleep 26 (2) (2003) 177–182.

[8] D.J. Buysse, C.F. Reynolds, III, T.H. Monk, et al., The Pittsburgh Sleep Quality Index: a new instrument for psychiatric practice and research, Psychiatry Res. 28 (2) (1989) 193–213.

[9] A. Germain, D.E. Moul, P.L. Franzen, et al., Effects of a brief behavioral treatment for late-life insomnia:Preliminary findings, J. Clin. Sleep Med. 2 (4) (2006) 403–406.

RECOMMENDED READING

R.R. Bootzin, P.M. Nicassio, Behavioral treatments of insomnia, in: M. Hersen, R.E. Eisler, P.M. Miller (Eds.), Progress in Behavior Modification, vol. 6, Academic Press, New York, NY, 1978, pp. 1–45.

J.D. Edinger, W.S. Sampson, A primary care "friendly" cognitive behavior insomnia therapy, Sleep 26 (2003) 177–182.

J.D. Edinger, W.K. Wohlgemuth, R.A. Radtke, et al., Dose–response effects of cognitive-behavioral insomnia therapy: a randomized clinical trial, Sleep 30 (2) (2007) 203–212.

C.A. Espie, S.J. Inglis, S. Tessier, L. Harvey, The clinical effectiveness of cognitive behaviour therapy for chronic insomnia: Implementation and evaluation of a sleep clinic in general medical practice, Behav. Res. Ther. 39 (2001) 60.

A. Germain, D.E. Moul, P.L. Franzen, et al., Effects of a brief behavioral treatment for late-life insomnia: preliminary findings, J. Clin. Sleep Med. 2 (2006) 407–408.

A.J. Spielman, P. Saskin, M.J. Thorpy, Treatment of chronic insomnia by restriction of time in bed, Sleep 10 (1987) 45–56.

Chapter 16

Using Bright Light and Melatonin to Reduce Jet Lag

Helen J. Burgess
Biological Rhythms Research Laboratory, Rush University Medical Center, Chicago, IL

PROTOCOL NAME

Using bright light and melatonin to reduce jet lag.

GROSS INDICATION

This is generally applicable to phase shifting the circadian clock in patients with circadian rhythm sleep disorders or winter depression.

SPECIFIC INDICATION

Bright light and melatonin can be used to reduce jet lag after crossing at least two time zones east or west.

CONTRAINDICATIONS

Bright light should probably not be used in:

- people with existing eye disease;
- people using photosensitizing medications.

Bright light can induce:

- migraines (in about one-third of migraine sufferers);
- mania (rare).

Melatonin should probably not be used in:

- people who are driving or operating heavy machinery (unless they have previously tested their response to melatonin and are taking <0.5 mg of melatonin);
- pregnant or nursing women (melatonin will transfer to the fetus/infant);
- women seeking to become pregnant;

Behavioral Treatments for Sleep Disorders. DOI: 10.1016/B978-0-12-381522-4.00016-X

- children (unless they suffer from a neurodevelopmental condition associated with extremely poor sleep);
- asthmatics and patients with gastrointestinal disease (melatonin may be inflammatory);
- patients using other medications (unless supervised by a physician).

RATIONALE FOR INTERVENTION

Rapid jet travel across multiple time zones produces a temporary misalignment between the timing of the central circadian clock and the desired sleep times in the new time zone. This circadian misalignment often leads to nighttime insomnia (early insomnia after flying east, late insomnia after flying west), daytime sleepiness, worsened mood, and gastrointestinal disturbances. Bright light and melatonin can be used to accelerate the shifting of the circadian clock such that the circadian misalignment is minimized and the severity and duration of jet lag are reduced.

STEP BY STEP DESCRIPTION OF PROCEDURES

Jet lag can be minimized with some preflight planning.

The first step is to estimate the timing of the minimum of your core body temperature rhythm ("T_{min}"). A general rule of thumb is that it occurs 3 hours before your habitual wake-up time [1].

The second step is to determine your flight schedule, including stopovers, direction of travel, when you would like to sleep at your destination, the time difference between home and your destination, and sunrise and sunset times at your destination (www.timeanddate.com is a useful website). When flying west, the circadian clock needs to shift later in time ("phase delay") to adjust to the new time zone. In general, when flying east the circadian clock needs to shift earlier in time ("phase advance") to adjust to the new time zone. However, eastward jet travel across eight or more time zones can be difficult to adjust to [2,3], and in this case the circadian clock will often phase delay.

The third step is to determine when to seek light and to avoid light to accelerate the shifting of your circadian clock. To phase delay, you need to seek light in at least the 4 hours before your T_{min} and avoid light in at least the 4 hours after your T_{min} [4]. To phase advance, you need to avoid light in at least the 4 hours before your T_{min} and seek light in at least the 4 hours after your T_{min} [4]. You can seek light by staying awake, by going outdoors and not wearing sunglasses, or by using a commercially available portable light box. You can avoid light by sleeping in a dark bedroom, staying indoors away from windows, wearing orange "blue blockers" glasses when inside, and wearing very dark sunglasses if you must go outside.

Studies of jet travelers who did not regulate their light exposure indicate people can phase delay up to 1.5 hours per day and phase advance up to 1 hour per day [2,3,5]. The more successful you are at seeking and avoiding light at the correct times, the more likely you will be able to phase delay about 2 hours per day and phase advance about 1.5 hours per day. Your success depends on having a flexible schedule, and, if you do not have a portable light box, good weather and reasonable temperatures that permit you to stay outside and receive light at the required times.

The fourth step is to consider if your schedule (including the required wake-up time to catch your flight) permits gradually shifting your sleep in the direction of travel in the days *before* your departure. This approach shifts your sleep and circadian clock together, and so does not produce circadian misalignment and jet lag [6,7]. Instead it reduces how much your circadian clock needs to shift on arrival, thereby reducing your jet lag. Preflight shifts are particularly beneficial for people traveling east, as preflight shifts increase your chances of getting bright light at the correct time on arrival, further facilitating phase advances. If you are traveling east, you will need to shift your habitual bed and wake times 1 hour earlier per day and maximize your bright light exposure in the first 3–4 hours after you wake up each morning. If you are traveling west, you will need to shift your habitual bed and wake times 1 hour later per day and maximize your bright light exposure in the 3–4 hours before your bedtime each night. Such a preflight regimen can phase advance the circadian clock 30–45 minutes per day [6], and phase delay the circadian clock by about 1 hour per day [8].

The fifth step is to consider taking melatonin to enhance your phase shifts to bright light. Phase advances in response to bright light can be further increased to about 1 hour per day if you take 0.5 mg of melatonin 10 hours before your T_{min} [7]. It is not yet known if phase delays in response to bright light can be further increased with melatonin.

The sixth step is to draw your jet lag plan containing all of the above elements. The jet lag plan should guide you on when to seek and avoid light, and can be stopped once you are sleeping well at night and performing well during the day in the new time zone.

Figures 16.1–16.3 display some examples of jet lag plans for a nonstop Los Angeles to Paris return flight. Los Angeles to Paris is an eastward flight across nine time zones. Such eastward flights are particularly difficult to adjust to, and phase delays often result.

Figure 16.1 shows a traveler, who normally sleeps 11 pm to 7 am in Los Angeles (T_{min} at 4 am) arriving in Paris without a preflight shift. As this traveler arrives in Paris in the early morning and moves through immigration, baggage claim and customs, and transits to her hotel, she is likely to receive significant bright light exposure immediately before her T_{min}. As phase advancing in these circumstances will be extremely difficult, this traveler instead plans to use this light exposure to help her phase delay. Even if she seeks and avoids light at the correct times, she is still likely to experience jet lag for 6–7 days, until her T_{min} falls into her desired sleep times.

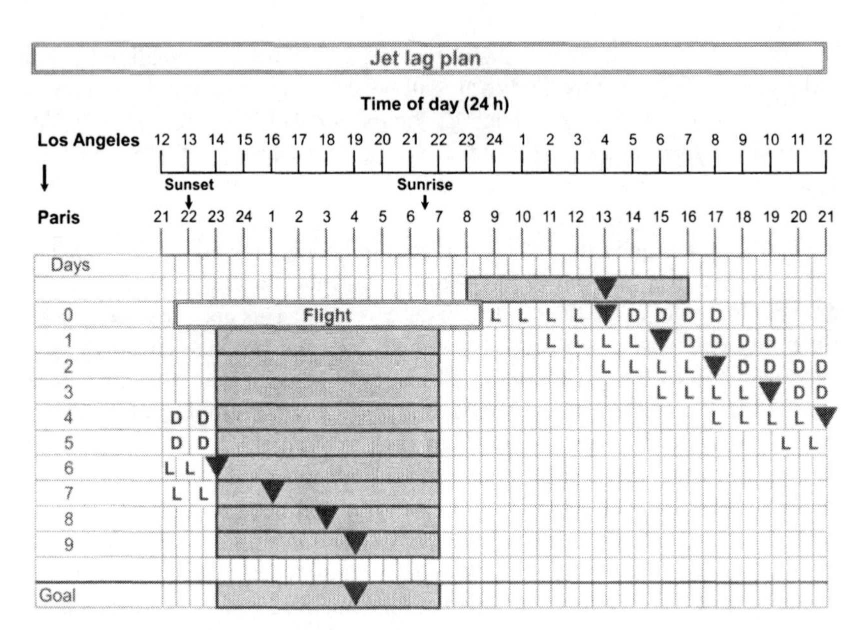

FIGURE 16.1 A jet-lag plan for a traveler who travels non-stop from Los Angeles to Paris with no preflight shift. The triangle represents the minimum of her core body temperature rhythm, T_{min}. L = when to seek light, D = when to seek dark.

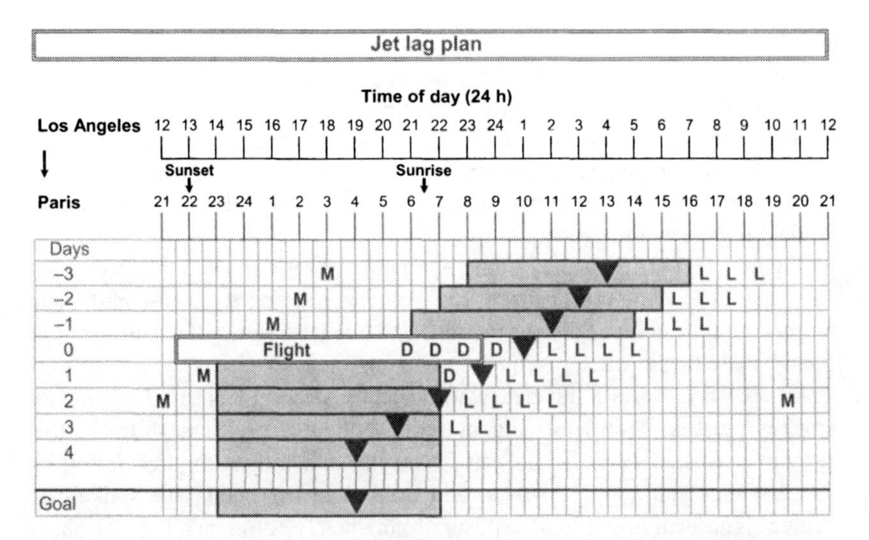

FIGURE 16.2 A jet-lag plan for a traveler who travels non-stop from Los Angeles to Paris with a 3-day preflight shift. The triangle represents the minimum of her core body temperature rhythm, T_{min}. L = when to seek light, D = when to seek dark, M = time to take 0.5 mg melatonin.

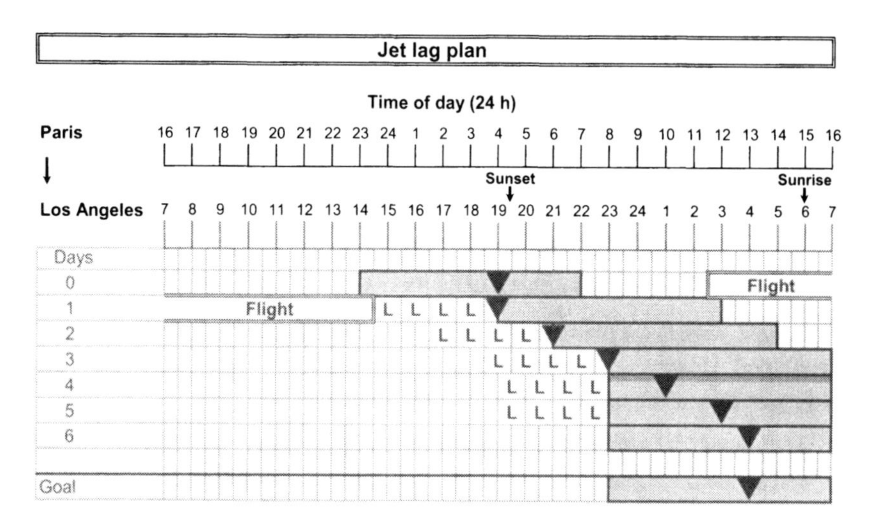

FIGURE 16.3 A jet-lag plan for a traveler who travels non-stop from Paris to Los Angeles with no preflight shift. The triangle represents the minimum of her core body temperature rhythm, T_{min}. L = when to seek light, D = when to seek dark.

Figure 16.2 shows the same traveler arrive in Paris after a 3-day preflight shift. In this case, the time interval during which she must avoid light after arrival in Paris is 3 hours shorter and she anticipates that by the time she transits to her hotel it will be time to seek light. After a quick shower, she sits outside with her laptop or good book to ensure she gets plenty of bright light. With this plan, she should experience jet lag for 3–4 days.

Figure 16.3 shows her return flight. This time, light exposure on her arrival in Los Angeles is beneficial and she has a flexible schedule such that at 7 pm she goes to sleep in a dark bedroom to ensure she avoids light after her T_{min}. With this strategy, she will likely experience jet lag for 3–4 days.

POSSIBLE MODIFICATIONS/VARIANTS

Jet lag will often worsen as we age. While older people can still phase shift as effectively to bright light as younger people [9], older people are more sensitive to circadian misalignment [10].

Morning types typically have earlier T_{min}s [11], and so may adjust better than most to eastward flights. Evening types typically have later T_{min}s [11], and so may adjust better than most to westward flights.

Commercially available light boxes vary in their size, portability, and wavelength. Generally, larger light boxes, which cover more of the visual field, are less aversive, but smaller light boxes are more portable. Current research suggests bright blue-light boxes are no more effective than bright white-light boxes [8,12].

Exposure to bright light does not have to be continuous for several hours in order to be effective. Intermittent light can still be effective in phase shifting the circadian clock [6,13], and people can take breaks from light exposure by going inside for short periods of time, or stepping away from the light box in order to shower, dress, and prepare meals. Nonetheless, the more exposure to bright light at the correct times, the better.

PROOF OF CONCEPT/SUPPORTING DATA/EVIDENCE BASE

More field studies on phase shifts to bright light and melatonin in jet travelers are needed. However, the results of three field studies indicate that bright light and melatonin at the correct times can help reduce jet lag:

- A study of 20 jet travelers reported that the more closely the travelers sought and avoided light at predetermined times, the less jet lag they reported [14].
- A study of 15 jet travelers showed that the use of bright light at predetermined times significantly reduced the severity of self-reported jet lag symptoms as compared to no bright light [15].
- A study of 6 jet travelers who flew eastward found that melatonin taken at the correct time accelerated phase shifts to the new time zone more than placebo [16].

REFERENCES

[1] J. Carrier, T.H. Monk, C.F. Reynolds, D.J. Buysse, D.J. Kupfer, Are age differences in sleep due to phase differences in the output of the circadian timing system?, Chronobiol. Int. 16 (1999) 79–91.

[2] T. Takahashi, M. Sasaki, H. Itoh, et al., Re-entrainment of circadian rhythm of plasma melatonin on an 8-h eastward flight, Psychiatry Clin. Neurosci. 53 (1999) 257–260.

[3] T. Takahashi, M. Sasaki, H. Itoh, et al., Re-entrainment of the circadian rhythms of plasma melatonin in an 11-h eastward bound flight, Psychiatry Clin. Neurosci. 55 (2001) 275–276.

[4] V.L. Revell, C.I. Eastman, How to trick mother nature into letting you fly around or stay up all night, J. Biol. Rhythms 20 (2005) 353–365.

[5] J. Aschoff, K. Hoffmann, H. Pohl, R. Wever, Re-entrainment of circadian rhythms after phase shifts of the zeitgeber, Chronobiologia 2 (1975) 23–78.

[6] H.J. Burgess, S.J. Crowley, C.J. Gazda, et al., Preflight adjustment to eastward travel: 3 days of advancing sleep with and without morning bright light, J. Biol. Rhythms 18 (2003) 318–328.

[7] V.L. Revell, H.J. Burgess, C.J. Gazda, et al., Advancing human circadian rhythms with afternoon melatonin and morning intermittent bright light, J. Clin. Endocrinol. Metab. 91 (2006) 54–59.

[8] M.R. Smith, C.I. Eastman, Phase delaying the human circadian clock with blue-enriched polychromatic light, Chronobiol. Int. 26 (4) (2009) 709–725.

[9] J.F. Duffy, J.M. Zeitzer, C.A. Czeisler, Decreased sensitivity to phase-delaying effects of moderate intensity light in older subjects, Neurobiol. Aging 28 (5) (2007) 799–807.

[10] M.L. Moline, C.P. Pollak, T.H. Monk, et al., Age-related differences in recovery from simulated jet lag, Sleep 15 (1992) 28–40.

[11] E.K. Baehr, W. Revelle, C.I. Eastman, Individual differences in the phase and amplitude of the human circadian temperature rhythm: with an emphasis on morningness–eveningness, J. Sleep Res. 9 (2000) 117–127.
[12] M.R. Smith, V.L. Revell, C.I. Eastman, Phase advancing the human circadian clock with blue-enriched polychromatic light, Sleep Med. 10 (2009) 287–294.
[13] D.W. Rimmer, D.B. Boivin, T.L. Shanahan, et al., Dynamic resetting of the human circadian pacemaker by intermittent bright light, Am. J. Physiol. 279 (2000) R1574–R1579.
[14] D.Z. Lieberman, An automated treatment for jet lag delivered through the internet, Psychiatric Serv. 54 (2003) 394–396.
[15] T. Lahti, J. Terttunen, S. Leppamaki, et al., Field trial of timed bright light exposure for jet lag among airline cabin crew, Int. J. Circumpolar Health 66 (4) (2007) 365–369.
[16] T. Takahashi, M. Sasaki, H. Itoh, et al., Effect of 3 mg melatonin on jet lag syndrome in an 8-h eastward flight, Psychiatry Clin. Neurosci. 54 (2000) 377–378.

RECOMMENDED READING

C.I. Eastman, H.J. Burgess, How to travel the world without jet lag, Sleep Med. Clin. 4 (2009) 241–255.
J. Waterhouse, T. Reilly, G. Atkinson, B. Edwards, Jet lag: trends and coping strategies, Lancet 369 (2007) 1117–1129.

Chapter 17

Using Bright Light and Melatonin to Adjust to Night Work

Helen J. Burgess
Biological Rhythms Research Laboratory, Rush University Medical Center, Chicago, IL

PROTOCOL NAME

Using bright light and melatonin to adjust to night work.

GROSS INDICATION

This protocol is indicated for people who want to work on a later schedule.

SPECIFIC INDICATION

This use of bright light and melatonin is specifically indicated for people who are working at least 2 consecutive weeks of night shifts, and particularly for workers engaged in high-risk work, such as nuclear power plant operators and health care workers.

CONTRAINDICATIONS

As the circadian system is slow to shift, phase shifting the circadian clock is not useful for people working for less than 2 consecutive weeks of night shifts, such as part of a rapidly rotating work shift schedule.

Bright light should probably not be used in:

- people with existing eye disease;
- people using photosensitizing medications.

Bright light can induce:

- migraines (in about a third of migraine sufferers);
- mania (rare).

Behavioral Treatments for Sleep Disorders. DOI: 10.1016/B978-0-12-381522-4.00017-1

Melatonin should probably not be used in:

- people who are driving or operating heavy machinery (unless they have previously tested their response to melatonin and are taking <0.5 mg of melatonin);
- pregnant or nursing women (melatonin will transfer to the fetus/infant);
- women seeking to become pregnant;
- children (unless they suffer from a neurodevelopmental condition associated with extremely poor sleep);
- asthmatics and patients with gastrointestinal disease (melatonin may be inflammatory);
- patients using other medications (unless supervised by a physician).

RATIONALE FOR INTERVENTION

The circadian systems of night workers do not usually adjust to working at night and sleeping during the day. Instead, the circadian clock continues to promote sleep at night and wakefulness during the day. Thus, night shift work is associated with poor performance and excessive sleepiness during the night shift and poor daytime sleep at home. While hypnotics may pharmacologically induce daytime sleep, and stimulants (caffeine, modafinil) may reduce excessive sleepiness during the night shift, studies show that circadian-induced sleepiness during night shifts remains high [1–3]. Furthermore, the health effects of the long-term use of these medications are unknown. Shift workers also have an increased risk for accidents, and for reproductive, cardiovascular, and gastrointestinal disorders and cancer [4–6]. Many of these negative results are likely due in part to the chronic circadian misalignment that is characteristic of night work [7].

This chronic circadian misalignment is largely due to inappropriate light exposure that keeps the circadian clock on a daytime schedule. Appropriately timed exposure to bright light at night, and avoidance of morning bright light, can facilitate a phase delay of the circadian clock such that the circadian system promotes wakefulness at night and sleep during the day.

STEP BY STEP DESCRIPTION OF PROCEDURES

The following steps are to reshape the pattern of light exposure to facilitate the circadian clock phase delaying, or shifting later, to adjust to night work and daytime sleep. Many of these steps are illustrated in Figure 17.1. Daytime sleep also needs to be protected.

1. Avoid morning light by wearing dark sunglasses that are approved for driving on the way home after the night shift [8].
2. Go to bed early after the night shift [8].

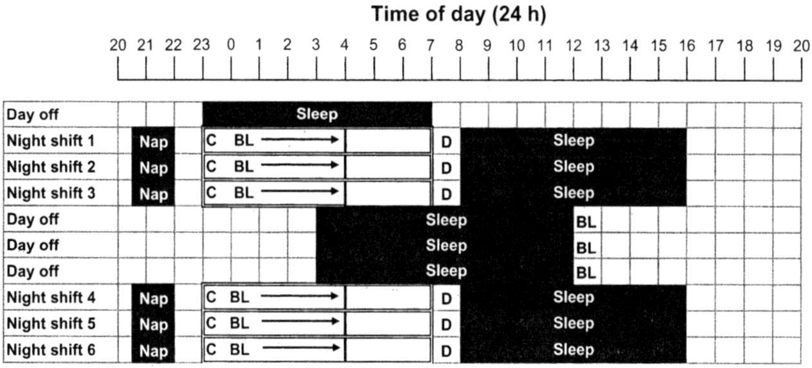

Time of day (24 h)

	20	21	22	23	0	1	2	3	4	5	6	7	8	9	10	11	12	13	14	15	16	17	18	19
Day off							Sleep																	
Night shift 1		Nap		C	BL →							D				Sleep								
Night shift 2		Nap		C	BL →							D				Sleep								
Night shift 3		Nap		C	BL →							D				Sleep								
Day off												Sleep					BL							
Day off												Sleep					BL							
Day off												Sleep					BL							
Night shift 4		Nap		C	BL →							D				Sleep								
Night shift 5		Nap		C	BL →							D				Sleep								
Night shift 6		Nap		C	BL →							D				Sleep								

FIGURE 17.1 A sample plan for a night worker who wants to sleep right after the night shift. This worker begins the night shifts unadjusted. A nap is taken before the night shifts to reduce sleep pressure, and some caffeine (C) can be taken in the first 2 hours of the night shift to improve alertness but not disrupt later daytime sleep. Bright light (BL) is used intermittently from the start of the night shift to 4 am. Bright light during the commute home is avoided with the use of dark sunglasses (D), and sleep occurs soon after the night shift in a dark bedroom. Sleep on subsequent days off remains late to stay adjusted to the night shift. Bright light after noon on days off can help the worker from sleeping too late if he or she does not want to regularly wake later than noon.

3. Maintain a light-tight bedroom. An inexpensive option is to tape black plastic over bedroom windows [8].
4. Reduce exposure to potential noise disturbances by turning off telephones, using a white-noise generator, and installing rugs over hardwood floors (if family members are home during the day).
5. If permissible, use a portable bright light box *at work until 4 am* [9]. The light box can be set up at your work station. You do not need to stare into the light box. Intermittent light exposure is still effective, so you do not have to sit in front of the light box the entire time [10,11]. Note the bright light will also keep you more alert [12].
6. Try to sleep on a late schedule on days off (e.g., 3 am to ~noon), as this will make for an easier transition back to night shifts [9].
7. If you have shifted too late and struggle to wake in the afternoons on your days off, half an hour of early afternoon bright light after 12 noon (from a light box or by going outside) will help shift you a little earlier [9].
8. If permissible, try napping in the few hours before or in the first half of a night shift to reduce sleep pressure [13,14]. This is especially useful before the first night shift. Give yourself some time to get over any grogginess (sleep inertia) upon waking.
9. To further improve alertness during the night shift, consider taking 200–450 mg of caffeine in the first 2 hours of the shift to improve alertness, but not disturb later daytime sleep [15].

POSSIBLE MODIFICATIONS/VARIANTS

As older people are more sensitive to circadian misalignment [16], they are likely to suffer even more from excessive sleepiness during the night shift and poor sleep during the day.

Morning types typically have more difficulty in adjusting to night shifts. Morning types have earlier circadian rhythms, and thus need to phase delay or shift their clocks more than evening types who are already on a later schedule [17]. A simulated night-shift study has shown that morning types are sleepier during night shifts [18].

Commercially available light boxes vary in their size, portability, and wavelength. Generally, larger light boxes, which cover more of the visual field, are less aversive, but smaller light boxes are more portable. Current research suggests bright blue-light boxes are no more effective than bright white-light boxes [19,20].

A potential criticism of the use of bright light to phase delay the circadian clock to adjust to night work and daytime sleep is that the time point of greatest sleepiness (normally around 4–6 am) may be shifted later to occur during the commute home [21]. This sleepiness may be further exacerbated by the use of dark sunglasses during the commute home. However, a study in real night workers suggest this occurs only temporarily as the time point of greatest sleepiness shifts later to occur after the commute home and well within the daytime sleep episode [11]. Thus, a few days of temporary sleepiness during the commute home (when driving is ill advised) needs to be balanced against permanent excessive sleepiness (and increased injuries and health risks associated with chronic circadian misalignment) if the circadian system is not shifted to facilitate good daytime sleep. Clearly, more research on morning driving performance in real night workers who are trying to shift later is required.

An alternative approach to adjust to night shifts is to phase advance or shift the circadian clock earlier to facilitate good sleep just prior to the night shift [22,23]. Sleeping just before going to work mimics what day workers typically do. In this case, morning bright light will facilitate a phase advance so there is no need for sunglasses during the commute home. A light box could be used *after 4 am* until the end of the shift. A high dose of melatonin (such as 3 mg) before going to sleep in the afternoon can help phase advance or shift the clock earlier [22,24], thereby facilitating the earlier onset of sleep. However, it is important to note that the feasibility and effectiveness of this alternative approach remains to be tested in real night workers.

Sometimes workers choose not to adjust their circadian clocks to night work in order to remain on a typical day schedule on their days off and thus most easily interact with their families, etc. In this case, naps, stimulants and hypnotics may be the only option.

PROOF OF CONCEPT/SUPPORTING DATA/EVIDENCE BASE

A study of nurses on permanent nights illustrated that the circadian systems in the majority of the nurses (25/30) had not phase delayed to adjust to the night shift [25]. The five nurses that were adjusted were exposed to less bright light in the morning and afternoon because they had darker bedrooms and stayed in bed longer.

Studies in real night workers, all nurses, have demonstrated the beneficial effects of light-based interventions on daytime sleep. In one study, bright light during the night shift increased total day sleep time by an average of 33 minutes [10]. Total sleep time further increased by 67 minutes when the nurses also wore dark sunglasses during their commute home. Similar improvements in night-time alertness were also observed. In a second study, nine nurses in a control group were instructed to go to bed 2 hours after the night shift, and slept in dark bedrooms [11]. Five of the nine nurses remained unadjusted to the night shift, and the group reported sleeping an average of 6.6 hours per night, which is typical of permanent night workers [26]. Ten nurses in the treatment group *also* wore dark sunglasses during their commute home and received bright light during the night shift. In this case, all 10 nurses adjusted to the night shift, and they reported sleeping an average of 7.3 hours per day (an extra 45 minutes of sleep per night) [27]. Simulated night-shift studies suggest that, for many young people, phase delaying the clock by about 5 hours or more can improve night-time performance so that they are close to baseline daytime levels [28]. More research measuring objective performance of real night workers during light-based interventions is needed.

Studies of real night-shift workers show that naps can improve performance and reduce accidents during the night shift without reducing daytime sleep quality, and are particularly effective for the first night shift [13,14].

To date, there is no strong evidence to support taking melatonin before daytime sleep that occurs *after* a night shift. In a study of nurses on the night shift, 0.5 mg of melatonin taken before daytime sleep helped less than one-third of the nurses phase delay to the daytime sleep schedule [29]. In terms of the hypnotic effects of melatonin, some placebo controlled studies in real night workers using relatively high doses (5–6 mg) have reported significant increases in the self-reported duration of daytime sleep of 26–56 minutes [30,31], but others report no such effect of melatonin [32]. Thus, more research is required to determine if such high doses of melatonin can improve objective measures of daytime sleep in real night workers.

REFERENCES

[1] P.K. Schweitzer, A.C. Randazzo, K. Stone, et al., Laboratory and field studies of naps and caffeine as practical countermeasures for sleep–wake problems associated with night work, Sleep 29 (2006) 39–50.

[2] J.K. Walsh, A.C. Randazzo, K.L. Stone, P.K. Schweitzer, Modafinil improves alertness, vigilance, and executive function during simulated night shifts, Sleep 27 (2004) 434–439.

[3] C.A. Czeisler, J.K. Walsh, T. Roth, et al., Modafinil for excessive sleepiness associated with shift-work sleep disorder, NEJM 353 (2005) 476–486.

[4] C.L. Drake, T. Roehrs, G. Richardson, et al., Shift work sleep disorder: prevalence and consequences beyond that of symptomatic day workers, Sleep 27 (2004) 1453–1462.

[5] A. Knutsson, Health disorders of shift workers, Occup. Med. 53 (2003) 103–108.

[6] K. Straif, R. Baan, Y. Grosse, et al., Carcinogenicity of shift-work, painting, and fire-fighting, Lancet Oncol. 8 (2007) 1065–1066.

[7] F.A. Scheer, M.F. Hilton, C.S. Mantzoros, S.A. Shea, Adverse metabolic and cardiovascular consequences of circadian misalignment, Proc. Natl. Acad. Sci. 106 (11) (2009) 4453–4458.

[8] C.I. Eastman, K.T. Stewart, M.P. Mahoney, et al., Dark goggles and bright light improve circadian rhythm adaptation to night-shift work, Sleep 17 (1994) 535–543.

[9] M. Smith, L. Fogg, C. Eastman, Practical interventions to promote circadian adaptation to permanent night shift work: Study 4, J. Biol. Rhythms 24 (2) (2009) 161–172.

[10] I.Y. Yoon, D.U. Jeong, K.B. Kwon, et al., Bright light exposure at night and light attenuation in the morning improve adaptation of night shift workers, Sleep 25 (2002) 351–356.

[11] D.B. Boivin, F.O. James, Circadian adaptation to night-shift work by judicious light and darkness exposure, J. Biol. Rhythms 17 (2002) 556–567.

[12] S.S. Campbell, D. Dawson, Enhancement of nighttime alertness and performance with bright ambient light, Physiol. Behav. 48 (1990) 317–320.

[13] M.T. Purnell, A.M. Feyer, G.P. Herbison, The impact of a nap opportunity during the night shift on the performance and alertness of 12-h shift workers, J. Sleep Res. 11 (2002) 219–227.

[14] S. Garbarino, B. Mascialino, M.A. Penco, et al., Professional shift-work drivers who adopt prophylactic naps can reduce the risk of car accidents during night work, Sleep 27 (2004) 1295–1302.

[15] J.K. Walsh, M.J. Muehlbach, P.K. Schweitzer, Hypnotics and caffeine as countermeasures for shiftwork-related sleepiness and sleep disturbance, J. Sleep Res. 4 (1995) 80–83.

[16] D.J. Dijk, J.F. Duffy, E. Riel, et al., Ageing and the circadian and homeostatic regulation of human sleep during forced desynchrony of rest, melatonin and temperature rhythms, J. Physiol. 516 (2) (1999) 611–627.

[17] S.J. Crowley, C. Lee, C.Y. Tseng, et al., Combinations of bright light, scheduled dark, sunglasses, and melatonin to facilitate circadian entrainment to night shift work, J. Biol. Rhythms 18 (2003) 513–523.

[18] N.A.J. Hilliker, M.J. Muehlbach, P.K. Schweitzer, J.K. Walsh, Sleepiness/alertness on a simulated night shift schedule and morningness–eveningness tendency, Sleep 15 (1992) 430–433.

[19] M.R. Smith, C.I. Eastman, Phase delaying the human circadian clock with blue-enriched polychromatic light, Chronobiol. Int. 26 (4) (2009) 709–725.

[20] M.R. Smith, V.L. Revell, C.I. Eastman, Phase advancing the human circadian clock with blue-enriched polychromatic light, Sleep Med. 10 (2009) 287–294.

[21] S.W. Lockley, Safety considerations for the use of blue-light blocking glasses in shift-workers, J. Pineal. Res. 42 (2) (2007) 210–211.

[22] K.M. Sharkey, C.I. Eastman, Melatonin phase shifts human circadian rhythms in a placebo-controlled simulated night-work study, Am. J. Physiol. 282 (2002) R454–R463.

[23] N. Santhi, D. Aeschbach, T.S. Horowitz, C.A. Czeisler, The impact of sleep timing and bright light exposure on attentional impairment during night work, J. Biol. Rhythms 23 (4) (2008) 341–352.

[24] H.J. Burgess, V.L. Revell, C.I. Eastman, A three pulse phase response curve to three milligrams of melatonin in humans, J. Physiol. 586 (2) (2008) 639–647.
[25] M. Dumont, D. Benhaberou-Brun, J. Paquet, Profile of 24-h light exposure and circadian phase of melatonin secretion in night workers, J. Biol. Rhythms 16 (2001) 502–511.
[26] J.J. Pilcher, B.J. Lambert, A.I. Huffcutt, Differential effects of permanent and rotating shifts on self-report sleep length: a meta-analytic review, Sleep 23 (2000) 155–163.
[27] F.O. James, E. Chevrier, D.B. Boivin, A light/darkness intervention to improve daytime sleep quality in night shift workers. Abstracts of the XVIth International Symposium on Night and Shiftwork, 2003, p. 100.
[28] M.R. Smith, L.F. Fogg, C.I. Eastman, A compromise circadian phase position for permanent night work improves mood, fatigue, and performance, Sleep 32 (11) (2009) 1481–1489.
[29] R.L. Sack, A.J. Lewy, Melatonin as a chronobiotic: treatment of circadian desynchrony in night workers and the blind, J. Biol. Rhythms 12 (1997) 595–603.
[30] S. Folkard, J. Arendt, M. Clark, Can melatonin improve shift workers' tolerance of the night shift? Some preliminary findings, Chronobiol. Int. 10 (1993) 315–320.
[31] I.Y. Yoon, B.G. Song, Role of morning melatonin administration and attenuation of sunlight exposure in improving adaptation of night-shift workers, Chronobiol. Int. 19 (2002) 903–913.
[32] M. James, M.O. Tremea, J.S. Jones, J.R. Krohmer, Can melatonin improve adaptation to night shift? Am. J. Emer. Med. 16 (1998) 367–370.

RECOMMENDED READING

H.J. Burgess, K.M. Sharkey, C.I. Eastman, Bright light, dark and melatonin can promote circadian adaptation in night shift workers, Sleep Med. Rev. 6 (2002) 407–420.

Part II

BSM Protocols for Adherence and Treatment of Intrinsic Sleep Disorders

Introduction

Mark S. Aloia
Division of Psychosocial Medicine, National Jewish Health, Denver, CO

Behavioral Sleep Medicine has become synonymous with Cognitive Behavioral Treatment for Insomnia (CBT-I). It is, however, truly much more, with a breadth and depth that deserves further attention. That is the goal of Part II of the book. This part will, for the first time, outline behavioral approaches to sleep disorders other than insomnia (e.g., obstructive sleep apnea and narcolepsy). It is not our intention to suggest that such interventions should be offered as first-line treatments for these disorders. Rather, we want to demonstrate that these treatments are options for some individuals for whom those mainstream therapies are less effective or palatable. These behavioral approaches are gaining acceptance. Research on them is becoming more prolific – and outcomes associated with them are impressive. The reader will find a straightforward approach to these interventions in the following pages.

Perhaps the second most common type of behavioral sleep intervention with adults is geared toward improving adherence to Positive Airway Pressure (PAP) treatment. PAP is an effective therapy for most patients with obstructive sleep apnea (OSA), but adherence rates are far poorer than we would hope. Recent studies suggest that the amount of PAP needed to change outcomes varies depending on the outcome measure being examined, although greater adherence seems to confer greater benefit in general. The chapters to follow will outline several approaches to improving adherence to PAP. The approaches represent the state of the science for behavioral interventions of poor adherence in general, and they are specifically geared toward PAP adherence. All of the authors recognize that behavioral factors dictate our approach toward caring for ourselves as a society. This begins with primary prevention, and continues to treatment adherence. Behavior is involved at every step, and these authors have demonstrated, through their work, that behavioral interventions are potentially powerful mechanisms of change. Some of these interventions have improved adherence upwards of 2 hours nightly. The chapters reflect an appreciation for the vast literature on theories of behavior change. Interventions are presented for individuals who have an anxiety response to the treatment, as well as for those who are simply ambivalent about treatment. One approach is taken out of a philosophy of treating chronic medical conditions – a new perspective we should consider when thinking about treating OSA. Group therapies are presented as well as individualized approaches. Approaches are often manualized or automated, allowing for easy dissemination. We are pleased to present all of these approaches, for the first time, in a single book.

We are breaking new ground in the study of Behavioral Sleep Medicine. This new ground does not ignore our strong history associated with CBT-I. Instead, it seeks to augment it and broaden our field to include behavioral approaches for other disorders and for the complex, behavioral, problem of poor adherence. Part II of the book could not only change the behavior of practicing clinicians; it could also generate additional interest in research associated with these behavioral techniques and problems. In any case, this part of the book highlights the new frontier of Behavioral Sleep Medicine. It is exciting, it is growing rapidly, and, we believe, it is an integral aspect of the future of our field.

Chapter 18

Motivational Enhancement Therapy

Motivating Adherence to Positive Airway Pressure

Shannon L. O'Connor Christian, Mark S. Aloia
National Jewish Health, Division of Psychosocial Medicine, Denver, CO

PROTOCOL NAME

Motivational Enhancement Therapy (MET): motivating adherence to Positive Airway Pressure (PAP) in obstructive sleep apnea.

GROSS INDICATION

This treatment can be employed with any user, or potential user, of PAP treatment as an approach to enhance adherence to treatment.

SPECIFIC INDICATION

This treatment modality has thus far been tested with patients who have been diagnosed recently with Obstructive Sleep Apnea (OSA) and who are judged to be good responders to PAP. A good responder is someone who exhibits the following on a PAP titration study: (1) AHI less than 10; (2) remission of snoring; (3) arousal index of less than 10; (4) PLM index of less than 15.

CONTRAINDICATIONS

This treatment modality may be less beneficial for patients with the following conditions:

- Presence of a serious medical condition (end stage renal failure, severe COPD, severe asthma), as these conditions may contribute to daytime sleepiness that does not improve with PAP treatment. Continued daytime sleepiness, despite adherence to PAP, could contribute to non-adherence to the device.
- History of or current diagnosis of a major psychiatric illness (including current substance abuse), with the *exception* of depression. Certain

Behavioral Treatments for Sleep Disorders. DOI: 10.1016/B978-0-12-381522-4.00018-3

psychiatric illnesses may interfere with a patient's ability to effectively participate in treatment.
- Notable cognitive impairment due to dementia or other causes that may interfere with the ability to engage effectively in the intervention.

RATIONALE FOR INTERVENTION

Despite the efficacy of PAP treatment in remediating many of the sequelae associated with OSA, adherence to PAP is poor. Approximately 25 percent of patients are estimated to discontinue treatment within the first year of use [1]. Patients with OSA are likely to fluctuate in both their willingness and their motivation to use treatment. As such, enhancing intrinsic motivation may be central in supporting adherence to PAP. Miller and Rollnick [2] developed Motivational Interviewing (MI), a counseling approach characterized by its client-centered and directive nature. The purpose of MI is to help people resolve their natural ambivalence about health behavior change in order for the behavior change to occur. Motivational Enhancement Therapy (MET) includes central components of motivational interviewing in that it is client-centered and it focuses on patients' perceived importance of change and their confidence that they can maintain a new behavior. Feedback sessions are included in which normative feedback is presented to the patient and discussed in a neutral, non-judgmental, and dispassionate manner. The feedback is designed to reinforce the patient's commitment to change, and to enhance the patient's level of self-efficacy (e.g., confidence that they can maintain the new behavior under difficult circumstances). "Elicit–Provide–Elicit" is a specific strategy used during feedback, which is designed to reduce the likelihood of patient denial and defensiveness. The therapist asks an open-ended question ("Elicit"), shares information ("Provide"), and follows up with another open-ended question ("Elicit") to learn the patient's reaction. Other key components of MET include adopting a curious, eliciting, and non-judgmental tone, calibrating the session to the patient's level of readiness to change, and exploring patient ambivalence about change. The desired result of this approach is the development of intrinsic motivation to use treatment and, therefore, enhanced long-term adherence.

STEP BY STEP DESCRIPTION OF PROCEDURES

There are two face-to-face sessions, 1 week apart, and a follow-up phone call at 1 month.

Session 1: Patient Assessment of PAP during Titration Night

Patients are asked about the experience of using PAP during the sleep study. This provides a starting point for learning about potential benefits and specific challenges experienced by them. The therapist reflects positive statements about PAP and empathizes when challenges are articulated, noting said challenges and positive statements to be used later in therapy.

Assessment of Motivation to Use PAP

The therapist asks patients to rate their motivation to use PAP on a scale of 1 to 10 (1 = doesn't want to use it at all; 10 = very much want to use it). It is imperative that the therapist uses a dispassionate tone so that accurate information is shared. The therapist tailors the visit based on the patient's stated level of motivation. Patients may also be asked why they feel their rating is not higher or lower. The question of why the rating is not higher should be asked first. The response represents the stated barriers to using PAP, and these can be used later in therapy. Perhaps more importantly, patients are asked why their rating is not lower. This is often more difficult for them to answer. Answers to this question represent the patient's own conceptualization of the benefits of treatment. These can also be used to support positive statements about PAP, and carefully challenge negative statements in future sessions.

Information Exchange: Video Clip of OSA Patient

A video clip of somebody experiencing apnea is shown to patients to illustrate what happens during episodes of apnea. After the video clip, they are asked for thoughts and feelings about the video and how the video might relate to them. This allows them to consider how apnea episodes may impact them personally. A personal focus is applied whenever possible.

Review of Patient's Pre-Treatment Polysomnography (PSG)

The therapist shares the patient's diagnostic PSG with him or her. The severity of apnea is made clear by placing the patient's AHI on a graph representing normal, mild, moderate, and severe ranges of apnea. The same type of graphic representation is provided for the patient's oxygen desaturation index (outlining normal and abnormal levels). Feedback is provided using the Elicit–Provide–Elicit strategy. Immediately after reviewing the information, patients are asked to share their thoughts and feelings about the graphs and how the results might relate to them.

Review of Symptoms

Patients are asked to specify the primary symptoms that led them to seek treatment. Typically, symptoms include mood, concentration, fatigue, and daytime sleepiness. In addition, medical and cognitive correlates of OSA that may not be apparent to patients are discussed (e.g., hypertension, cardiovascular risk, etc.). The tone of the exchange is neutral in order to provide the patients with relevant information while allowing them to weigh the importance of the information to themselves personally.

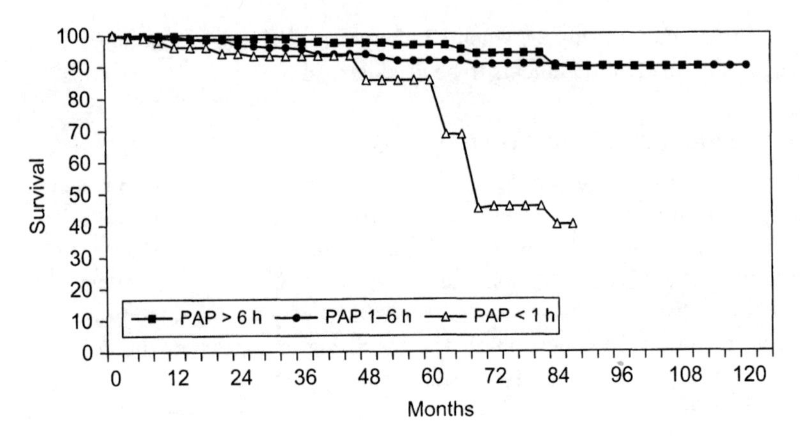

FIGURE 18.1 Kaplan-Meier cumulative survival rates according to categories of PAP compliance. Cumulative survival rates in the PAP > 6h group were significantly higher than in the PAP 1 1h group ($p < 0.00005$). Cumulative survival rates in the PAP 1–6h group were significantly higher than in the PAP < 1h group ($p = 0.01$). Cumulative survival rates were not different in the PAP > 6h group and the PAP 1–6h group ($p = 0.11$). *Graph used with permission from the publisher: Campos-Rodriquez, F., Pena-Grinan, N., Reyes-Numez, N., De la Cruz-Moron, Il, Perez-Ronchel, J., De la Vega-Gallardo, F. and Fernandez-Palacin, A. (2005)* [3]. *Mortality in obstructive sleep apnea-hypopnea patients treated with positive airway pressure.* Chest, *128, 624–633.*

Review of Mortality Graph

A graph that shows cardiovascular morbidity and mortality rates according to PAP use (<1 hour; 1–6 hours; >6 hours) over a period of 0–120 months is shown to the patient (see Figure 18.1 for an example). The graph illustrates the significantly higher cumulative survival rates for those who use PAP >6 hours and those who use it 1–6 hours as compared with those who use it <1 hour. Patients are asked for thoughts and feelings about the graph and the degree to which they perceive it as applying to them. This exchange offers an opportunity for patients to reflect upon the consequences of using or not using PAP over the long-term. As with all feedback, the Elicit–Provide–Elicit process is used.

Following is an example of the interchange that might accompany a review of Figure 18.1.

Positive Response

Therapist: This graph shows the results from a study illustrating the relationship between amount of CPAP use and the likelihood of having a significant heart problem, like a heart attack or a stroke. Individuals who use CPAP 6 hours or more each night fare the best – they live longer than people who use it only 1–6 hours per night. People who have sleep apnea but don't use CPAP at all have significantly greater mortality risk than those who use CPAP for the recommended time or those who use it for 1–6 hours per night. What do you make of these results?

Patient: Wow! That's a big difference – the one line is way down there, and other two, well, they become the same line over here, after a while. It really makes me think. My parents both died of heart attacks and, like I mentioned, I'm already worried about my high blood pressure. It makes me think twice about my apnea and whether it's related to my blood pressure. Wow, I just can't believe the difference.

Therapist: You're really surprised to see the difference that CPAP can make in your health.

Patient: Yes. It just makes me think that I'd really better use it because I don't want to miss out on my watching my grandkids grow up, and if this thing will help with my health, I'll do it. I want to be one of the people on this top line here.

Therapist: You're already concerned about your blood pressure, and knowing that CPAP can make a difference for you makes you even more certain that you want to use it regularly just like the people on the top line of the graph.

Negative Response

Therapist: This graph shows the results from a study illustrating the relationship between amount of CPAP use and the likelihood of having a significant heart problem, like a heart attack or a stroke. Individuals who use CPAP 6 hours or more each night fare the best – they live longer than people who use it only 1–6 hours per night. People who have sleep apnea but don't use CPAP at all have significantly greater mortality risk than those who use CPAP for the recommended time or those who use it for 1–6 hours per night. What do you make of these results?

Patient: I really don't think this applies to me. The study was probably done on people sicker than me, or people with worse apnea. Besides, I don't have any heart problems now and I don't even have a family history.

Therapist: So this study doesn't even apply to you and you don't really see that it is pertinent to how you approach treatment for your apnea?

Patient: Yes. I mean, I can see how it might work for some people who have heart problems, but that's not me.

Therapist: So, you see the value in the treatment where the heart is concerned, but it's not necessary for you because you don't have a heart problem, right?

Patient: Well, I wouldn't say treatment is not necessary, but my heart is fine.

Therapist: Ok, let me restate that. Treatment may be beneficial for you, but for reasons other than your heart.

Patient: Yes, that's right.

Therapist: Great, let me tell you more about CPAP.

Review of Titration PSG and Comparison to Diagnostic PSG

The patient has a personalized review of the effectiveness of PAP based on his or her PSG data (diagnostic and titration). Special attention is given to the degree to which AHI and oxygen desaturation are improved with the use of PAP. As in the previous feedback section, normative values are used for comparison. The primary goal is to enhance patient self-efficacy by demonstrating that patients are capable of treating their OSA with PAP.

Negotiate a Plan Based on the Patient's Readiness and Confidence

To evaluate patients' confidence and readiness to initiate treatment, they are asked the extent to which they will be able to use PAP for 5+hours/night. Subsequently, patients are asked to set achievable, specific goals by identifying steps related to PAP use. The goals should be based on their readiness and confidence at the time of *this* visit. Goals are better set low than high, to allow them to be reachable and to enhance self-efficacy. Patients are asked to note daily improvements in patient-specific areas of concern so that any changes that result from PAP use are duly noted.

Summary

The therapist provides a summary of the session with highlights of the take-home message, including: (1) patient concerns about health related to having untreated OSA; (2) patient reaction to feedback on the PSG; (3) medical conditions the patient may be at risk for with untreated OSA; (4) benefits the patient experienced after using PAP; (5) motivation to use PAP; (6) patient goals. The importance of Session 2 is emphasized, and is subsequently scheduled for 1 week after the mask fitting.

Session 2: Patient's Subjective Appraisal of Adherence to PAP

The patient is asked to provide an estimate of the frequency and duration of PAP use over the previous week. This provides a starting point for understanding the patient's experience of using the device during the first week of treatment. The therapist empathizes with difficulties and reinforces positive aspects of PAP. If the patient denies any changes due to PAP use, the therapist normalizes the fact that changes and benefits may be noticed over a period of time.

Values Assessment

To begin the values assessment exercise, patients are asked to share tangible goals and activities related to daily living, and to share what is most important to them (e.g., having a nice place to live, spending time with family, being more active). The therapist encourages the patient to discuss three or more areas in order to select a suitable area for discussion. The therapist initiates a discussion of values in order to build a discrepancy between the patient's current status and aspired status with regards to the stated goal and its relation to apnea. The patient is asked to address: (1) the extent to which PAP might help with achieving the goal; (2) the extent to which PAP might hinder the goal; (3) the chances (scale 0–100) that the goal will be achieved if PAP is not used or is used less than 5 hours/night; (4) the chances (scale 0–100) that the goal will be achieved if PAP is used 5+ hours/night. After a short summary, the therapist reflects the patient's goals and highlights the discrepancy between current sleep apnea and the patient's broader values/goals.

Decisional Balance Exercise

This section includes a motivational enhancement technique designed to explore pros and cons of adherence to PAP. The therapist asks the patient to provide the downsides of using PAP, followed by the upside of using it. After summarizing, the therapist engages in a volley of reflections in an effort to explore the patient's ambivalence about using PAP. Overall, the therapist highlights ambivalence, normalizes this ambivalence as a natural part of this process, and expresses empathy. The therapist guides the patient through any ambivalence about using PAP, with the goal of its ultimate resolution.

The following is an example of an interchange that might occur during the decisional balance exercise.

Therapist: I would like to understand the full picture about what using CPAP has been like for you. First, let's start with your thoughts on what you think the costs of or the downsides are about using CPAP.

Patient: Well, the tubing is the biggest hindrance. It's tied to the machine, so rolling around to get comfortable in bed is just really hard. I normally start out on my stomach and move to my back and side, and I just don't have the same freedom as I did before when I'm trying to get comfortable so I can fall asleep.

Therapist: It interferes with your freedom and your comfort in several ways.

Patient: Exactly. My throat gets dried out, too. I wake up about 1 or 1:30 am and my throat is so sore I have to suck on a piece of candy or get some water to make the soreness go away. I have to go through the whole process of taking off the mask and getting the candy or water, and then getting the darn thing back on. It's just a pain.

Therapist: Not only is it hard to get comfortable to fall asleep at night, you can't even sleep through until the morning sometimes because your throat is so dried out. It's a hassle.

Patient: Yes, that's right.

Therapist: How about the other side – what do you think are some *good* things or the upsides of using CPAP?

Patient: I hope it will help bring down my blood pressure so I can get off this medication. I don't like being on the medication, but I am concerned about my health. And there are other potential health benefits, like having more energy and being more alert. One thing I struggle with now is that I can't sit down in the evening and read something that's sort of boring without falling asleep. Right now I just get by with not reading much at night, but I'd like to be able to read if I wanted to do that.

Therapist: Having good health and being alert are important to you, and CPAP may give you more freedom with how you spend your time, like being able to read in the evening.

Patient: Yes.

Therapist: So on the one hand, you don't like CPAP because you find it uncomfortable in several ways and it's frustrating to try to get comfortable to fall asleep; on the other hand, you like CPAP because you want to improve your blood pressure and to be more alert and have more energy. It sounds as if you are being pulled in two directions; what do you make of this?

Patient: Well, when I think about it, my health is way more important than being able to sleep on my stomach. It's just a hassle and I wish I didn't have to use it, but when I compare the two, my health is much more important to me.

Review of Feedback on Reaction Time

The patient is given a graph illustrating his or her reaction time off-treatment, which is based on AHI off-treatment. This is done in cases where reaction time is assessed before and after treatment. AHI pre- and post-treatment is covered in a previous assessment session. The patient is told how this reaction time equates to reaction times calibrated to alcohol use and an inferred risk for motor vehicle accidents. The Elicit–Provide–Elicit process is used when exploring the patient's thoughts about the graph. The therapist communicates with a non-judgmental tone and empathizes throughout the exchange. Ongoing reflections assist the patient with processing the information.

Information Exchange: PAP Benefits for Health and Functioning

The therapist shares information about the medical benefits of sleep apnea treatment (e.g., lower blood pressure, decreased risk of heart attack) and how treatment is associated with improvements in daily functioning (e.g., increased alertness/productivity). The therapist provides a menu of options to the patient, who is asked to select the areas that are most relevant for him or her. A discussion of these areas then ensues. In addition, the therapist reviews medical-related concerns previously identified in Session 1 to help the patient link stated concerns with medical benefits identified in this section. Reflections and empathy are used throughout this section.

Information Exchange: Cognitive Benefits of Sleep Apnea Treatment

The therapist shows the patient a graph which illustrates the relative increase in vigilance performance for those who use PAP ≥4 hours a night compared with those who use PAP <4 hours a night, over a 6-month period of time (see Figure 18.2 for an example). The graphs indicate that greater use of PAP increases vigilance from initial use to 3 months, with continued increases from 3 to 6 months. The patient is asked to share any thoughts and concerns. The therapist reinforces insight about the importance of PAP use, and empathizes with stated patient concerns.

Assess Patient Motivation and Confidence

The patient is asked to rate, on a 10-point scale, (1) motivation for treatment, (2) motivation to use PAP 5+ hours/night, and (3) confidence to

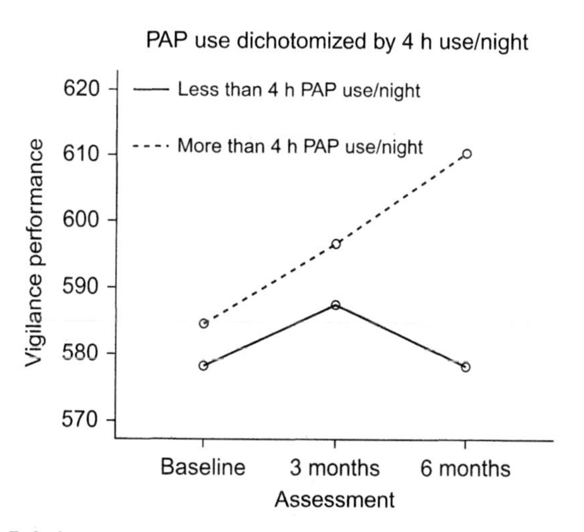

FIGURE 18.2 Relative increases in vigilance performance for Good (≥4 h/night) versus Poor (<4 h/night) CPAP users over time.

implement treatment. The patient is asked why each rating was chosen, why a lower rating was not chosen, and what will need to occur for a higher rating to be given. This section helps clarify the patient's level of motivation and confidence, and potential factors that may interfere with PAP use.

The following is an example of a potential interchange that might occur while conducting the scaling exercise.

Therapist: How motivated or ready are you to treat your sleep apnea? Rate your motivation or readiness on a scale of 0—10, with 0 being not at all motivated and 10 being extremely motivated.

Patient: Probably a 7 or an 8.

Therapist: What would have to happen for you to move up to a higher number, like a 9 or a 10?

Patient: Well, I'm sort of nervous about it, it's equipment, I'm not technologically oriented or adept, and you young people know what you are doing. Us old folks, it's just new and intimidating.

Therapist: So you are a little bit nervous about the equipment itself?

Patient: Yes, if it doesn't work, what I'll be able to do about it. So I think if I knew what to do or who to call if I had a problem, I'd be a 9 or a 10.

Therapist: What makes you a 7 or 8 and not a lower number like 4 or 5?

Patient: Well, I want to feel better, and I think the purpose is that I'll feel better if I use it. And I know that it may be hard, but I'm the kind of person that sticks with things. I had knee surgery a while ago and it was tough, but I stuck with the therapy and everything that I was supposed to do and I'm good to go now. I think I can be successful with this because I'll stick with it.

Therapist: So you had success after your knee surgery and you are seeing some parallels between knee surgery and what you had to do and using the CPAP?

Patient: Yes, exactly.

Therapist: OK, so you feel like you might not know what to do if something went wrong and if you knew who to call when there was a problem, you'd be even more motivated and ready to tackle your sleep apnea?

Patient: Exactly.

Explore and Identify Experienced or Anticipated Barriers to PAP Use

The therapist tailors this section to the patient's stated motivation from the previous section. The therapist explores experienced and anticipated barriers the patient raised during the session (e.g., decisional balance sheet) in an effort to highlight any remaining areas of concern. The patient is asked to consider creative ways to problem solve areas of concern and to identify steps to support the routine use of PAP.

Renegotiate a Plan Based on Readiness and Confidence

The therapist helps the patient to renegotiate goals based on his or her stated readiness and confidence to use PAP. Patient goals from Session 1 are reviewed, barriers are identified, and positive steps to remediate difficulties are discussed. The patient is encouraged to notice all changes, even subtle ones, that result from PAP use. In addition, the patient is asked to consider additional resources to help achieve the stated goals.

Wrap Up and Results

The therapist summarizes the session, including:

1. Patient concerns about symptoms of untreated OSA
2. Potential barriers to PAP use
3. Patient benefits from PAP use
4. Current patient motivation and confidence
5. Specific steps the patient will take with regards to PAP use
6. The patient's ultimate goal
7. Additional resources the patient has identified that can be helpful.

Phone Call

Patient Self-Report of PAP Use

The therapist summarizes major points from Session 2, including the patient's stated goals. The patient is asked about the frequency of PAP use for the previous week, the greatest number of hours of use, and the lowest number of hours of use. The therapist asks the patient to reflect on the nights in which he or she was able to use PAP 5+ hours (and PAP <5 hours/night) and to identify supports (and barriers) to PAP use. In addition, the patient is asked to reflect on both scenarios (PAP use ≥5 hours, PAP use <5 hours) and to share the presence or absence of symptoms the next day. The therapist maintains a nonjudgmental attitude and a dispassionate tone, empathizing with the patient's difficulties and reflecting the patient's motivational statements.

Building Confidence to Use PAP

The therapist asks the patient to rate confidence on a 10-point scale, queries why a higher number was not chosen, and asks what needs to happen for confidence to increase. The therapist lists various situations and asks the patient to rate the confidence level in using PAP regularly ("not at all", "somewhat", "very"). The situations are ones typically faced by PAP users (increased time getting ready for bed; mask discomfort; side effects; feeling closed in; feeling embarrassed; traveling; concern about disrupting a bed partner). The patient's unique concern is included in the list, as well. The patient is asked to develop a concrete plan to address each item to which the reply was "not at all confident". Upon completing the section, the patient is asked to identify a concern or challenge, other than sleep apnea, that he or she was able to overcome successfully. The therapist facilitates the patient's application of strategies used for the other problem to the issue of adherence in the use of PAP (e.g., internal motivation, external support).

Summarize Session

The therapist summarizes the patient's motivation and strategies to use PAP regularly, and how he or she intends to build confidence in using PAP.

POSSIBLE MODIFICATIONS WITH VARIANTS

Modifications can be made with regard to the specific information discussed with the patients, and any personal feedback can be employed and tied to potential PAP use. One such modification presented above involves performance testing before and after treatment. This is a powerful way of demonstrating real changes with treatment on a personal level. The tenets of MET, however, must remain constant. Among them, the Elicit–Provide–Elicit process must be used when dealing with situations in which defenses might be raised by the information provided to the patient.

PROOF OF CONCEPT/SUPPORTING DATA/EVIDENCE BASE

PAP is an effective treatment for patients diagnosed with OSA, and greater PAP use is thought to optimize clinical benefits. However, adherence rates to PAP are notoriously low in most studies, making interventions designed to increase adherence clinically useful.

Preliminary data support the value of utilizing intervention strategies to increase patient adherence – specifically those designed to increase intrinsic motivation and patient self-efficacy, such as MET [4]. In a study comparing the efficacy of brief MET therapy, education (ED), and standard care (SC), both the ED and MET interventions demonstrated effects over SC at 3 months. In a more careful analysis of the data, it was noted that MET worked best for patients who demonstrated ambivalence about treatment. This was defined as those patients who used between 2 and 5 hours a night within the first week of treatment. These individuals gained significantly over SC in their use of PAP over the course of a year. ED was no better than SC in these patients. Self-efficacy was also improved in these individuals compared to the other groups. However, at 6 months, only MET demonstrated efficacy over SC. Other studies have noted the importance of self-efficacy as a predictor of adherence to PAP, but no other studies have yet been conducted using MET therapy.

REFERENCES

[1] N. McArdle, G. Devereux, H. Heidarnejad, et al., Long-term use of PAP therapy for sleep apnea/hypopnea syndrome, Am. J. Resp. Crit. Care Med. 159 (4) (1999) 1108–1114.
[2] W.R. Miller, S. Rollnick, Motivational Interviewing: Preparing People to Change Addictive Behaviors, Guildford Press, New York, NY, 1991.
[3] F. Campos-Rodriquez, N. Pena-Grinan, N. Reyes-Nunez, et al., Mortality in obstructive sleep apnea-hypopnea patients treated with positive airway pressure, Chest 128 (2005) 624–633.
[4] M.S. Aloia, K. Smith, J.T. Arnedt, et al., Brief behavioral therapies reduce early PAP discontinuation rates in SAS: preliminary findings, Behav. Sleep Med. 5 (2) (2007) 89–104.

RECOMMENDED READING

M.S. Aloia, J.T. Arnedt, R.L. Riggs, et al., Clinical management of poor adherence to CPAP: Motivational enhancement, Behav. Sleep Med. 2 (4) (2004) 205–222.
M.S. Aloia, K. Smith, J.T. Arnedt, et al., Brief behavioral therapies reduce early PAP discontinuation rates in SAS: preliminary findings, Behav. Sleep Med. 5 (2) (2007) 89–104.
W.R. Miller, S. Rollnick, Motivational Interviewing: Preparing People to Change Addictive Behaviors, Guildford Press, New York, NY, 1991.
S. Rollnick, P. Mason, C. Butler, Health Behavior Change: A Guide for Practitioners, Churchill Livingstone, London, 1999.
J.O. Prochaska, C.A. Redding, K.E. Evers, The transtheoretical model and stages of change, in: K. Glanz, F.M. Lewis, B.K. Rimer (Eds.), Health Behavior and Health Education, Jossey-Bass, San Francisco, CA, 1997.

Chapter 19

Exposure Therapy for Claustrophobic Reactions to Continuous Positive Airway Pressure

Melanie K. Means, Jack D. Edinger
Department of Veterans Affairs Medical Center and Duke University Medical Center, Durham, NC

PROTOCOL NAME

Exposure therapy for claustrophobic reactions to Continuous Positive Airway Pressure (CPAP).

GROSS INDICATION

Exposure therapy is indicated for individuals with sleep apnea who are unable to tolerate CPAP devices due to anxiety reactions.

SPECIFIC INDICATION

Some patients prescribed CPAP therapy for sleep-related breathing disorders experience claustrophobia, anxiety, or panic symptoms related to wearing the mask (feeling restricted) and/or tolerating the air pressure (feeling suffocated). Exposure therapy is indicated for such individuals.

CONTRAINDICATIONS

Absolute contraindications for CPAP exposure therapy are unknown. It is reasonable to presume that this intervention would hold similar contraindications as exposure therapy for other anxiety disorders. Such contraindications may include unstable psychiatric symptoms (e.g., substance use, post-traumatic stress disorder, suicidal/homicidal ideation, psychosis), inability to maintain a therapeutic relationship, or economic/domiciliary instability [1].

Behavioral Treatments for Sleep Disorders. DOI: 10.1016/B978-0-12-381522-4.00019-5

RATIONALE FOR INTERVENTION

In order to understand the treatment needs of patients who present with claustrophobic reactions to CPAP, it seems useful to consider first the etiology and mechanisms that perpetuate such reactions. Claustrophobia is a form of specific phobia that entails extreme anxiety and panic elicited by situations such as tunnels, elevators, or other settings in which the individual experiences a sense of being closed in or entrapped. According to Rachman and Taylor [2], claustrophobia is composed of two "core" fears: fear of restriction, and fear of suffocation. Traditionally, the development of such fears has been explained by the two-factor model described by Mowrer [3]. This model, which evolves from the early work of Pavlov [4], proposes that fear reactions such as claustrophobia are initially acquired by classical conditioning and then are maintained by operant conditioning. The classical conditioning involves the learning of associations between an unconditioned stimulus (UCS) and a conditioned stimulus (CS). Typically, the UCS is a stimulus that evokes danger or discomfort – reactions that are called unconditioned responses (UCRs). A conditioning occurs when the CS is paired with the UCS over one or more trials, and through this association the CS comes to produce conditioned responses (CRs) that mimic the UCRs. Under proper circumstances, the CS–UCS link tends to decay over time as the CS is presented in the absence of the UCS (extinction). However, when a fear such as claustrophobia develops, this process of extinction is blocked because the person quickly learns the fear can be reduced or prevented by avoiding or escaping the CS that causes the CR. This avoidance behavior reduces anxiety in the short-term, but prevents extinction from occurring – thereby maintaining the phobia over time. Of course, learning history, personal belief systems, emotional processing, and other cognitive factors may be involved in the classical and operant conditioning of a phenomenon such as claustrophobia and contribute to the fear response [5,6].

Because CPAP requires the patient to breathe pressurized air through a nasal or full-face mask strapped to the head, it is not difficult to understand how this treatment can tap into fears of suffocation and restriction. In some patients, this therapy may elicit memories of the original UCS or set of circumstances that elicited the claustrophobic response to CPAP. For example, we have seen military veterans who report traumatic, near suffocation experiences while wearing gas masks during their military training. For them, CPAP elicits memories of such experiences, resulting in a phobic-like fear and avoidance of the CPAP device. In contrast, some patients appear to develop claustrophobic reactions de novo, specifically in response to an unpleasant experience while using CPAP. For example, some patients may awaken from sleep feeling as though they are not getting enough air from CPAP, and experience frightening feelings of suffocation. This anxiety reaction may be exacerbated by nasal congestion experienced either as a side effect of the CPAP or due to other causes (sinus problems, respiratory infections, etc.). Such experiences may serve as a "one-trial" classical conditioning paradigm that sets the stage for CPAP avoidance and consequent perpetuation of the anxiety via operant conditioning. In either case, such difficulties tend not to remit spontaneously, and require targeted intervention.

The treatment of choice for specific phobias, including claustrophobia, is exposure therapy [7]. Exposure therapy describes a variety of techniques wherein the phobic individual confronts the feared object or situation either imaginally or in real life (in vivo). Typically, a hierarchy of fearful situations ranging from least to most anxiety-provoking is generated by the individual. Under the guidance of a therapist, the individual is supported in experiencing these feared situations in a gradual manner, and over time the anxiety decreases. The effectiveness of exposure therapy stems from learning to tolerate and manage anxiety without the need to escape or avoid the phobic stimulus, thereby permitting extinction to occur. The emotional processing of the fear is facilitated by fear activation (exposure to the phobic stimulus) in the context of incompatible information that there is no negative outcome and the individual is safe [6]. In addition to reducing fear, exposure therapy increases the individual's perception of control over fear [8]. Exposure-based therapies, particularly in vivo exposure, produce robust and durable treatment effects for specific phobias [7,9].

Exposure therapy for CPAP emerged as a means of breaking the link between anxiety (triggered by CPAP as the CS) and the avoidance response [10]. A deconditioning process based on those used for specific phobias is employed so that CPAP loses it value as a CS for anxiety and avoidance. This goal is achieved through the gradual re-exposure of the patient to CPAP in a structured manner so as to extinguish the link between CPAP as the CS, and the UCS that led to the initial problematic response. Admittedly, this link is often a symbolic one in that CPAP was never associated with the original UCS but merely mimics it and elicits memories of it. Nonetheless, graded exposure to CPAP under therapeutic guidance helps eliminate this link and foster CPAP tolerance. Most likely, exposure therapy results in both a classical deconditioning of CPAP-related anxiety as well as significant subtle cognitive processing or reframing such that the CPAP device comes to be viewed as a safe, anxiety-free, and potentially rewarding activity.

STEP BY STEP DESCRIPTION OF PROCEDURES

Exposure therapy for CPAP-related claustrophobia is a short-term behavioral intervention that typically can be delivered effectively in one to six sessions over 1–3 months [10–12]. Because there is no scientific evidence delineating specific treatment components that yield the most effective outcomes, this section describes our typical clinical protocol which we have found to be successful with military veterans.

The components of each therapy session are outlined in Box 19.1. The purpose of the first session is not only to implement the exposure intervention, but also to conduct an assessment and clinical history, evaluate the patient's knowledge of sleep apnea and CPAP therapy, and cultivate the therapeutic

Box 19.1 Exposure Therapy Session Components

Initial Session (Session 1)

- Assessment and history
  - Claustrophobia
  - CPAP therapy
- Patient education on sleep apnea and CPAP therapy
- Build therapeutic rapport and trust
- Implementation of exposure therapy
  - Presentation of treatment rationale
  - Establish exposure hierarchy
  - Goal setting/homework

Follow up Sessions (Sessions 2–6)

- Assess adherence to homework
  - Monitor progress
    - Patient self-report
    - Objective CPAP data
- Problem-solve obstacles
- Conduct in-session exposure trial (if indicated)
- Provide feedback and support regarding CPAP use

relationship. The session typically begins with asking patients to describe their experiences with CPAP thus far, which renders information about their perception of the problem. Obtaining information on which elements of CPAP therapy (e.g., tolerating air pressure, having the mask on the face, having the mask strapped over the head) the patient finds most distressing is informative. An assessment of claustrophobia in other situations and the presence of other anxiety disorders assists in conceptualizing the problem. As part of the assessment, it may be useful to collect baseline measures of variables such as claustrophobia (see Chasens et al. [13] for adaptation of a claustrophobia questionnaire for use with apnea patients) or daytime sleep propensity (e.g., the Epworth Sleepiness Scale [14]) that can be used to monitor treatment progress. It is often helpful to assess patients' knowledge and understanding of both sleep apnea and CPAP therapy. This information can be used to correct any misunderstandings and foster motivation to engage in CPAP therapy.

The first step in implementing the exposure protocol is presenting the treatment rationale, which is arguably the most important step in ensuring the success of the exposure intervention. Most patients will present to treatment having already developed a strong association between the CPAP device and emotional distress (anxiety, claustrophobia), such that they are avoiding CPAP entirely and are reluctant to try the device again. We typically explain to patients that the purpose of treatment is to help them adapt to CPAP gradually through a series of "small steps" and practice. In this way, they can learn to overcome their discomfort with the device and use it successfully. Patients may benefit from both an understanding of how their CPAP intolerance developed and a "normalization" of their problem through an explanation that claustrophobic reactions to CPAP are common. They may be reassured to learn that their problem is treatable, and that they can reap the rewards of sleep apnea treatment.

Once the patient understands the treatment rationale and accepts the exposure intervention, the CPAP exposure steps are presented. We have developed a standard exposure therapy patient handout (Figure 19.1) that presents a hierarchy of steps from least anxiety-provoking to most. Although we have found this hierarchy to be sufficient for many patients, individualizing the protocol for some patients is indicated. To break the association between night-time attempts at using CPAP and claustrophobic reactions, we typically instruct patients to discontinue CPAP at bedtime during the initial stages of exposure treatment. Many patients are relieved by this instruction. In most cases, the exposure intervention itself can be enacted at home by the patient, per the patient handout. We emphasize regular daily CPAP practices in the home environment, starting with short periods of time (5–10 minutes) and gradually

The goal of these steps is to help you become more comfortable with CPAP while you are awake so that you can learn how to sleep easily with CPAP. For now, do not try wearing CPAP during sleep until you are comfortable with it during the daytime. If your machine has a RAMP button, you may use this function to keep the pressure at a low level during practices.

1. Turn the CPAP airflow ON. Hold mask over your nose, and practice breathing with machine on while awake. While you are doing this, keep your mouth closed and breathe regularly through your nose. Start with short periods of time (1–5 min) and gradually build up to longer periods of time.

2. Turn the CPAP airflow ON and wear the mask over your nose with the straps on your head. Practice breathing with CPAP on while awake. Wear CPAP for longer periods of time until you can have it on for 15–20 min comfortably.

3. Take a nap during the day with CPAP machine and mask on. It is not important whether you fall asleep or not – the goal is to rest comfortably in your bed with the CPAP on.

4. Wear CPAP at night when you go to sleep.

If you experience claustrophobia or uncomfortable feelings, go to previous step until comfortable. Then proceed to next step.

FIGURE 19.1 Sample patient handout describing exposure steps for home practice.

increasing length of practice (up to 20–30 minutes). Patients are instructed to cease practice if anxiety rises to an uncomfortable level. It may be helpful for patients to self-monitor their level of anxiety before and after practice sessions (see Zayfert and Becker [8] for a handout that can be used for this purpose). Patients are encouraged to proceed at their own pace and to reintroduce CPAP at bedtime only when they have increased their comfort with this device. Thus, the session concludes with a discussion of homework and goals regarding the home CPAP practice, along with an assessment of any obstacles or barriers to enacting the treatment recommendations at home. A follow-up session is scheduled for approximately 2 weeks to evaluate progress. CPAP machines are equipped with internal software that records CPAP use on a removable card, and patients are asked to bring this card to their next session in order to monitor progress.

Follow-up sessions provide an opportunity to evaluate progress, address problems, and conduct additional exposure therapy if needed. The session begins with a patient report of progress. Successes are reinforced through supportive comments, and obstacles are addressed as needed. The CPAP card is read during the session, which permits the patient to receive immediate feedback regarding treatment progress. Because the CPAP card displays the time of day and length of time CPAP was used, this information provides a direct and objective measurement of adherence to homework. Many patients who are practicing diligently with CPAP respond positively to seeing their efforts displayed on the CPAP report. When the CPAP report indicates that the patient engaged in CPAP exposure practices infrequently or not at all, the focus of the session becomes obstacles towards homework adherence. In some cases, the hierarchy may need to be modified or re-negotiated. Other individuals respond well to setting goals and rewards to improve adherence to home practice. For example, one patient set a goal of practicing with CPAP at home 5 days a week for 3 weeks. When this goal was met, he rewarded himself by dining at his favorite steakhouse.

If the patient continues to report claustrophobic reactions while using CPAP at home, or does not seem to be making progress through home practice, more intensive therapeutic guidance and an in-session exposure trial are indicated. The patient is asked to bring his or her CPAP equipment to the session. We have developed the custom of first asking patients to apply their CPAP as they do at home. This request evolved from our observations that, for some patients, "claustrophobia" is caused by an incorrectly applied or fitted mask. We have seen patients who, despite receiving CPAP training from our nursing staff and a home care company, were applying the mask upside down or adjusting the straps incorrectly. Correcting these errors in mask application resolved the claustrophobia. Along these same lines, claustrophobia can sometimes be ameliorated by trying an alternative mask style, and this observation bespeaks the importance of close follow-up by an experienced treatment team to resolve such problems expediently.

We begin the in-session exposure trial with the patient seated in a chair. Many patients report increased feelings of claustrophobia while reclined in bed compared to sitting, probably in part due to obesity-related breathing restriction in a supine position. By explaining each step of the procedure at the outset, the therapist engenders the patient's trust and confidence. When exposure therapy is used for other anxiety disorders, the importance of the therapeutic relationship is well-recognized [8,15]. It is also critical that the patient maintain a sense of control during the exposure process [8,15]. To this end, we permit the patient to hold and remove the mask during the entire procedure and demonstrate how to remove the mask quickly if needed. Adjustments to mask fit are made only after the patient gives permission to be touched. Depending on the degree of CPAP-related claustrophobia, the patient will be asked to start at a level that induces anxiety at a tolerable level. For some individuals, this may be as brief as holding the mask over their nose for a few seconds at a time at the lowest pressure of 4 cm/H_2O (as per manufacturers' guidelines, we never ask patients to wear the CPAP mask unless the air pressure is on). The patient is encouraged to keep the mask in place until the anxiety subsides. Asking the patient to rate his or her anxiety level on a scale of 0–100 provides a method of measuring anxiety levels during the session. The patient sets the pace and progresses through the additional hierarchy steps during the same or subsequent sessions. Because we provide the exposure therapy in the context of a sleep laboratory, we have the advantage of also observing the patient using CPAP while reclined on a bed. With sufficient exposure, it is not unusual for the patient to fall asleep during a session. As the patient becomes increasingly comfortable with CPAP, it is important to increase tolerance of the CPAP pressure to the therapeutic level. In-session successes are strongly reinforced through verbal feedback from the therapist. Patients are often surprised at their progress, and develop a sense of confidence, mastery, and self-efficacy.

One of the risks of exposure therapy is creating an increase in anxiety symptoms if the exposure proceeds too quickly [8,16]. Although CPAP exposure is by design an uncomfortable process for the patient, our patients have not reported any adverse outcomes thus far. This observation may be attributable to the fact that patients exert total control over their level of CPAP exposure. Additionally, it is possible that patients for whom the anxiety level was too uncomfortable dropped out of treatment altogether. Although we have observed treatment successes with challenging patients, exposure therapy requires patients to be motivated and committed.

Once patients complete the exposure protocol and are using CPAP at home successfully, they may find it easier to maintain successful CPAP use with ongoing support and feedback about their increasing CPAP use provided by the device's internal adherence monitoring software. Follow-up visits may be spaced at increasing intervals (e.g., 3 months, 6 months, 12 months), or as needed.

POSSIBLE MODIFICATIONS/VARIANTS

There is a variety of modifications and variants that may increase treatment success for certain individuals. Alternative exposure protocols for adults [11] and children [17,18] have been published. The CPAP exposure protocol also can be modified and implemented prophylactically to prevent anticipated claustrophobia. For example, prior to the diagnosis of sleep apnea, some patients express a concern about being able to tolerate CPAP on the night of their sleep study. These individuals often benefit from the opportunity to try CPAP gradually before their sleep study. In addition, we have employed the exposure treatment successfully with other types of positive airway pressure delivery systems (e.g., auto-CPAP, BiPAP, etc.). Although we routinely prescribe home CPAP practice, this may not be necessary for treatment success if exposure is conducted in session [11].

The implementation of relaxation training may be indicated for patients who are unable to reduce their level of anxiety sufficiently during the exposure protocol. In such cases, it may be beneficial to cultivate relaxation through therapeutic techniques such as relaxation training, visualization, or deep breathing prior to initiating the exposure therapy. Once the patient becomes adept at relaxing, the exposure therapy can be initiated. This technique can help patients learn how to manage anxiety and use CPAP while in a relaxed state.

A number of additional therapeutic strategies may enhance the exposure treatment. As an adjunctive intervention, cognitive-behavioral therapy techniques can be useful both in challenging patient beliefs or thoughts that may be interfering with the exposure therapy and in helping the patient develop positive coping statements [8,11]. As an example, many claustrophobic patients, upon applying CPAP, think, "I can't breathe. I am suffocating." Helping the patient recognize this automatic thought and substitute it with a helpful thought (such as, "I can breathe easily and freely with CPAP") can reduce anxiety. Because exposure therapy involves discomfort to the patient, difficulties with adherence, attendance, and motivation should be anticipated. Such problems can be addressed through direct therapeutic discussion, or other techniques such as behavioral contracts, goal setting, or the use of rewards.

PROOF OF CONCEPT/SUPPORTING DATA/EVIDENCE BASE

Claustrophobia is a commonly reported side effect of CPAP therapy, and may lead to treatment abandonment. Almost one-third of sleep apnea patients endorse CPAP-related claustrophobia [13,19]. In a large sample of newly diagnosed sleep apnea patients, CPAP-related claustrophobia was perceived as one of the largest deterrents to CPAP therapy, with less than half of patients reporting that they would use CPAP if they felt claustrophobic [20]. Kribbs and colleagues [19] assessed side effects of CPAP therapy and discovered that claustrophobia was the only side effect that discriminated CPAP adherence;

low CPAP adherers were more likely to report problems with claustrophobia than high adherers. Similarly, Chasens et al. [13] found that sleep apnea patients recruited from multiple North American sleep centers were more than twice as likely to have low CPAP adherence if they scored high on a claustrophobia questionnaire. Interestingly, claustrophobia scores decreased over the 3-month treatment period, which, the authors note, may reflect a naturalistic exposure to CPAP.

To date, there have been no randomized controlled trials of exposure therapy targeting CPAP-related anxiety. However, the utility of this intervention is suggested by individual case studies [10,11] and case series reports [12,21]. In our retrospective case series study [12], patients with CPAP-related claustrophobia attended between one and six exposure sessions with a behavioral sleep psychologist. At post-treatment (an average of 15 weeks after the final therapy session), patients used CPAP on a greater percentage of nights and for more hours per night compared to pre-treatment. Effect size calculations for CPAP adherence variables revealed a large effect of treatment. Furthermore, neither patient characteristics, nor number of treatment sessions, nor length of the follow-up period predicted exposure treatment response.

The individual case studies mentioned above provide a glimmer of optimism that treatment gains endure long term, both at 6 months [10,11] and 6 years after treatment of CPAP-related claustrophobia [10]. Unfortunately, these case studies relied on patient self-report of CPAP use, which notoriously overestimates objectively measured adherence.

For pediatric sleep apnea patients, graded exposure techniques incorporated as part of a behavioral treatment package have shown promise in promoting CPAP acceptance and adherence, even for children with developmental delay and/or cognitive impairment [17,18]. In these studies, however, it is impossible to disentangle the influence of the exposure technique per se from the other behavioral package components.

CPAP exposure therapy is a promising intervention that is both clinically appealing and easy to implement. However, this intervention is lacking rigorous scientific evaluation; the overall state of the research support is weak, suffering from uncontrolled trials and small sample sizes. Future studies with randomized controlled trials, larger sample sizes, objective measures of CPAP adherence, and long-term outcomes are needed. Studies would also benefit from formalizing the diagnosis of CPAP-related claustrophobia, standardizing measures of claustrophobia, and further investigating treatment drop-outs and predictors of outcome. Additionally, the extant published reports have used an in vivo exposure protocol without the use of relaxation [10–12]. Thus, it remains to be determined whether the addition of relaxation training improves outcomes, at least for some individuals. Measures of treatment enactment are needed to assess adherence to assigned home practice, and its influence on outcome. Finally, there is virtually no information on whether gender or other demographic variables influence treatment response. Despite these limitations,

CPAP-related exposure therapy has become a routine part of our clinical sleep services due to its high demand and rewarding clinical outcomes.

REFERENCES

[1] W.F. Flack Jr., B.T. Litz, T.M. Keane, Cognitive-behavioral treatment of war-zone-related posttraumatic stress disorder: a flexible, hierarchical approach, in: V.M. Follette, J. Ruzek, R.F. Abueg (Eds.), Cognitive-Behavioral Therapies for Trauma, Guilford Press, New York, NY, 1998, pp. 77–99.

[2] S. Rachman, S. Taylor, Analyses of claustrophobia, J. Anxiety Disord. 7 (4) (1993) 281–291.

[3] O.H. Mowrer, Learning Theory and Behavior, John Wiley, New York, NY, 1960.

[4] I.P. Pavlov, Lectures on Conditioned Reflexes, International Publishers, New York, NY, 1928.

[5] B.J. Cox, S. Taylor, Anxiety disorders: Panic and phobias, in: T. Millon, P.H. Blaney, R.D. Davis (Eds.), Oxford Textbook of Psychopathology, Oxford University Press, New York, NY, 1999.

[6] E.B. Foa, M.J. Kozak, Emotional processing of fear: Exposure to corrective information, Psychol. Bull. 99 (1986) 20–35.

[7] K.B. Wolitzky-Taylor, J.D. Horowitz, M.B. Powers, M.J. Telch, Psychological approaches in the treatment of specific phobias: a meta-analysis, Clin. Psychol. Rev. 28 (6) (2008) 1021–1037.

[8] C. Zayfert, C.B. Becker, Cognitive-Behavioral Therapy for PTSD: A Case Formulation Approach, Guilford Press, New York, NY, 2007.

[9] Y. Choy, A.J. Fyer, J.D. Lipsitz, Treatment of specific phobia in adults, Clin. Psychol. Rev. 27 (3) (2007) 266–286.

[10] J.D. Edinger, RA. Radtke, Use of in vivo desensitization to treat a patient's claustrophobic response to nasal CPAP. Sleep, J. Sleep Res. Sleep Med. 16 (7) (1993) 678–680.

[11] C.S. McCrae, P.T. Ingmundson, Using graduated in vivo exposure to treat a claustrophobic response to nasal continuous positive airway pressure: Hispanic male veteran associates nasal mask with gas masks worn during combat, Clin. Case Stud. 5 (1) (2006) 71–82.

[12] M.K. Means, J.D. Edinger, Graded exposure therapy for addressing claustrophobic reactions to continuous positive airway pressure: a case series report, Behav. Sleep Med. 5 (2) (2007) 105–116.

[13] E.R. Chasens, A.I. Pack, G. Maislin, et al., Claustrophobia and adherence to CPAP treatment, Western J. Nurs. Res. 27 (3) (2005) 307–321.

[14] M.W. Johns, A new method for measuring daytime sleepiness: The Epworth Sleepiness Scale, Sleep 14 (1991) 540–545.

[15] R. Noyes Jr., R. Hoehn-Saric, The Anxiety Disorders, Cambridge University Press, New York, NY, 1998.

[16] J.H. Jaycox, E.B. Foa, Obstacles in implementing exposure therapy for PTSD: Case discussions and practical solutions, Clin. Psychol. Psychother. 1996 (3) (1996) 176–184.

[17] K.L. Koontz, K.J. Slifer, M.D. Cataldo, C.L. Marcus, Improving pediatric compliance with positive airway pressure therapy: the impact of behavioral intervention, Sleep 26 (8) (2003) 1010–1015.

[18] J.C. Rains, Treatment of obstructive sleep apnea in pediatric patients: Behavioral intervention for compliance with nasal continuous positive airway pressure, Clin. Pediatr. 34 (10) (1995) 535–541.

[19] N.B. Kribbs, A.I. Pack, L.R. Kline, et al., Objective measurement of patterns of nasal CPAP use by patients with obstructive sleep apnea, Am. Rev. Respir. Dis. 147 (4) (1993) 887–895.

[20] T.E. Weaver, G. Maislin, D.F. Dinges, et al., Self-efficacy in sleep apnea: Instrument development and patient perceptions of obstructive sleep apnea risk, treatment benefit, and volition to use continuous positive airway pressure, Sleep 26 (6) (2003) 727–732.

[21] I. Casas, M.D. de la Calzada, M. Guitart, A. Roca, Diagnosis and treatment of the phobia due to treatment with air using nasal continuous pressure, Revista de Neurologia 30 (6) (2000) 593–596.

RECOMMENDED READING

E.R. Chasens, A.I. Pack, G. Maislin, et al., Claustrophobia and adherence to CPAP treatment, Western J. Nurs. Res. 27 (3) (2005) 307–321.

K.L. Koontz, K.J. Slifer, M.D. Cataldo, C.L. Marcus, Improving pediatric compliance with positive airway pressure therapy: The impact of behavioral intervention, Sleep 26 (8) (2003) 1010–1015.

C.S. McCrae, P.T. Ingmundson, Using graduated *in vivo* exposure to treat a claustrophobic response to nasal continuous positive airway pressure: Hispanic male veteran associates nasal mask with gas masks worn during combat, Clin. Case Stud. 5 (1) (2006) 71–82.

M.K. Means, J.D. Edinger, Graded exposure therapy for addressing claustrophobic reactions to continuous positive airway pressure: A case series report, Behav. Sleep Med. 5 (2) (2007) 105–116.

Chapter 20

Sleep Apnea Self-Management Program

Carl Stepnowsky
University of California, San Diego, CA
VA San Diego Healthcare System, San Diego, CA

PROTOCOL NAME

Sleep apnea self-management program.

GROSS INDICATION

This program is indicated for patients with Obstructive Sleep Apnea (OSA) who are prescribed Continuous Positive Airway Pressure (CPAP) therapy.

SPECIFIC INDICATION

The Sleep Apnea Self-Management Program (SASMP) was designed to be incorporated into existing clinical care processes, particularly ones that include both diagnostic and treatment initialization services. SASMP provides basic education about diagnostic testing, sleep apnea, and CPAP therapy.

CONTRAINDICATIONS

Because of its focus on providing basic education about sleep testing, sleep apnea, and CPAP therapy, the SASMP in its current format does not provide a specific intervention related to claustrophobia. The reader is referred to a systematic desensitization protocol for those patients with clinically significant claustrophobia related to CPAP therapy.

RATIONALE FOR INTERVENTION

Treating OSA as a Chronic Disease

The acute and the chronic illness models each emphasize different characteristics in the conceptualization of disease [1]. Acute illness is typically

Behavioral Treatments for Sleep Disorders. DOI: 10.1016/B978-0-12-381522-4.00020-1

characterized by abrupt or rapid onset, limited duration, a predominant cause (usually), a commonly accurate diagnosis and prognosis, and a high cure rate. In contrast, chronic illness is typically characterized by gradual onset, lengthy or indefinite duration, multivariate causation (which may change over time), and a focus on functional status rather than individual diagnoses. In addition, cure of chronic illness is unlikely, and long-term management of symptoms and disease consequences is often necessary. Historically, OSA has been treated as an acute illness, as evidenced by interventions developed in an attempt to "cure" OSA through interventions that alter the anatomy of the airway through surgery, oral appliances, and even medications. However, OSA would be better characterized as a chronic illness, based on its disease characteristics.

CPAP has emerged as the most effective form of therapy for OSA, but, unlike previous "curative" treatments, CPAP therapy is designed to *manage* apnea, not to cure it. CPAP is an aid that must be worn throughout each night in order to provide maximal benefit. OSA is a chronic illness that can often be managed by the affected patient on a night-to-night basis. As such, OSA is an excellent target for behavioral intervention to improve long-term self-management.

What is Chronic Disease Self-Management?

Because CPAP can be considered, in part, a behavioral intervention that requires self-management, the large literature on chronic disease self-management provides guidance for developing behavioral approaches for OSA patients. Self-management can be defined broadly as a systematic behavioral approach to help patients with chronic conditions participate actively in self-monitoring of symptoms or physiologic processes, decision-making (i.e., managing the disease or its impact, based on self-monitoring), and problem-solving [2]. Chronic disease self-management programs primarily focus on three content areas: (1) disease, medication, and health management; (2) role management; and (3) emotional management [3].

Why Implement a Self-Management Program for Sleep Apnea Patients?

There are a number of reasons why a self-management approach might be appropriate for OSA patients who are prescribed CPAP therapy. First, qualitative research has demonstrated that OSA affects multiple aspects of an individual's health-related quality of life, including (1) managing OSA symptoms, CPAP side effects, and weight loss (i.e., health management); (2) maintaining work performance, social contacts, and family relationships (i.e., role management); and (3) dealing with symptoms of depression and anxiety (i.e., emotional management) [4–7]. The similarities between the problems reported by OSA patients and the content areas of the self-management approach are remarkable. Using qualitative methods such as focus groups and discourse analysis, these studies repeatedly show that one of the core issues with which the sleep apnea patient must contend is problem-solving (i.e., how best to manage problems within each of the content areas) [6]. Thus, one of the core features of self-management programs is problem-solving.

Second, self-management programs are conducted in a group format and can utilize lay leaders, thereby potentially augmenting pre-existing clinical and support services. Limited health care resources often prevent patients from receiving optimal follow-up care. Patients who participate in the self-management group can spend maximal time and effort learning new skills and building confidence to manage their condition – time that health care professionals cannot efficiently spend with patients in typical clinical settings. In a sense, the group self-management approach attempts to cost-efficiently "intensify" clinical support and follow-up for sleep apnea patients.

A self-management approach appears to be well suited as an alternative method for helping to introduce CPAP therapy to the OSA patient. The SASMP was developed based on the original Chronic Disease Self-Management Program (CDSMP) [8], and is considered a disease-specific self-management program.

STEP BY STEP DESCRIPTION OF PROCEDURES

Background

Physical Setting and Presentation Type

SASMP is best delivered in a comfortable conference room with adequate lighting and seating. An overhead projector connected to a computer with CPAP software is an ideal way to present the material in an electronic format. While it is not necessary to implement SASMP using electronic audio-visual equipment, this was the format in which it was initially evaluated. The original CDSMP was quite successful without the use of electronic audio-visual equipment. Each site will have to consider the resources available to them, and the needs of their audience. For a more detailed discussion of presentation options, please see the section below on audio-visual presentation variants.

The room and number of chairs should be able to accommodate the anticipated number of patients and their spouses or significant others who help support their medical issues. The table should be of sufficient size to hold a CPAP unit and its accessories for each patient. In addition, the room should be outfitted with enough electrical power strips to accommodate the expected number of CPAP units, preferably with the strips located on the top of the table for ease of use.

Group Size

Ideally, groups are run with a minimum of three patients and a maximum of six patients. Because SASMP was designed to include instruction on sleep diagnostic studies as well as initial CPAP set-up, groups larger than six become unwieldy and lose their effectiveness when performed with only one leader. Please see the section below on possible modifications/variants for more information. Group sessions with two patients can be run, but they tend to lose the peer support aspect that comes from slightly larger groups.

Number and Timing of Sessions

The SASMP consists of four weekly sessions of about 1–2 hours each, depending on the session and the make-up of the group. We initially considered a timing schedule that allowed for increasing the time between sessions, but we found that (1) patients' attendance decreased as the sessions progressed, and (2) patients said that they needed the follow-up sessions to occur earlier in the treatment initialization process. Therefore, we designed the program to comprise four weekly sessions. One variation to consider when designing the program is the timing and content of the first session. As group members are first introduced to home sleep testing and basic education about sleep apnea during Session 1, scheduling the second session only a week after the first requires rapid sleep scoring, and is not practical for labs unable to provide this service. Whether or not to allow for more time between Sessions 1 and 2 will vary based on the needs of the end-user. We found it best to conduct Session 2 (CPAP set-up) and the two follow-up sessions using 1-week time intervals.

SASMP Sessions

Session 1: Sleep Apnea and Sleep Testing

Session 1 is focused on introducing sleep apnea and home sleep testing. Sleep apnea is introduced via a 7-minute video, followed by a short question and answer session. Because this program was designed to be used in a setting that utilizes home sleep testing, the majority of the time for this session is spent discussing the specifics of the home sleep equipment, including a description of the equipment used, its justification and purpose, and how to use it. Time is also spent discussing what will happen next in terms of sleep study scoring, and the phone call that patients will receive with the results of their sleep studies. At this point, patients are undiagnosed. The next three sessions will be dedicated to those patients who are diagnosed with sleep apnea and prescribed CPAP therapy.

Session 2: Getting Started on CPAP Therapy

The agenda for Session 2 includes a general review of sleep apnea and of sleep apnea as a chronic disease, followed by an introduction to self-management and a review of CPAP therapy.

Review of Sleep Apnea

This module comprises a review of sleep apnea and its consequences. It begins with a definition and discussion of apnea and hypopneic events, and includes a short video (90 seconds) of a patient who is experiencing several apneic events while undergoing a sleep study. The goal of the video is to show the patients what sleep apnea looks and sounds like. While the bed partners can often describe sleep apnea in great detail, we found that it is very rare for an OSA patient to be familiar with the symptoms of the disease. While one variation on this would be to include a component of the patient being videotaped (or audiotaped) to help personalize this experience, the time and effort for such an endeavor is usually outside the scope of a program designed to have wide applicability.

Next is a module on sleep study results. This module begins with an explanation of how a sleep study is scored, including sharing screenshots from an actual study. The calculation and interpretation of the Apnea-Hypopnea Index (AHI) follows, and includes a review of commonly used AHI thresholds. This module provides patients with a good understanding of this metric, allowing them to better track their progress on CPAP. We have found that a patient having this knowledge is critical to fostering collaborative decision-making between patient and provider.

The last topic included in the sleep apnea review is a recap of common OSA symptoms, divided into night-time and daytime symptoms to emphasize the potential effect that OSA has on patients' lives. It is helpful to discuss each group member's symptoms as a way of personalizing the symptoms and aiding understanding of the effect of those symptoms on quality of life and functioning. Through such discussion, participants gain understanding of common OSA symptoms, which helps them to better track and assess changes in their own symptoms during CPAP therapy.

Concluding with a question and answer period for any remaining questions and comments about the material covered so far in the session provides an opportunity for those who may not have been engaged previously to more easily participate. Because this program is conducted in group format, group dynamic issues often arise – for example, how to handle patients who may dominate the conversation, who choose not to participate (and what strategies may help encourage participation), and who may detract from the group process (e.g., question the existence of sleep apnea; question the validity of treatment). It should be noted here that patients are not required to participate, and that individual decisions on extent of participation are respected. For patients who may want to dominate the conversation, providers are given instruction on group-leading techniques that can be helpful.

Sleep Apnea as a Chronic Disease

The next module in Session 2 covers sleep apnea as a chronic disease. The key characteristics of acute and chronic diseases are discussed. Typically, to make the distinction between acute and chronic disease more striking, a broken arm or leg is used as an example of an acute disease in contrast to chronic disease. This module is included to help answer many of the common questions about sleep apnea (e.g., How long have I had it? How long do I need to use CPAP? What other treatments are available? Why isn't there a pill or medication I can take for sleep apnea?) We also include this module to lay the foundation for how the patients might consider approaching their sleep apnea care, as well as any other chronic conditions they may have. It is quite common for sleep apnea patients to have hypertension, diabetes, or other chronic conditions.

Sleep Apnea Self-Management

The third section of Session 2 builds upon the previous section, which provided participants with an approach to chronic disease management, emphasizing their active participation and a collaborative relationship with their provider in making treatment decisions. The following keys to successful sleep apnea self-management are discussed: (1) understanding sleep apnea; (2) understanding how CPAP manages sleep apnea on a nightly basis; (3) the importance of troubleshooting problems with CPAP therapy, such as monitoring symptoms and working collaboratively with the healthcare team; and (4) increasing the benefits while reducing the problems of using CPAP. This last point is discussed openly and honestly. We have found that overemphasizing CPAP therapy's potential benefits without adequately discussing the difficulty of using CPAP can set unrealistically high expectations, potentially resulting in treatment failure. This point is crucial. Because the goal is to help patients to get to an adequate CPAP use level, we have found patients have the best chance for success when they are able to anticipate common problems and know how to handle those problems. We have a tool to measure this called the Decisional Balance Index, which is a relative weighting of the pros and cons of using CPAP. Earlier research has shown that, to the extent that pros outweigh the cons, CPAP is used more. While there is no "magic bullet" to treatment adherence for CPAP or any other medical treatment, we have found the Decisional Balance Index to be a very useful tool for monitoring progress.

To emphasize the potential benefits of CPAP, we next discuss the sleep apnea symptom cycle, using an interactive graphic (see Figure 20.1) that shows how sleep apnea can lead to disrupted, non-restorative sleep, which can then lead to a whole host of consequences such as sleepiness/low energy, anger/frustration/irritability, depressive symptoms, stress/anxiety, weight gain, and back around to increased sleep apnea levels. We emphasize that this chain is meant to illustrate the cycle that is common to sleep apnea sufferers. It is also important to note that this symptom cycle can "downward spiral", and patients may experience some portion of it at some time in their lives. We also talk about the timeframe during which patients may have experienced sleep apnea, with some participants discussing how they may have been affected since childhood, while others experience few or no symptoms until adulthood.

Next is a graphic showing how this "downward spiral" of symptoms may be reversed with treatment of OSA. We discuss how the key to successful treatment is a significant reduction in the number of apneas and hypopneas each

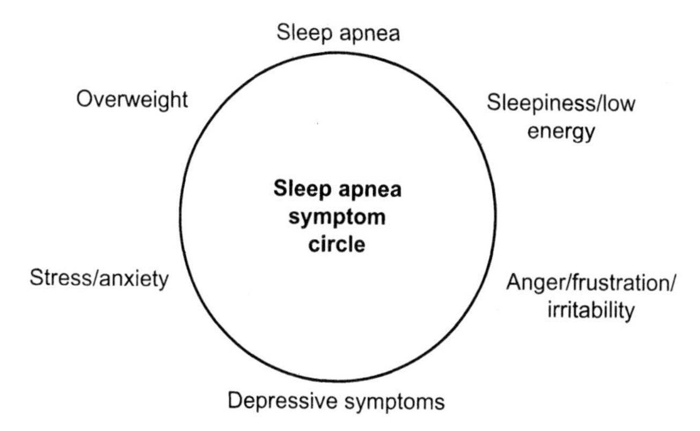

FIGURE 20.1 Symptom Cycle Graphic.

night to within a normal range. We re-emphasize the idea that the goal of CPAP therapy is to help get below 10 events per hour, and ideally to less than 5 per hour of sleep, per CPAP metrics. We then describe several positive changes in symptoms that are likely relevant to patients' lives, including moving from daytime sleepiness to daytime alertness; from being irritable to being more calm; from having morning headaches to not having them; from having difficulty with concentration to being more focused; from having hypertension to perhaps having reduced need for medications; and generally from having reduced quality of life to improved quality of life. Along with this discussion of the hope and benefits of CPAP therapy, it is important to acknowledge that the range of perceived benefit varies. Some patients experience a relatively dramatic effect in the first several days of CPAP therapy, for others it may take weeks or months, and some may never experience notable benefit. Another key point to make is that CPAP can only help with sleep apnea and the problems that sleep apnea causes. Patients may have other significant medical issues that make it difficult to experience the described benefits of successfully treating OSA. However, it will be important to track the benefits perceived so that patients can make the best decision about whether to continue with CPAP therapy.

The program then transitions from review and discussion of OSA to the "how" of CPAP therapy and symptom management. The "how" points out that sleep apnea management includes three steps: (1) using CPAP every night as prescribed, (2) engaging in good sleep hygiene, and (3) considering making health behavior changes, including dietary changes and increasing physical activity. The "how" of using CPAP is discussed more fully in the next module, when we introduce and provide instruction on using the CPAP equipment. Engaging in good sleep hygiene is then reviewed (see Chapter 3 for more in-depth discussion of how sleep hygiene issues may be approached). Within the context of SASMP, we emphasize those factors that are applicable to OSA patients. The goal is to lay the foundation for the next session, in which we will talk about those sleep hygiene recommendations each patient may want to integrate into his or her care plan.

CPAP Introduction and Instruction

The first module included in this section of Session 2 is a review of what happens to the airway when snoring, when having an apneic event, and when breathing normally. It is shown that CPAP provides continuous positive airway pressure, and effectively works as an airway "splint" to hold the airway open at night while breathing. To help emphasize the uniqueness of the positive airway pressure mechanism of action, the group engages in discussion about the throat being multi-functional (e.g., for breathing, eating, and talking). No other treatment currently exists that matches the effectiveness of positive airway pressure therapy. Patients are then shown an interactive diagram of CPAP working to emphasize its effectiveness in holding the airway open, as well as to introduce the components of CPAP therapy.

The next module focuses on the specifics of CPAP therapy. The first topic covers what is considered the correct "dose" of therapy, and includes a discussion of pressure versus time on therapy. How to obtain the appropriate pressure is also explained, as is the possibility that air pressure may need to be adjusted up or down, depending on a number of factors. Time on therapy is covered both as (1) how CPAP is prescribed (i.e., to be used all night, every night, including naps) and (2) the ideal use level (i.e., that which results in clinically important changes). We then discuss the full range of schedules used to get patients started on CPAP, from those individuals who are able to use CPAP all night, every night, to those who use a tapered, gradual schedule. We emphasize the importance of not getting frustrated when problems happen, and that it is often a 2- to 3-week process for most patients. We note that it is important to keep an eye out for any problems or issues related to the mask/interface, head straps, and air leakages.

The next topic, the specifics of CPAP therapy, is presented using a slide on working with the healthcare team. The "Take PART" message is utilized, and is based on the idea of (1) preparing a written list of concerns and questions for each visit or interaction with their provider, (2) asking any relevant questions, (3) repeating back any key points so any potential miscommunications can be corrected, and (4) taking action [9].

During the final part of this session, the actual CPAP set-up is explained, after which each patient is fitted for a mask, and the group learns how to use and care for their CPAP units.

Session 3: First Week on CPAP Therapy

The agenda for Session 3 includes sleep apnea self-management, review of the patients' experiences during their first week on CPAP (benefits and problems experienced), and problem-solving, fatigue management, and action planning.

To provide a framework under which the program and session are operating, the keys to sleep apnea self-management are reviewed: (1) understanding sleep apnea; (2) understanding how CPAP manages sleep apnea on a nightly basis; (3) the importance of troubleshooting problems with CPAP therapy, such as monitoring symptoms and working collaboratively with the healthcare team; and (4) increasing the benefits of, while reducing the problems associated with, using CPAP.

The session immediately moves to a review of what benefits patients may have experienced during the first week. Whether using a PowerPoint presentation or a flip-chart, an ongoing list of benefits is written down so that all group members can see them and add to them. It is not uncommon to get a fairly sizable list after only 1 week of therapy, including such items as "more rested", "no need to sleep in", "fewer headaches", "more energy during the day", and "fewer bathroom trips at night".

The next step is to review the problems that patients experienced, once again using a list to keep track of the items offered by the group members.

Once a list of the group's problems with CPAP is made, the next step is to begin the process of problem-solving. The leader reviews the concept of problem-solving, and gives some examples that are encountered in everyday life. Then the leader makes the transition to discussing problem-solving for sleep apnea patients specifically, and for managing chronic illnesses in general. Table 20.1 provides the problem-solving steps. This discussion is followed by an exercise during which each participant reports on how much he or she is using CPAP. Each patient then describes one key problem he or she would like the group's help in solving. This format is used because patient-generated topics tend to be more relevant to the group.

Once the group members discuss their specific CPAP and sleep apnea problems, and possible solutions, the rest of the session is dedicated to reviewing their action plans and then discussing strategies for managing fatigue and sleepiness, as well as weight management and sleep apnea.

TABLE 20.1 Problem-Solving Steps

Identify the problem
List ideas to solve the problem
Select one method to try
Assess the results
Substitute another idea (if the first didn't work)
Utilize other resources
If need be, accept that the problem may not be solvable now

Because sleepiness is so common in this patient group, the program spends considerable time talking about its various causes, how to identify it, how to track it over time, and, finally, ways to deal with it.

The next topic, weight management, is relevant to a substantial number of sleep apnea patients. The group reviews the link between weight and sleep apnea, and the potential benefit of weight loss on OSA. If patients are interested in pursuing weight management, they are encouraged to talk to their providers about developing a plan. A general introduction to, and discussion of, the role weight management plays in SASMP follows, but is not pursued for individual patients as part of this program.

The final topic for Session 3 is action planning. Action planning is a behavioral technique that allows participants to write down a specific action that can be realistically accomplished within a short time period, often 1 week. Such planning is performed in the same way as described by the CDSMP [9]. There are several key characteristics to action planning: (1) the chosen action needs to be something the individual *wants* to do, (2) the action needs to be reasonable or doable, and lastly, (3) the action needs to address a behavior (i.e., something you do, such as exercising more) and not a goal (i.e., lower weight). Ideally, the chosen behavior is closely related to OSA management, but it does not have to be. A key feature of action planning is that it helps to build confidence that the patients can take actions and thereby build self-efficacy. A behavior is something that can be responsive to the following questions: What? How often? How much? When? Walking is a good example of a behavior, as it can provide answers to those four questions.

Leaders provide an action-planning handout to group members so they can write down their individual plans. Once the leader reviews and leads the group through a sample plan, a volunteer is asked to present his or her own idea for an action plan. The group can offer suggestions to help refine the plan. Once the first individual goes through his or her plan, the leader goes around the table so that the other members can verbalize their own action plans.

Session 4: Second Week on CPAP Therapy

The agenda for Session 3 includes feedback/problem-solving; review of first 2 weeks on CPAP (benefits and problems experienced); CPAP download review; action-planning and problem-solving; and looking back and planning for the future.

The fourth and final session begins with tasks similar to those in Session 3, starting with a review of the benefits that the group members experienced and then listing these benefits. As in the previous session, group members generate this list via brainstorming. In addition, some discussion of each problem is appropriate, especially if it helps the individuals to better understand how treating sleep apnea helps their daily functioning. For example, improved recall of dreams might be indicative of more REM sleep, so the point might be made that this is a sign that the patient is experiencing fewer breathing events while sleeping, resulting in less disruption to sleep and greater ability to experience deeper levels of sleep. If the leader saved the benefit list from last week, sometimes it is useful to compare the two lists to show that more benefits were obtained after another week on CPAP therapy. Then, as in the previous week's session, the group generates a list of the problems they experienced with CPAP. This list can also be compared to the previous week's list.

The next module is focused on *CPAP data download review*. This requires some pre-planning on the part of the group leader, as he or she needs to decide whether to use PowerPoint or a handout. If using PowerPoint, the appropriate equipment should be available in the meeting room. If using handouts, they should be printed out prior to the meeting. Regardless of the method, individual members should be asked to volunteer to share personal data with the group if they are comfortable doing so. It should be emphasized that this is completely voluntary. Our experience has been that, by this point, the group members have usually developed a rapport with each other, and most do agree to share their data. Key points to review with the group members concerning their downloaded data include help with interpretation of the key data values, such as amount and timing of use, apnea-hypopnea index, and amount of mask leak. The goal of such discussion is to foster better understanding of how well CPAP is working for each group member, and what can be done to help improve CPAP for each person.

Once the download review is done, the program moves back to troubleshooting and problem-solving of any outstanding problems. Oftentimes, this is already done in the context of the download review. However, this review presents another opportunity for group members to gain further assistance with any residual problems they may be having. These final two sessions are geared toward helping patients overcome any problems with using CPAP, because even when things are going well, most patients tend to benefit from further guidance and instruction on their CPAP therapy. While CPAP appears to be a straightforward therapy, with the advent of new features (e.g., variants on pressure settings, humidification, auto-start for airflow, pressure ramping), it takes time and effort to help the patients find the settings that work best for them.

The session then moves away from the specific details of sleep apnea and CPAP therapy, and goes back to the larger picture. Reviewing the larger goals of SASMP helps foster group members' self-management skills. We review the three main tasks of self-management: (1) taking care of health problems, (2) carrying out normal activities, and (3) managing any emotional changes that may occur. The group discusses how, for sleep apnea patients, these changes tend to occur slowly over time, and that with CPAP therapy, the hope is that patients' activities that have been reduced or stopped can slowly be increased as time goes on. The group then reviews the symptom cycle, and offers hope that CPAP can begin to reverse the downward spiral. The importance of working collaboratively with sleep providers, as well as maintaining contact, is emphasized.

The last module concerns *looking back and planning for the future.* By this point in the program, most group members have a good understanding of sleep apnea, how it affects their lives, how CPAP works, and how they can best use CPAP to manage their sleep apnea. We ask them what their goals are for their health, and what steps they would like to take to achieve those goals. They are asked to consider what other aspects of their health and life they would like to begin to address. The action plans from the previous session are reviewed, and action planning is offered as but one method they can use to help achieve behavior change.

POSSIBLE MODIFICATIONS/VARIANTS

Audio-Visual Presentations: Electronic vs Non-electronic

While the original SASMP intervention utilized electronic audio-visual presentations, one variation that might be necessary for some groups is to use paper. This is possible if the following changes are made. Patient handouts can be printed and provided as a replacement for the PowerPoint slides. For important concepts, the original Chronic Disease Self-Management Program relied on large-sized paper flip-charts and black marker. Finally, patient-specific CPAP download data can be provided to the group members in paper format as well.

Group Size

As stated in the previous section, our experience has been that SASMP is best conducted with a minimum of three patients and a maximum of six patients. The group can be done with fewer, but group peer support is reduced. We have found, as have other group medical sessions, that the peer support is a valuable aspect of this intervention. Given that CPAP instruction becomes unwieldy, groups are limited to six or less. One variation that may be novel is to split Session 2 into two groups, and then bring all of the follow-up members together for Sessions 3 and 4. While the numbers may approach 12 (and higher if spouses or significant others are included), the clear benefit is a large patient-to-provider ratio. We have found that, on follow-up, there are many questions that are common across patients, and answering these questions in a group format can be an efficient use of a provider's time. That said, the downside of this approach is that patients make more equipment requests as they learn more about other masks or accessories. These additional requests may or may not be clinically indicated, and may or may not be consistent with local policies. We have found that the peer pressure can exert a non-trivial influence. However, we have found that clear local policies on mask replacement and/or a savvy, experienced provider can handle these issues. It must be remembered that the goal of the self-management approach is to allow the patients to get to such a point of knowledge and understanding that they can work collaboratively with the provider and understand the clinical decision-making so that they can essentially "self-manage" their sleep apnea on a daily basis, and consult with the provider on an as-needed basis.

Leader Type and Number

Two key issues not discussed above are leader type and the number of leaders. The CDSMP utilizes lay leaders, and primarily takes place outside of health care systems. It is truly a community-based, peer-led program. The SASMP was designed to take place within the health care system as part of clinical care processes, and therefore is based on being led by a sleep provider. The original SASMP intervention utilized one respiratory therapist as its leader. There might be several variants to the intervention as designed. To run more participants through, it might be co-led by two sleep providers at each session. In that case, the number of participants could potentially be doubled, though this would require a large conference room and may begin to lose some of the intimacy of a small group. Alternatively, slighter larger groups might be run with one primary leader and one secondary provider, who would be present during the sleep recording and CPAP set-up time periods, when a second person would clearly be needed.

Another alternative might be to include a peer co-leader who is a diagnosed sleep apnea patient who was successful with CPAP therapy. Clearly, the advantage of the CDSMP was its utilization of peer leadership, and while health professionals like to think they have the answers, there is something powerful about connecting with peers on health issues. That said, a peer co-leader might be best utilized during Sessions 3 and 4, when more time is dedicated to getting used to CPAP therapy than in Sessions 1 and 2.

PROOF OF CONCEPT/SUPPORTING DATA/EVIDENCE BASE

The sleep apnea self-management program draws from the Chronic Disease Self-Management Program (CDSMP) [8], which is one example of a formalized self-management program, developed and evaluated at the Stanford University School of Medicine Patient Education Research Center [8,10]. This program has an over 20-year track record of studying how best to manage multiple aspects of chronic diseases [11,12]. Taught by trained lay and professional leaders, CDSMP is a course that educates patients, and promotes behavior change related to symptom management, medication and complex medical regimen adherence, and maintenance of functional ability. CDSMP utilizes multiple activities to teach health management skills, including role playing, "lecturettes", brainstorming sessions, and action plans [9]. A key feature of the program is peer leadership – people who are themselves living with chronic illness lead, teach, role-model, and share life experiences with the CDSMP participants. CDSMP has been shown to improve symptom management, self-rated health-related quality of life, and communications with medical staff, and to reduce physician visits and hospitalizations [12]. Successful disease-specific variants of the CDSMP include programs for HIV/AIDS [13,14], arthritis [15,16], and low back pain [17].

Initial pilot research on a small group of sleep apnea patients found that the SASMP resulted in 5.5 hours per night of CPAP use over the first month of therapy [18]. In a significantly larger study, SASMP resulted in an additional 1.1 hours of CPAP use over a 6-month time period relative to the Usual Care group [19]. The amount of time required by SASMP is four ~1.5-hour sessions, which includes instructional time on home sleep testing and CPAP instruction. If one estimates the time spent on sleep recording and CPAP set-up conservatively at 2 hours, this would suggest that the SASMP uniquely takes about 4 hours of time. Because this is in a group setting that averages between three and six patients (and we can conservatively use four as an average), one could estimate that SASMP requires about 1 unique extra hour per patient. From a planning perspective, one could weigh the costs and benefits of implementing such a program versus spending 1 extra hour per patient on an individual face-to-face basis using current staffing levels. It would seem reasonable that some clinics or sleep providers could find that time, or replace current intervention time with this program. Importantly, this program was designed to be used by clinics and sleep providers.

REFERENCES

[1] H. Holman, K. Lorig, Perceived self-efficacy in self-management of chronic disease, in: R. Schwarzer (Ed.), Self-Efficacy: Thought Control of Action, Hemisphere Publishing Corporation, Washington, DC, 1992, pp. 305–323.

[2] P. Shekelle, Evidence Report and Evidence Based Recommendations: Chronic Disease Self-Management for Diabetes, Osteoarthritis, Post-Myocardial Infarction Care, and Hypertension, RAND, Santa Monica, CA, 2003.

[3] J. Corbin, A. Strauss, Unending Work and Care: Managing Chronic Illness at Home, Josey-Bass Publishers, San Francisco, CA, 1988.

[4] W.W. Flemons, Measuring health related quality of life in sleep apnea, Sleep 23 (Suppl 4) (2000) S109–S114.

[5] W.W. Flemons, M.A. Reimer, Development of a disease-specific health-related quality of life questionnaire for sleep apnea, Am. J. Respir. Crit. Care Med. 158 (2) (1998) 494–503.

[6] D. Veale, G. Poussin, F. Benes, et al., Identification of quality of life concerns of patients with obstructive sleep apnoea at the time of initiation of continuous positive airway pressure: A discourse analysis, Qual. Life Res. 11 (4) (2002) 389–399.

[7] T.E. Weaver, L.M. Laizner, L.K. Evans, et al., An instrument to measure functional status outcomes for disorders of excessive sleepiness, Sleep 20 (10) (1997) 835–843.

[8] K.R. Lorig, D.S. Sobel, P.L. Ritter, et al., Effect of a self-management program on patients with chronic disease, Eff. Clin. Pract. 4 (6) (2001) 256–262.

[9] K. Lorig, H. Holman, D.S. Sobel, et al., Living a Healthy Life with Chronic Conditions, second ed., Bull Publishing Company, Boulder, CO, 2000.

[10] K.R. Lorig, D.S. Sobel, A.L. Stewart, et al., Evidence suggesting that a chronic disease self-management program can improve health status while reducing hospitalization: A randomized trial, Med. Care 37 (1) (1999) 5–14.
[11] K. Lorig, V. Gonzalez, The integration of theory with practice: A 12-year case study, Health Educ. Q. 19 (3) (1992) 355–368.
[12] K. Lorig, H. Holman, Self-management education: History, definition, outcomes, and mechanisms, Ann. Behav. Med. 26 (1) (2003) 1–7.
[13] A.L. Gifford, D. Laurent, V. Gonzales, et al., Pilot randomized trial of education to improve self-management skills of men with symptomatic HIV/AIDS, J. Acquir. Immune Defic. Syndr. Hum. Retrovirol. 18 (2) (1998) 136–144.
[14] A.L. Gifford, K. Lorig, D. Laurent, V. Gonzales, Living Well with HIV and AIDS, Bull Publishing Co., Palo Alto, CA, 2000.
[15] K.R. Lorig, R.G. Kraines, B.W. Brown, Jr., N. Richardson, Outcomes of self-help education for patients with arthritis, Arthritis Rheum. 28 (6) (1985) 680–685.
[16] K.R. Lorig, P.D. Mazonson, H.R. Holman, Evidence suggesting that health education for self-management in patients with chronic arthritis has sustained health benefits while reducing health care costs, Arthritis Rheum. 36 (4) (1993) 439–446.
[17] M. Von Korff, J.E. Moore, K.R. Lorig, A randomized trial of a lay person-led self-management group intervention for back pain patients in primary care, Spine 23 (23) (1998) 2608–2615.
[18] C.J. Stepnowsky, J.J. Palau, A.L. Gifford, S. Ancoli-Israel, A self-management approach to improving continuous positive airway pressure adherence and outcomes, Behav. Sleep Med. 5 (2) (2007) 131–146.
[19] C. Stepnowsky, T. Zamora, Effect of a self-management intervention on CPAP adherence and treatment efficacy, Sleep 32 (Abstract Supplement) (2009) A225.

RECOMMENDED READING

K. Lorig, H. Holman, D.S. Sobel, et al., Living a Healthy Life with Chronic Conditions, second ed., Bull Publishing Company, Boulder, CO, 2000.
C. Gordon, T. Galloway, Review of Findings on Chronic Disease Self-Management Program (CDSMP) outcomes: physical, emotional & health-related quality of life, healthcare utilization and costs, J. Epidemiol. Community Health 62 (2008) 361–367.
C.J. Stepnowsky, J.J. Palau, A.L. Gifford, S. Ancoli-Israel, A self-management approach to improving continuous positive airway pressure adherence and outcomes, Behav. Sleep Med. 5 (2) (2007) 131–146.

Chapter 21

Cognitive Behavioral Therapy to Increase Adherence to Continuous Positive Airway

Model I: Psycho-education

Delwyn Bartlett

Medical Psychology, Sleep & Circadian Group, Woolcock Institute of Medical Research, Glebe, NSW, Australia

University of Sydney, NSW, Australia

PROTOCOL NAME

Cognitive behavioral therapy to increase adherence to continuous positive airway: psycho-education.

GROSS INDICATION

This model is used to provide information about obstructive sleep apnea (OSA); to educate the patient on the most effective treatment, continuous positive airway pressure (CPAP); and to educate the individual on the medical and psychiatric risks when OSA is not treated.

SPECIFIC INDICATION

Most sleep laboratories provide basic information about OSA, and then introduce patients to the numerous CPAP machines and masks available on the market. Anecdotal evidence suggests that many patients come away from these sessions feeling confused and unsure of what health benefits they will actually achieve from using a CPAP machine when it seems both foreign and personally invasive.

Research has shown that between 18 and 24 percent of patients diagnosed with OSA will not even rent or buy a CPAP machine, and, of those who do use CPAP, 50 percent will not be using it at 30 months [1]. Many other CPAP patients remain intermittent users only, with positive physical improvements, such as reduced daytime sleepiness or improved neurocognitive performance being difficult to assess. Hence, there is an overwhelming need to improve both the uptake

Behavioral Treatments for Sleep Disorders. DOI: 10.1016/B978-0-12-381522-4.00021-3

and adherence to CPAP therapy with a simple psycho-educational intervention that can be used by most staff members working in a sleep laboratory.

CONTRAINDICATIONS

There are few initial contraindications for the use of psycho-education to enhance adherence to CPAP. Even the patient with a previous history of claustrophobia can be slowly guided until he or she learns to feel comfortable with the mask. This takes time as the patient learns to manage the equipment, knowing that the control comes from gaining confidence with use.

Other more physical difficulties, such as sinusitis, leaks, skin irritations, etc., can be overcome in most instances, provided that the patient seeks help and is heard by sleep laboratory staff. For some groups, there may be a cultural barrier to the uptake and adherence of CPAP.

RATIONALE FOR INTERVENTION

Previous research employing predominantly behavioral interventions for CPAP adherence has been somewhat equivocal, with some effective outcomes, such as increasing CPAP usage by 2 hours per night [2]. However, some other interventions have been very labor intensive, which is a negative factor when considering the economic costs of running such a program.

More recently a pilot study [3] of 100 patients found that a 2×1-hour session cognitive behavior therapy (CBT) intervention which also included mask fitting and machine information resulted in increased uptake (only 4 patients in the treatment group did not take up CPAP compared with 15 in the mask-fitting only group). There was a significant difference in hours of nightly usage, with 37 patients using CPAP for >4 hours and 24 patients using it for >6 hours compared with the mask-fitting group, where 15 used CPAP for >4 hours and 7 used it for >6 hours. These pilot study data then formed the basis for what has now become our "treatment as usual", which consists of a psycho-education intervention to enable patients to better understand the risks of untreated OSA and how they can use CPAP on a nightly basis.

STEP BY STEP DESCRIPTION OF PROCEDURES

Patients who have been diagnosed with OSA are booked for a psycho-education session prior to undergoing their CPAP titration study. This can be done on the day of their titration study, or within the week prior to it.

The 30- to 40-minute education session is presented in a group setting with three or four patients, and run by a psychologist. In this format, however, a sleep technologist and/or CPAP therapist can run such a session. This is an interactive session, and patients are encouraged at the beginning of the session to ask questions throughout the presentation. Patients can also bring their partners to the education sessions.

The psycho-education intervention includes a slide presentation which has been designed to present factual information on the following:

- Normal sleep and sleep staging
- Hours of sleep and opportunity to sleep
- What is Obstructive Sleep Apnea?
- What happens to the airway with the development of OSA?
- What happens to other systems in the body with untreated OSA, with particular emphasis on the cardiovascular system?
- How safe is anyone on the road with an untreated OSA individual driving?
- What were the triggers for the individuals in the group seeking medical treatment?
- What is CPAP?
- What does CPAP do?
- What are the sleep stage changes that are likely to occur when CPAP is being used on a regular basis?
- Realistic expectations of the process of learning to use CPAP
- Other health factors/benefits, such as weight loss
- Side effects of using CPAP associated with seasonal temperature changes (too hot, too cold)
- The role of the patient's partner – what does the partner think of CPAP? Does the CPAP machine make more noise than the loud snoring and witnessed apneas? What to do if the patient is still snoring …
- Seeking help and asking questions after the titration study, both in the early days of treatment and later.

This slide presentation is predominantly educational, but also contains a strong cognitive component designed to promote positive outcomes that can and will occur with nightly CPAP usage.

This session needs to be presented in a way that promotes discussion, emphasizing that all questions are important, since a patient may be asking a question that someone else in the group wanted to ask but did not feel confident to do so. Patients need to be listened to, and their questions answered in an empathetic way.

Emphasis is placed *on the options* that CPAP gives the patient in terms of general health, safety at work, safety on the road, and having more energy for partners, family members, and friends. By not using CPAP these options are reduced, and the patient can again experience isolation with increased sleepiness, loss of energy, and lowered mood.

Using CPAP means that it is ***safe*** for the patient to go to sleep at night through all the stages of sleep.

Patient autonomy promotes that the patient is in charge of the treatment and can take off the mask and stop the machine at any chosen time. The patient needs to know that he or she is able to set the boundaries while still understanding that this treatment is the best option at this point in time.

This is a very useful way of introducing the patient to the practical aspects of using CPAP.

Handling of the mask(s) is an important component of the adaptation process. Patients are encouraged to hold their CPAP masks on their faces in neutral situations, such as watching television. Such practiced behaviors increase mask-handling confidence, but help the patient to realize how important it is to make CPAP use just another aspect of healthy daily living.

Patterns of CPAP use are also discussed, such as patients having "one night off" a week, which then becomes "two to three nights off", until usage is reduced to only one or two nights, where little perceived benefit is the likely outcome.

Realistic expectations about using CPAP require exploration, and need to be discussed in detail. Anecdotal evidence from running these education groups suggests those patients in the group who state that CPAP is going to "cure" all aspects of health problems are often the ones who stop using, or become intermittent users.

Technical aspects of the mask, the machine and how the patient manages any difficulties are discussed. An important message here is that there is no **one** answer that applies to technical and physical difficulties that arise when using CPAP. The patient is encouraged to "own" his or her equipment and to be responsible for it, and, when it is not working or other difficulties arise, then action needs to come from the patient in seeking help. This is about the patient's health and well being.

EDUCATIONAL MATERIALS

A copy of the slide presentation is given.

The CPAP Action Booklet is a booklet designed to be a reference for patients regarding what OSA is, what CPAP does, sleep hygiene measures, and care of CPAP mask and machine.

The Relaxation Booklet includes simple breathing exercises to reduce any anxiety with initial use of the CPAP mask. An easily accessible acupuncture pressure point on the wrist is shown, which can be a useful adjunct as the ramp is working.

REFERENCES

[1] L. Grote, J. Hedner, R. Grunstein, H. Kraiczi, Therapy with CPAP: incomplete elimination of sleep related breathing disorder, Eur. Respir. J. 16 (2000) 921–927.

[2] C.J. Hoy, M. Venelle, R.N. Kingshott, et al., Can intensive support improve continuous positive airway pressure use in patients with sleep apnea/hypopnea syndrome? Am. J. Respir. Crit. Care Med. (1999) 159–1100.

[3] D. Richards, D.J. Bartlett, K. Wong, et al., Increased adherence to CPAP with a group cognitive behavioral treatment intervention: a randomized trial, Sleep 30 (5) (2007) 635–640.

Chapter 22

Cognitive Behavioral Therapy to Increase Adherence to Continuous Positive Airway

Model II: Modeling

Delwyn Bartlett
Medical Psychology, Sleep & Circadian Group, Woolcock Institute of Medical Research, Glebe, NSW, Australia
University of Sydney, NSW, Australia

PROTOCOL NAME

Cognitive behavioral therapy to increase adherence to continuous positive airway: modeling.

GROSS INDICATION

The diagnosis of obstructive sleep apnea (OSA) can be overwhelming and even confusing for many patients, especially if the gold standard treatment of continuous positive airway pressure (CPAP) is only briefly explained. At one level CPAP is often thought of as being difficult and cumbersome, whilst for other patients there is a perception that using CPAP is similar to being on a life support system! This latter view of treatment can, paradoxically, lead to outright rejection of CPAP. Few patients have the opportunity to explore what CPAP does, and the long-term positive health benefits of using it.

SPECIFIC INDICATION

Social cognitive theory and the use of modeling gives the opportunity to correct distorted beliefs about OSA and CPAP through the presentation of positive real-life CPAP users' experiences, and how it relates to the person.

Social cognitive theory (SCT) relates to constructs that describe how humans make choices. Perceptions and expectations derived from past experiences influence how a person acts. The provision of accurate information enhances new

Behavioral Treatments for Sleep Disorders. DOI: 10.1016/B978-0-12-381522-4.00022-5

learning experiences, and can correct faulty or irrational beliefs through exposure to positive stimuli. *Self-efficacy* is a key component of this process, and relates to a belief in one's ability to accomplish a specified behavior by setting realistic goals; *outcome expectations* relate to the belief that using, for example, CPAP will produce a successful outcome and benefits [1]; therefore, the experience of using realistic models (real life CPAP users) telling their story encompasses this model. Previous research with a small randomized intervention study ($n = 12$) [2] based on self-efficacy and decisional balance found improved adherence to CPAP, and a larger study ($n = 100$) found improving self-efficacy resulted in improved uptake and nightly adherence to CPAP compared with the simple provision of CPAP machine information and mask fitting alone [3].

CONTRAINDICATIONS

There is no evidence at present to suggest specific negative outcomes to using modeling in relation to promoting CPAP use. However, the real-life CPAP users need to be representative of both genders and a wide range of ages in order to challenge stereotypical images that individuals with OSA are middle-aged overweight men. For some groups there may be a cultural barrier to the uptake and adherence of CPAP that may or may not be addressed by the choice of models.

STEP BY STEP DESCRIPTION OF PROCEDURES

The modeling is presented in a group setting. The modeling component of CPAP education can be undertaken at a time independent of the titration study. However, the aim is to present this component BEFORE the patient has his or her CPAP titration study. Partners are encouraged to join the session, and are recruited to join the team (as the support person, consistent with the SCT idea to enhance social support to optimize behavior change) consisting of the patient/partner and clinicians. Anecdotal experience suggests that having the partner present enables the treatment to become a "family affair", where the health and well being of the patient is the primary outcome. Following from this, when patients experience any difficulties with the day-to-day realities of using CPAP, their partner is more likely to encourage them to stay with the treatment. Another incentive for the patient is the lack of snoring and apneas in the shared bed. When partners are not able to come to the session, the provision of written material is a useful way of helping them understand the treatment and be involved in the treatment process. Underlying this process is the need to encourage patients to explain the handouts and information booklets to the absent partner.

Knowledge is an important underlying premise in SCT; therefore, the following listed components become an integral part of forming the basis of a successful outcome:

- Understanding and information about normal sleep and sleep staging.
- What OSA is, and how individuals often struggle to manage during the daytime with excessive sleepiness when it remains untreated.

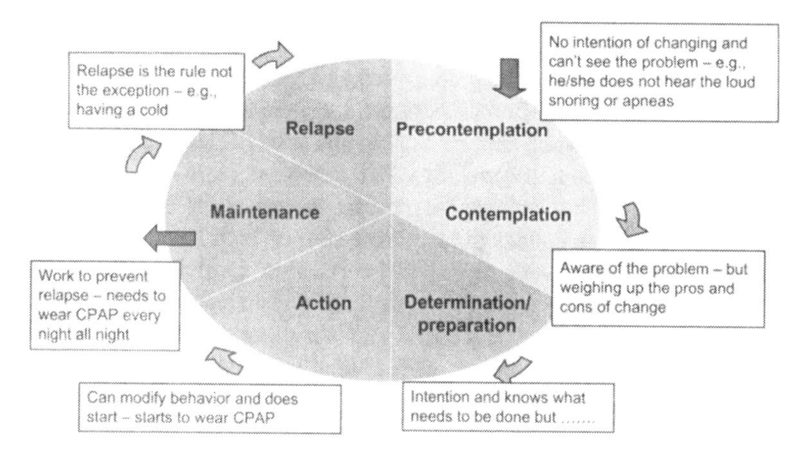

FIGURE 22.1 **Stages of change model.**

- Cardiovascular disease and other health risks associated with untreated OSA.
- What CPAP is, what it does, and what the benefits of using CPAP are.
- The cognitive component investigates what the patient is currently thinking in relation to the diagnosis of OSA and the information he or she has at present in relation to the suggested treatment with CPAP therapy.
- *Stages of Change from the Transtheoretical Model*™ are introduced in this setting as a pie-chart slide (see Figure 22.1). This multidimensional approach is presented on a continuum where each pie segment represents a category or stage of change. There are pros and cons for each stage.

  Precontemplation is the stage when there is no intention of change, such as the loud snorer who sees that it is not his or her problem and can't see what all the fuss is about!

  Contemplation, sometimes called "fence sitting", suggests there is some recognition there may be a problem with the snoring/apneas, and there may be a need to do something about it. This change is often triggered by the bed partner moving out of the shared bed.

  Preparation is about a change in both intention and behavior. A consultation with the Primary Care Physician (PCP) re. the snoring/apneas is an example of the patient showing that he or she understands the problem and is now prepared to take some action. This is likely to be followed up with referral to a sleep specialist, and a diagnostic sleep study will be undertaken.

  Action relates to how the patient modifies his or her behavior, experience, and/or environment to make the necessary change. This category/change stage is explained by the huge changes individuals need to instigate to make CPAP treatment work for them. It is learning about OSA, learning about CPAP and what it does, undergoing a titration study, and being committed to this new treatment for at least a specific time period. Learning to seek help, to overcome all the physical and psychological obstacles that often arise in the early days and weeks of using CPAP, is an important component of change in this category.

Maintenance is about undertaking CPAP treatment for at least 6 months. Another component, though not necessarily stated in this approach, is the need for the patient to take ownership of both having OSA and the undertaking that this treatment intervention gives health and life choices. There is also a need continually to update and seek help when there are mask/machine problems. Many patients let this part of the process slip and do not bother, as it is time consuming and difficult at times to keep this up. A key message here is that no question or problem is insignificant.

Relapse needs to be seen as normal, as it is generally not possible to use the mask/machine all the time. What is important is what the patient does during a relapse period, and how he or she can get back on track again when, for example, the cold/flu/traveling has been resolved.

- How willing the patient is to undertake this treatment, and what the level of his or her motivation is (scale 1–10). What factors would increase motivation?
- Confidence (self-efficacy) levels are discussed (scale 1–10) at onset. CPAP at the very least is different from anything the patient has ever experienced before, and it is difficult for many patients to adapt to using it. The objective is to set realistic levels and slowly increase confidence with the use and with problem-solving methods. Confidence is generally increased with competence in managing the mask and machine.

These basic components of CPAP education (Model I) need to be presented before the modeling component (Model II). An understanding of CPAP is crucial to be able to identify with the models in a video.

Key Components of a Modeling Video

- Example of successful CPAP usage. We used four different people in our video: a younger woman with a baby, a 30-something man, an older woman and an older man discussing very different but eventually successful CPAP outcomes.
- Relevant CPAP users that are representative of the wider community.
- A genuine story, and perhaps consideration of a more amateur video to emphasize this, compared with using actors in a more professional presentation.
- Content – how does/would the story apply to the average OSA patient? Does it/would it influence motivation? Does it contain key messages in relation to treatment and adherence?
- Perseverance – overcoming all the physical difficulties. These include problems with sinusitis, leaks, skin irritations, possible noise, etc. These

factors need to be discussed within the modeling framework, as these quite usual difficulties require *early intervention and perseverance*. The emphasis is placed on the patient that if CPAP is not working then it is important to get help or a small difficulty can become a large problem.

- Self-efficacy – a clear example of a patient believing that he or she can have a successful outcome using CPAP, even though there may have been considerable difficulties to overcome.
- Outcome expectations – an example of a patient believing that the treatment is necessary for good health, which enables him or her to persevere for a number of weeks and months to attain the desired outcome of ease of usage and relief of symptoms.
- Choice – this is similar to self-efficacy in many ways, but is often an easier way of working toward the same outcome. Using CPAP as the best treatment for the patient at this time is a choice, and it is also the patient's choice to use CPAP all night, every night. The patient can also choose to take the mask off whenever he or she decides to – all these points encourage autonomy, and help to address some issues of claustrophobia.

Discussion Following the Video Presentation

- What did the patients most relate to in the video?
- Of the CPAP stories, which model was the one that they felt represented how it might be for them?
- What enabled the CPAP users on the video to maintain the treatment even when it was difficult?
- Did the concept of the Stages of Change Model make more sense to them after the video?
- What would keep them involved in their CPAP treatment, and where do they currently see themselves in this model?
- What would help the patient to move onto the next stage? Long term, how would the patient maintain "maintenance"?
- How will the patient deal with relapse?

CASE STUDY: ONE PATIENT'S JOURNEY IN LEARNING TO USE CPAP

The Intervention

Following the educational intervention, Peter stated that from that session he understood the effectiveness of CPAP for OSA, but that many individuals found it very difficult and stopped using it. He was determined to succeed, and stated that "failure was not an option" for him. He also stated that he would adapt to using CPAP, and he would find solutions to whatever problems might arise.

The first experience of using CPAP: At the mask-fitting session immediately following the education, Peter felt that breathing with the mask might be difficult. He decided to sit on the edge of the bed with the mask on his face, taking it on and off as he became used to the minimum pressure of 4-cm H_2O pressure. He still found it strange and quite difficult, but again stated to himself that he could and would succeed. This is an example of a patient with high self-efficacy enabling him to recognize the challenge and manage it. However, individuals with low self-efficacy can also learn to meet such challenges and gain confidence in their decisions.

Problems Encountered

Peter's first problem was "pain in the back of his nasal passage near the top of his throat". Upon reflection, he felt that he had a respiratory infection on the night of his CPAP titration study which continued to be very uncomfortable for him until he sought help and was given a humidifier.

Peter's second problem was irritation from the cold air as he started to use CPAP in winter. The humidifier helped, but he then needed to put the heater on in his bedroom, which is not what most people do in his home country of Australia in the winter time. Increased electricity costs were the result for him, and he has stated that he will investigate alternatives for next winter, such as using a heated tube which would be less expensive compared with a room heater. Here again he persevered and found at least an initial solution, with the option of looking for other alternatives next winter.

Peter's third problem was the discomfort from the CPAP pressure. The ramp was useful initially, but he still felt uncomfortable at sleep onset. He then stated that he resolved this problem by sheer perseverance, and one morning, 3 weeks after he started using CPAP, he woke with the mask still on his face and felt totally at ease with the 9 cm of H_2O pressure. It felt normal for him – something that had been difficult and strange initially had become "normalized" into his daily life.

Peter's fourth problem was a skin irritation from the mask. He understood that his prescribed pressure stopped the apneas, and the mask needed to be firm against his face to seal possible leaks; however, it also made his nose tender. On his CPAP titration study, he had started off using a nasal pillow which "did not give off any air pressure", but halfway through the night he woke with pain around his nostrils and then used a nasal mask. He then bought a nasal pillow so that he could alternate between the nasal mask and the nasal pillows, stating that over time he feels his nostrils will "toughen up" and he will then not have to deal with the issue of pressure on his skin and face. Again, his perseverance enabled him to find a workable solution where he was able to achieve relative comfort, a good seal, and the future goal of "toughened nostrils".

Peter's fifth problem was what he described as the "psychological reaction to discomfort of the mask". He, like many CPAP users, would wake and remove his mask, and then fall back to sleep without replacing his mask. He decided that he had to remind himself every night that CPAP was essential for his health. He "needed to avoid sleep apnea because of the increased risk of heart disease and stroke!" His previously high blood pressure was a reminder that he could not afford to sleep without his CPAP machine. He then decided that he would not take the mask off unless he was properly awake and ready to get out of bed in the morning. He reminded himself of this frequently. He called these affirmations and behavior changes "mental adjustments", and then added that it was his decision to use CPAP. He had, at this stage, taken "ownership" of his sleeping disorder and the treatment.

Peter used a wonderful metaphor to describe his CPAP journey. He stated that "adjusting to CPAP was like adapting to a new pair of shoes". It may hurt for a while as your feet hurt from the pressure and friction because you are not used to it. With perseverance, the shoes wear in and your feet adjust and toughen up. Those thoughts helped him to accept and adapt to CPAP.

For Peter, using CPAP reduced his feelings of chronic fatigue. He was also aware that there were some days that he did not feel good even when he used CPAP. However, on the few nights when he did not use CPAP he felt terrible, which reminded him of how he had felt every day before he started using CPAP. It was worth working through the discomfort and the trials and effort required to master CPAP.

REFERENCES

[1] A. Bandura, Social Learning Theory, Prentice Hall, Englewood Cliffs, NJ, 1977.
[2] M. Aloia, M. Lina Di Dio, M. Ilniczky, et al., Improving compliance with nasal CPAP and vigilance in older adults with OSAHS, Sleep Breath 5 (2001) 13–21.
[3] D. Richards, D.J. Bartlett, K. Wong, et al., Increased adherence to CPAP with a group cognitive behavioral treatment intervention: a randomized trial, Sleep 30 (5) (2007) 635–640.

Chapter 23

The Avoidance of the Supine Posture during Sleep for Patients with Supine-related Sleep Apnea

Arie Oksenberg
Sleep Disorders Unit, Loewenstein Hospital-Rehabilitation Center Raanana, Israel

PROTOCOL NAME

Positional therapy: the avoidance of the supine posture during sleep for patients with supine-related sleep apnea.

GROSS INDICATION

This therapy is mainly suitable for patients with supine-related sleep apnea (positional patients) who have most of their breathing abnormalities concentrated in the supine posture, and in whom while sleeping in the lateral postures (and sometimes in the prone posture) the amount of breathing abnormalities is significantly reduced to a non-pathological level.

SPECIFIC INDICATIONS

Originally, this therapy was first suggested for Obstructive Sleep Apnea (OSA) patients with Apnea Hypopnea Index (AHI) in the supine posture double or more than that Index in the non-supine postures.

Specifically, this therapy is recommended for:

- Patients with any type of breathing abnormality during sleep – mainly obstructive, but also mixed or central apnea (with or without Cheyne-Stokes breathing); and also for patients with upper airway resistance syndrome who suffer most of their breathing abnormalities while sleeping in the supine posture and in whom, by sleeping in other positions, the amount of these events is reduced to a non-pathological level – i.e., AHI < 5 or at least AHI < 10

Behavioral Treatments for Sleep Disorders. DOI: 10.1016/B978-0-12-381522-4.00023-7

- Patients without sleep apnea but with snoring (primary snoring) that is confined mainly to the supine posture
- Patients who have not succeeded with Continuous Positive Airway Pressure (CPAP), an oral device, or any other treatment, and mainly have breathing abnormalities in the supine posture.

A crucial issue for positional patients is that the severity of the disease is related mainly to the *sleep time spent (or not spent) in the supine posture.*

CONTRAINDICATIONS

Positional therapy is not recommended for:

- Patients who for any reason (shoulder problems, or any other physical disability that interferes with their sleep in the lateral position) cannot avoid the supine posture during sleep
- Positional patients who prefer to sleep in the supine posture
- Non-positional patients who have many breathing abnormalities in the supine and lateral postures as well; for these patients CPAP is the treatment of choice, since they also suffer from a more severe disease
- Positional patients who continue to snore loudly and perhaps have also events of flow limitation while sleeping in the lateral postures.

RATIONALE FOR INTERVENTION

If a sleep apnea patient has mainly apneas and hypopneas in the supine posture, but when sleeping in the lateral positions or prone posture these breathing abnormalities disappear or are markedly reduced to a non-pathological level, it is almost intuitively obvious that this patient should avoid the supine posture during sleep. It is not clear, however, how the patient should accomplish this task during sleep. In order to avoid this posture during sleep, and thereafter to learn how to sleep only in the other postures (mainly the lateral posture), it becomes important to find a simple behavioral therapy for this purpose.

The prevalence of positional OSA patients (patients who have most of their sleep-related breathing abnormalities in the supine posture) is high. In a large study including 574 consecutive OSA patients diagnosed by polysomnography in a Sleep Disorders Unit, it was found that 55.9 percent had at least twice as many breathing abnormalities during sleep in the supine posture compared to the lateral position [1]. The prevalence of positional patients was much higher in mild to moderate OSA patients (ranging from 65–69 percent) than in severe OSA. Recently, we have expanded these findings in 2077 OSA patients [2], and others [3,4] have corroborated these results despite using a stricter definition of positional OSA.

The high prevalence of positional OSA in the less severe forms of OSA is important, because mild OSA patients are less likely to succeed with CPAP [5] and therefore might be good candidates for positional therapy. Furthermore, since mild OSA patients make up the vast majority of OSA patients [6], if this form of therapy were successful it could be used by a considerable number of OSA patients [7].

Another point worth mentioning is that the supine posture during sleep not only increases the frequency of apnea/hypopnea events, but also increases the severity of these events. The length of the apnea events, the degree of desaturation, the severity of the tachy-bradycardia changes after the apnea events and the lengths of the accompanying arousals are all more severe in the supine position than in the lateral position [8]. Thus, adopting the lateral posture during sleep (positional therapy) can improve not only the frequency but also the nature of these breathing abnormalities.

The deleterious effect of the supine posture during sleep appears to be important also in patients with central sleep apnea with or without Cheyne-Stokes breathing. Four studies [9–12] in stroke and heart-failure patients have provided evidence showing that these types of breathing abnormalities are more prevalent in the supine than in the lateral position. Therefore, adopting the lateral position during sleep may represent a new and valuable behavioral approach for the treatment of breathing abnormalities during sleep in these patients. However, this topic requires further and extensive investigations.

STEP BY STEP DESCRIPTION OF PROCEDURES

Positional therapy can be achieved by different means. It does not matter which method is used to avoid patients sleeping on their back. Moreover, it is important that patients find the right technique for themselves – the most comfortable and effective technique, which they feel is best. This issue is very important, since patients must use it for a relatively long period of time (at least several weeks) – hopefully, until they learn to avoid the supine posture without using the technique.

The bottom line of any variation of this therapy is that whenever patients roll onto their back or try to roll onto their back during sleep, a device will immediately correct their position, or be so uncomfortable that it encourages sleeping in the lateral posture.

Some positional devices and techniques are described below:

- *The tennis ball technique* [13]. A tennis ball is placed into a pocket of a wide cloth band or belt attached around the waist so that the ball lies in the center of the patient's back. When patients roll onto their back, the pressure of the ball will cause them instinctively to roll back onto their side again. Some may use a T-shirt with a long vertical pocket holding three or four tennis balls along the back; this is perhaps less likely to slip out of place during sleep.
- *An alarm system* [14]. This momentarily wakes patients whenever they lie on their back, and has been used successfully.

- *The Sleep Positioner* [15]. This device consists of a rectangular-shaped foam block, surrounding a hard cylindrical core, which is secured to the patient's back by elastic straps.
- *The Positioner* [16]. This consists of a soft vest made of cotton tricot with a zip in front, woven straps that attach to a board via Velcro® fasteners, and a pillow that is placed on top of the board. When correctly adjusted, the straps make it impossible for patients to roll over to the supine position, but allow them to turn onto either side.
- *The BPOD unit* [17]. Located on the chest midline, this detects the position of the sleeper. If patients remain on their back for more than a user-selected delay (typically 2.5 s), the unit delivers a vibratory stimulus to them via a buzzer also located on the chest. This annoys sleepers enough to make them change to a lateral or prone posture.
- *Thoracic anti-supine* band (TASB) [18]. This comprises two equal lengths of cotton stockinette-covered 6-mm foam rubber with 25-mm Velcro® sewn-on attachments at each end. The band length is the measurement from the base of the xiphisternum, round the left side of the chest, over the sixth thoracic spinous process, between the midpoints of the scapulae and across the right shoulder to the point on the tenth rib in the mid-clavicular line. A polystyrene ball (8- or 10-cm in circumference, depending on the subject's size) is inserted inside the stockinette such that it is positioned between the scapulae at the level of the sixth thoracic vertebra. The two short ends are draped over the shoulders and front-fastened with Velcro over the two long ends.
- *The supine position prevention vest* [19]. The vest is made of linen, with a half cylindrical piece of hard foam in its dorsal part.
- *The Zoma positional sleeper* [20]. This is a 12- by 5.5- by 4-inch device made of lightweight semi-rigid foam. It is contained in a backpack-type material with a Velcro® elastic belt. The device is worn on the back, with the elastic belt brought around each side of the patient and secured anteriorly.
- *The vest-type design* [21]. This device is of a vest-type design with a connected controller. In the vest-like part, two air chambers are installed in parallel on the left and right sides of the back. During sleep, one of the chambers is inflated to prevent the supine position, and then deflated after a pre-specified time while the other chamber is inflated.

Improving Patients' Acceptance of Positional Therapy

Since your patients may be amused at the suggestion of this form of therapy and might not take you seriously, you should show them just how striking the positional effect is for them personally. For this purpose, it is important to show a clear summary graph of the polysomnographic data containing the most valuable information for easy understanding by the patient.

Figure 23.1 shows a summary graph which includes in parallel the hypnogram, sleep markers, time scale, SaO_2 levels, heart-rate changes, snoring sounds in a calibrated mode (40–80 dB), apnea/hypopnea episodes and

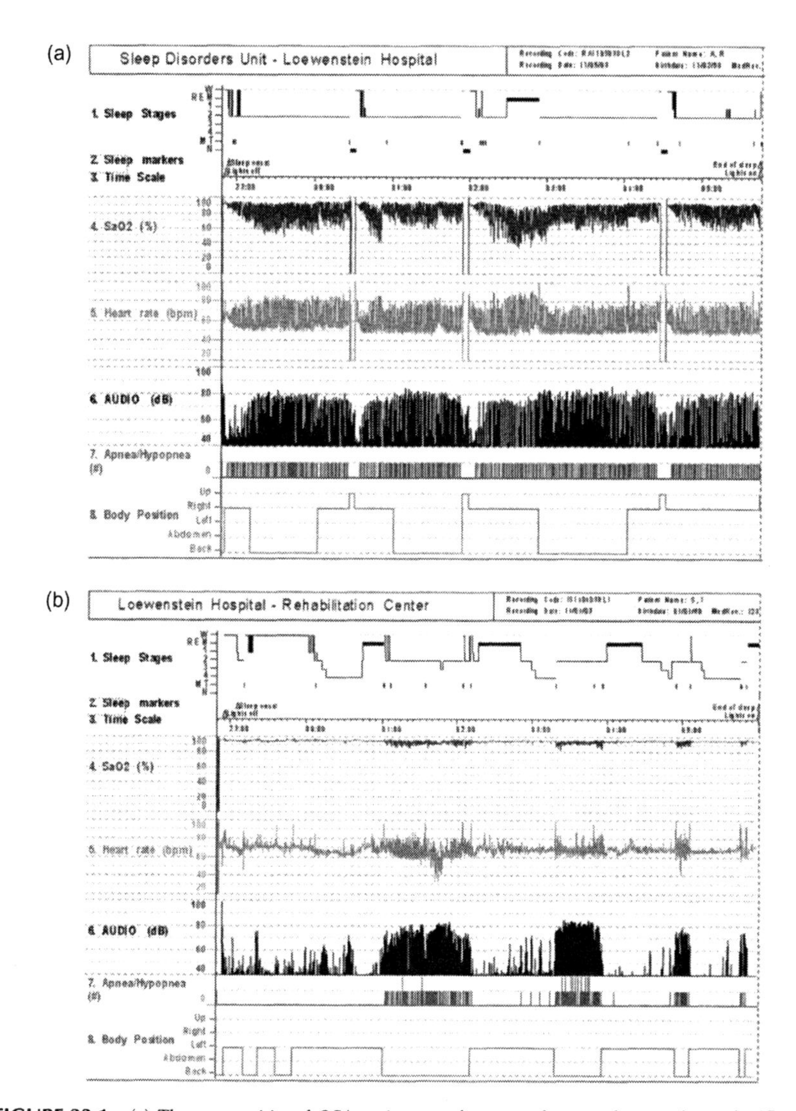

FIGURE 23.1 (a) *The non-positional OSA patient*: continuous and severe desaturations, significant cyclic variations in heart rate, constant and loud snoring, and a high number of apneas/hypopneas appear independent of body position. (b) *The positional OSA patient*: Desaturations, cyclic variations in heart rate, loud snoring, and apneas/hypopneas appear almost exclusively in the supine position. Reproduced with permission from A. Oksenberg, Positional and non-positional obstructive sleep apnea patients, Sleep Med. 6 (2005) 377–378.

duration, and changes in body postures for a particular patient. We also show the patient samples of the same summary graphs for another individual with a very clear positional effect, and for one with no positional effect [22]. This makes it very easy for the patient to understand immediately the effect that body position has on breathing abnormalities during sleep.

In addition, we manufacture tennis-ball belts. A belt is offered to patients if they express interest. Thus, patients receive a complete explanation of the results of the sleep evaluation test and, if accepted, they go home with a very simple, non-invasive, cheap, and hopefully effective form of treatment.

POSSIBLE MODIFICATIONS/VARIANTS

Elevated Posture

At least three reports [23–25] have provided data demonstrating the effect of elevated posture of the head and upper body for the improvement of breathing abnormalities during sleep. In one of these reports, a shoulder-head elevation pillow (SHEP) was used. The SHEP was designed to standardize the elevated posture at 60° above the horizontal. In this study [25], only 29 percent (4/14) achieved success (AHI $\leq$ 10), and 21 percent (3/14) a partial success (AHI > 10 <16). However, in a previous study of 13 OSA patients [23], AHI was reduced from 48.9 $\pm$ 5.4/h supine to 19.6 $\pm$ 6.9/h in an elevated posture of about 60° from horizontal.

It should be mentioned that very severe OSA patients, as well as some patients with overlap syndrome (OSA+COPD), frequently argue that the seated position or reclined posture are the best postures for sleep. They claim that it is easiest to breathe in these postures. Unfortunately, no research has been done to address this topic.

Knee-up Posture

There has been one case report [26] and one study [27] where new posture was evaluated as a treatment for apnea. The larger study examined 24 patients with OSA, who were asked to sleep with a foam wedge under their knees, providing approximately 60° of elevation, while sleeping supine. Although the results did not show a robust effect, in some patients this maneuver improved the AHI and the Desaturation Index. The mechanism underlying this improvement is unknown, but since this position allows for a greater displacement of the diaphragm during expiration, the net effect becomes an increase in lung volumes, which may induce a decrease in pharyngeal resistance.

Head Extension

A cervical pillow which promotes head extension similar to that used in cardiopulmonary resuscitation (CPR) to create an open airway in an unconscious victim was used in two small studies with mild–moderate OSA patients (12 and 18 patients each) [28,29]. A significant trend toward improvement, despite spending more time in the supine position and having similar amounts of REM sleep, was found. The mechanism by which the cervical pillow improves sleep-disordered breathing in patients with mild to moderate OSA is most likely the increased cross-sectional area of the airway associated with head extension.

PROOF OF CONCEPT/SUPPORTING DATA/EVIDENCE BASE

Proof of Concept

As reported earlier [30], the spouses of habitual snorers and obstructive sleep apnea patients were probably the first to identify the effect of body position on these breathing abnormalities many years ago. Indeed, in a short letter published in *Chest* in 1984 [31], under the title "Patient's wife cures his snoring", there is confirmation of the above statement. In the letter, his wife wrote:

In regard to my husband's sleep apnea-snoring problem, after we talked to you, I invented a method to prevent my husband from sleeping on his back. I sewed a pocket into the back of a T-shirt and inserted a hollow, lightweight plastic ball (about the size of a tennis ball). I fastened one side of the pocket with safety pins so that the ball can be removed to launder the shirt. It's working beautifully. In about two days, I could see a vast improvement in his energy level, alertness, and interest in life. He no longer falls asleep while sitting straight up in a chair, and the quiet, snoreless nights are great. I thought that this information might be helpful to other patients with similar problems.

Moreover, when one asks the spouses of habitual snorers and OSA patients about the possible effect of body position on these sleep-related breathing disturbances, it is quite common to hear some of the following descriptions: "Doctor, my husband snores so loudly when he sleeps on his back that I am sure that the snores are heard by our neighbors", or "At the beginning he used to snore only when he slept on his back, but now he snores, and snores loudly, in all body positions, and when he sleeps on his back he seems to have breathing pauses lasting a few seconds at a time". All these descriptions suggest that body position plays an important role in breathing functions during sleep. Furthermore, in one of the first articles published on breathing abnormalities during sleep, Gastaut et al., in 1966 [32], mentioned the aggravating effect of the supine posture on sleep apnea. Moreover, in one of the first published reports on snoring treatment, positional therapy was mentioned [33].

Supporting Data

Most of the data related to this topic were published in the 1980s, and the majority of studies were reported only in abstract form. In published manuscripts, the number of patients has been very small. Most of this information could be found in our previous report [30], but it is important to mention the first two abstracts published in 1982, which reported a marked improvement in OSA patients' condition simply by shifting them from their back to the lateral position during sleep [34,35], and mentioning, perhaps for the first time, the tennis ball technique as a method of avoiding the supine posture during sleep.

Here, two of three patients were followed for 8 months and 2 years, respectively, and a marked reduction in the number of apneas was objectively seen at follow-up. However, in 1948 Robin mentioned that "a cotton reel sewn into the back of the pajamas is efficacious" for snoring treatment [33].

Another very important contribution to the field comes from the work of R. Cartwright, who published her earliest two papers on the topic in *Sleep*: the first, in 1984, showed the effect of the supine posture on OSA severity [36], and the second, in 1985, demonstrated preliminary data on the effect of positional therapy [14]. An alarm system was used to avoid the supine position in 10 moderately obese positional OSA patients. While wearing the alarm, the Apnea Index of seven patients remained within or near normal limits (AHI ≤ 10). On the follow-up night, with only an instruction to maintain the lateral posture, five patients remained significantly improved. In another study, the alarm system was used continuously for 8 weeks in 20 positional patients [37]. All patients had less than 5 minutes of supine sleep on the night when the alarm device was used, but on a subsequent night, without the alarm, only 11 patients (55 percent) had less than 5 minutes of supine sleep. In the other nine patients (45 percent) supine sleep time ranged from 11.5 to 172 minutes, and five of them (25 percent of the whole group) still slept for about 1–3 hours in the supine posture.

It would appear from these and another comparative study [38] that about two-thirds of patients will successfully learn to avoid the supine posture with or without the use of a device, but the other one-third of patients will require the continuous use of some type of device in order to avoid, successfully, the supine position during sleep.

Jokic et al. [39] compared 2 weeks of positional therapy with 2 weeks of CPAP in 13 mildly obese positional OSA patients. CPAP treatment was more effective than positional therapy in reducing respiratory events and preventing desaturation, but the treatments had similar efficacy in terms of sleep quality, daytime sleepiness, mood, quality of life, and daytime functioning. The results of this study suggest that one could offer positional patients a short trial with positional therapy followed by a short trial of CPAP, or vice versa. They could then be given the opportunity to choose the best therapy for themselves, based on their own experience. This perhaps will be reflected in better compliance.

Skinner et al. [18] compared the efficacy of CPAP vs the thoracic anti-supine band (TASB) for avoiding the supine posture during sleep in 20 positional patients with mild to moderate OSA. After 1 month of treatment, CPAP was more effective than TASB for the decrease in AHI. Treatment success (AHI ≤ 10) was achieved in 13/18 patients with TASB, and in 16/18 patients with CPAP. No significant differences in sleep efficiency or subjective responses were observed between treatments.

Recently, Permut et al. [20] also compared the effectiveness of positional therapy (using the Zzoma positional sleeper) vs CPAP in 38 mild to moderate positional patients with an AHI < 5 in the non-supine posture, and concluded that positional therapy is equivalent to CPAP in normalizing the AHI, with similar effects on sleep quality and nocturnal oxygenation.

We have previously [13] assessed the use of positional therapy, using the tennis ball technique (TBT), during a 6-month period in 78 consecutive positional OSA patients. Of the 50 patients who returned the questionnaire, 19 (38 percent) (Group A) said they were still using the TBT, and 12 (24 percent) (Group B) said they had used it initially and stopped using it within a few months, but were still avoiding the supine position during sleep. Nineteen patients (38 percent) (Group C) stopped using the TBT within a few months but did not learn how to avoid the sleep supine posture. Patients still using the TBT showed a significant improvement in their self-reported sleep quality and daytime alertness, and a decrease in snoring loudness. Age appears to be the only parameter that significantly differentiated between patients who complied and those who did not comply with this form of therapy: patients who complied were older than patients that did not comply with this therapy. The main reason for patients stopping the use of the TBT in Group C was that using it was uncomfortable.

A recent Australian long-term (2.5 years) follow-up study [40] of compliance with TBT gave quite disappointing results. The same questionnaire that we used [13] was sent to 108 patients prescribed TBT at the Adelaide Institute for Sleep Health between July 2004 and March 2008, and 67 (62 percent) patients replied to the questionnaire. Of these, 4 (6.0 percent) reported they were still using TBT; 9 (13.4 percent) were no longer using TBT but claimed to have learned to avoid the supine position during sleep; and 54 (80.6 percent) were neither using TBT nor avoiding the supine posture. Similar to our results [13], the main reason for stopping TBT use was that it was too uncomfortable (34/54 patients). Based on these results, the authors correctly concluded that

although tennis ball devices are simple, cheap, and ostensibly effective forms of positional therapy, most positional OSA patients prescribed them become non-compliant and untreated in the long-term, primarily because of the intrinsic discomfort associated with such therapies. Thus, improved therapeutic options appear to be needed for this important group.

An important new study [41] searching for the best position for overcoming snoring and sleep apnea in 16 mild to moderate positional patients showed that a 30° rotation from supine to lateral and 20 mm elevation of the upper trunk with moderate support (60–70 mm) of the cervical vertebrae were effective at reducing snoring. For sleep apnea, a rotation >40° from supine to lateral, with higher levels of cervical vertebrae support, with head tilting (>70 mm) and scapula support (30 mm) were recommended for an AHI reduction >80 percent. This study clearly shows that not only the body posture but also the head/neck/upper trunk position influences the upper airway in the occurrence of snoring and sleep apnea during sleep. In supporting of this concept, Ono et al. [42] showed, several years ago, that the cross-sectional area in the retroglossal region was significantly increased in both the supine with the head rotated and lateral recumbent positions.

Tanaka et al. [43], in a new retrospective study of 213 severe OSA patients, found that the lateral AHI was considered to have a stronger influence on subjective daytime sleepiness (ESS) than the supine AHI. In mild to moderate OSA patients, no significant correlation was found between ESS and total AHI, or AHI at any position. These results suggest that in severe OSA patients with very high supine AHI, the degree of daytime sleepiness severity will be related to the lateral AHI. If the lateral AHI is very high and similar to the supine AHI, the daytime sleepiness will be very high too; however, on the contrary, if the lateral AHI is relatively low, it is expected that the subjective daytime sleepiness will be less severe.

Evidence Base

Unfortunately, the research on the effect of positional therapy on sleep-related breathing abnormalities lacks good clinical trials. Most of these investigations are not controlled, randomized studies; they include few patients and short-term follow-up.

In our study [13], we referred to this issue and stated:

It is ironic that in spite of the fact that every sleep laboratory in the world records the body position changes during all polysomnographic evaluations, in most cases these data are not being used for anything except for being mentioned in the report. Most of the reviews on sleep apnea therapy either mention this form of therapy in a superficial way or do not mention it at all. This in spite of the fact that over half the OSA patients are positional including over 60% of the mild OSA patients which are the majority of the patients with OSA. One could ask why it is that this kind of therapy has not been investigated more thoroughly and used more frequently. Unfortunately there is a good reason for this. This topic totally lacks good randomized, controlled studies. Most of the studies in this area are small, non-randomized, uncontrolled and short term. If large randomized, controlled and long-term studies would be carried out, we may find that changing the body posture during sleep, a relatively simple behavioral maneuver, may have a powerful therapeutic effect on many sleep apnea patients, and may thus help avoid the deleterious health and behavioral consequences of this disease.

Without question, until good research on this topic is carried out, the real therapeutic value of this behavioral therapy will be debatable.

SUMMARY

Positional therapy – the avoidance of the supine posture during sleep – is simple, inexpensive, and could represent an effective form of therapy for positional patients with sleep-related breathing abnormalities who have a non-pathologic AHI in the lateral posture. However, until large, randomized, controlled and long-term studies are performed, the real therapeutic value of this behavioral therapy will be debatable.

REFERENCES

[1] A. Oksenberg, D.S. Silverberg, E. Arons, H. Radwan, Positional vs nonpositional obstructive sleep apnea patients. Anthropomorphic, nocturnal polysomnographic and multiple sleep latency test data, Chest 112 (1997) 629–639.

[2] A. Oksenberg, E. Arons, S. Greenberg-Dotan, et al., The significance of body posture on breathing abnormalities during sleep: data analysis of 2077 obstructive sleep apnea patients, Harefuah 148 (2009) 304–309, 351, 360.

[3] M.J. Mador, T.J. Kufel, U.J. Magalang, et al., Prevalence of positional sleep apnea in patients undergoing polysomnography, Chest 128 (2005) 2130–2137.

[4] W. Richard, D. Kox, C. den Herder, et al., The role of sleep position in obstructive sleep apnea syndrome, Eur. Arch. Otorhinolaryngol. 263 (2006) 946–950.

[5] L. Rosenthal, R. Gerhardstein, A. Lumley, et al., CPAP therapy in patients with mild OSA: implementation and treatment outcome, Sleep Med. 1 (2000) 215–220.

[6] T. Young, M. Palta, J. Dempsey, et al., The occurrence of sleep-disordered breathing among middle-aged adults, N. Engl. J. Med. 328 (1993) 1230–1235.

[7] A. Oksenberg, D.S. Silverberg, Avoiding the supine posture during sleep for patients with mild obstructive sleep apnea, Am J Respir Crit Care Med. (2009). 180:101(letter); author reply 101–2.

[8] A. Oksenberg, Y. Khamaysi, D.S. Silverberg, A. Tarasiuk, Association of body position with severity of apneic events in patients with severe nonpositional obstructive sleep apnea, Chest 118 (2000) 1018–1024.

[9] A. Oksenberg, E. Arons, D. Snir, et al., Cheyne-Stokes respiration during sleep: a possible effect of body position, Med. Sci. Monit. 8 (2002) CS61–CS65.

[10] C Sahlin, E. Svanborg, H. Stenlund, K.A. Franklin, Cheynes-Stokes respiration and supine dependency, Eur. Resp. J. 25 (2005) 829–833.

[11] I. Szollosi, T. Roebuck, B. Thompson, M.T. Naughton, Lateral sleeping position reduces severity of Central Sleep Apnea/Cheyne-Stokes respiration, Sleep 29 (2006) 1045–1051.

[12] S. Joho, Y. Oda, T. Hirai, H. Inoue, Impact of sleeping position on central sleep apnea/ Cheyne-Stokes respiration in patients with heart failure, Sleep Med. 11 (2010) 143–148.

[13] A. Oksenberg, D.S. Silverberg, D. Offenbach, E. Arons, Positional therapy for obstructive sleep apnea patients: a 6-month follow-up study, Laryngoscope 116 (2006) 1995–2000.

[14] R.D. Cartwright, S. Lloyd, J. Lilie, H. Kravitz, Sleep position training as treatment for sleep apnea syndrome: a preliminary study, Sleep 8 (1985) 87–94.

[15] P. Freebeck, D. Stewart, Compliance and effective therapy for positional apnea, Sleep Res. 24 (1995) 236.

[16] H. Loord, E. Hultcrantz, Positioner – a method for preventing sleep apnea, Acta Otolaryngologica (2007) 861–888.

[17] http://4sleep.us/product.html

[18] M.A. Skinner, R.N. Kingshott, S. Filsell, D.R. Taylor, Effect of the "tennis ball technique" vs CPAP in the management of position dependent obstructive sleep apnea syndrome, Respirology 13 (2008) 708–715.

[19] J.T. Maurer, B.A. Stuck, G. Hein, et al., Treatment of obstructive apnea with a new vest preventing the supine position, Dtsch Med. Wochenschr 128 (2003) 71–75.

[20] I. Permut, M. Diaz-Abad, W. Chatila, et al., Comparison of positional therapy to CPAP in patients with positional obstructive sleep apnea, J. Clin. Sleep Med. (2010) (in press).

[21] J.H. Choi, J.H. Park, J.H. Hong, et al., Efficacy study of a vest-type device for positional therapy in position dependent snorers, Sleep and Biol. Rhythms 7 (2009) 172–180.

[22] A. Oksenberg, Positional and non-positional obstructive sleep apnea patients, Sleep Med. 6 (2005) 377–378.

[23] D.R. McEvoy, D.J. Sharp, A.T. Thornton, The effect of posture on obstructive sleep apnea, Am. Rev. Respir. Dis. 133 (1986) 662–666.

[24] A.M. Neill, S.M. Angus, D. Sajkov, R.D. McEvoy, Effects of sleep posture on upper airway stability in patients with obstructive sleep apnea, Am. J. Respir. Crit. Care Med. 155 (1997) 199–204.

[25] M.A. Skinner, R.N. Kingshott, D.R. Jones, et al., Elevated posture for the management of obstructive sleep apnea, Sleep Breath 8 (2004) 193–200.

[26] S. Geer, L.B. Straight, D.A. Schulman, D.L. Bliwise, Effect of supine knee position on obstructive sleep apnea, Sleep Breath 10 (2006) 98–101.

[27] D.L. Bliwise, D. Irbe, D.A. Schulman, Improvement in obstructive sleep apnea in the supine "knees-up" position, Sleep Breath 8 (2004) 43–47.

[28] C.A. Kushida, S. Rao, C. Guilleminault, et al., Cervical positional effects on snoring and apneas, Sleep Res. Online 2 (1999) 7–10.

[29] C.A. Kushida, C.M. Sherrill, S.C. Hong, et al., Cervical positioning for reduction of sleep disordered breathing in mild-to-moderate OSAS, Sleep Breath 2 (2001) 71–78.

[30] A. Oksenberg, D.S. Silverberg, The effect of body posture on sleep-related breathing disorders: facts and clinical implications, Sleep Med. Rev. 2 (1998) 139–162.

[31] Editor's note, Patient's wife cures his snoring, Chest 85 (1984) 582.

[32] H. Gastaut, C.A. Tassinari, B. Duron, Polygraphic study of the episodic diurnal and nocturnal (hypnic and respiratory) manifestations of the Pickwickian syndrome, Brain Res. 2 (1966) 167–186.

[33] I.G. Robin, Snoring, Proc. R. Soc. Med. 41 (1948) 151–153.

[34] E.I. Jackson, H.S. Schmidt, Modification of sleeping position in the treatment of obstructive sleep apnea, Sleep Res. 11 (1982) 149.

[35] N.B. Kavey, S. Gidro-Frank, D.E. Sewitch, The importance of sleeping position and a simple treatment technique, Sleep Res. 11 (1982) 152.

[36] R.D. Cartwright, Effect of sleep position on sleep apnea severity, Sleep 7 (1984) 110–114.

[37] R. Cartwright, Home modification of sleep position for sleep apnea control, in: L Miles, R. Broughton, (Eds.), Clinical Evaluation and Physiological Monitoring in the Home and Work Environment, Raven Press, Palo Alto, 1990, pp. 123–129.

[38] R.D. Cartwright, R. Ristanovic, F. Diaz, et al., A comparative study of treatments for positional sleep apnea, Sleep 14 (1991) 546–552.

[39] R. Jokic, A. Klimaszewski, M. Crossley, et al., Positional treatment vs. continuous positive airway pressure in patients with positional obstructive sleep apnea syndrome, Chest 115 (1999) 771–781.

[40] J.J. Bignold, G. Deans-Costi, M.R. Goldsworthy, et al., Poor long-term patient compliance with the tennis ball technique for treating positional obstructive sleep apnea, J. Clin. Sleep Med. 5 (2009) 428–430.

[41] J.B. Lee, J.H. Park, J.H. Hong, et al., Determining optimal sleep position in patients with positional sleep-disordered breathing using response surface analysis, J. Sleep Res. 18 (2009) 26–35.

[42] T. Ono, R. Otsuka, T. Kuroda, et al., Effects of head and body position on two- and three-dimensional configurations of the upper airway, J. Dent. Res. 79 (2000) 1879–1884.

[43] F. Tanaka, H. Nakano, N. Sudo, C. Kubo, Relationship between the body position-specific apnea-hypopnea index and subjective sleepiness, Respiration (2009) (in press).

RECOMMENDED READING

J.J. Bignold, G. Deans-Costi, M.R. Goldsworthy, et al., Poor long-term patient compliance with the tennis ball technique for treating positional obstructive sleep apnea, J. Clin. Sleep Med. 5 (2009) 428–430.

R.D. Cartwright, S. Lloyd, J. Lilie, H. Kravitz, Sleep position training as treatment for sleep apnea syndrome: a preliminary study, Sleep 8 (1985) 87–94.

R.D. Cartwright, R. Ristanovic, F. Diaz, et al., A comparative study of treatments for positional sleep apnea, Sleep 14 (1991) 546–552.

E. Chang, G. Shiao, Craniofacial abnormalities in Chinese patients with obstructive and positional sleep apnea, Sleep Med. 9 (2008) 403–410.

Editor's note, Patient's wife cures his snoring, Chest 85 (1984) 582.

H. Gastaut, C.A. Tassinari, B. Duron, Polygraphic study of the episodic diurnal and nocturnal (hypnic and respiratory) manifestations of the Pickwickian syndrome, Brain Res. 2 (1966) 167–186.

S. Isono, A. Tanaka, T. Nishino, Lateral position decreases collapsibility of the passive pharynx in patients with obstructive sleep apnea, Anesthesiology 97 (2002) 780–785.

S. Joho, Y. Oda, T. Hirai, H. Inoue, Impact of sleeping position on central sleep apnea/Cheyne-Stokes respiration in patients with heart failure, Sleep Med. 11 (2010) 143–148.

R. Jokic, A. Klimaszewski, M. Crossley, et al., Positional treatment vs. continuous positive airway pressure in patients with positional obstructive sleep apnea syndrome, Chest 115 (1999) 771–781.

C.H. Lee, H.W. Shin, D.H. Han, et al., The implication of sleep position in the evaluation of surgical outcomes in obstructive sleep apnea, Otolaryngol. Head Neck Surg. 140 (2009) 531–535.

J.B. Lee, J.H. Park, J.H. Hong, et al., Determining optimal sleep position in patients with positional sleep-disordered breathing using response surface analysis, J. Sleep Res. 18 (2009) 26–35.

M.J. Mador, T.J. Kufel, U.J. Magalang, et al., Prevalence of positional sleep apnea in patients undergoing polysomnography, Chest 128 (2005) 2130–2137.

M.J. Mador, Y. Choi, A. Bhat, et al., Are the adverse effects of body position in patients with obstructive sleep apnea dependent on sleep stage?, Sleep Breath 14 (2010) 13–17.

R.D. McEvoy, D.J. Sharp, A.T. Thornton, The effects of posture on obstructive sleep apnea, Am. Rev. Respir. Dis. 133 (1986) 662–666.

A. Oksenberg, D.S. Silverberg, The effect of body posture on sleep-related breathing disorders: facts and clinical implications, Sleep Med. Rev. 2 (1998) 139–162.

A. Oksenberg, D.S. Silverberg, E. Arons, H. Radwan, Positional vs nonpositional obstructive sleep apnea patients. Anthropomorphic, nocturnal polysomnographic and multiple sleep latency test data, Chest 112 (1997) 629–639.

A. Oksenberg, D.S. Silverberg, Avoiding the supine posture during sleep for patients with mild obstructive sleep apnea, Am. J. Respir. Crit. Care Med. 180 (2009). 101(letter); author reply 101–102.

A. Oksenberg, D.S. Silverberg, D. Offenbach, E. Arons, Positional therapy for obstructive sleep apnea patients: a 6-month follow-up study, Laryngoscope 116 (2006) 1995–2000.

A. Oksenberg, Y. Khamaysi, D.S. Silverberg, A. Tarasiuk, Association of body position with severity of apneic events in patients with severe nonpositional obstructive sleep apnea, Chest 118 (2000) 1018–1024.

T. Ono, R. Otsuka, T. Kuroda, et al., Effects of head and body position on two- and three-dimensional configurations of the upper airway, J . Dent. Res. 79 (2000) 1879–1884.

I. Permut, M. Diaz-Abad, W. Chatila, et al., Comparison of positional therapy to CPAP in patients with positional obstructive sleep apnea, J. Clin. Sleep Med. (2010) (in press).

D.A. Pevernagie, A.W. Stanson, P.F. Sheedy, II, et al., Effects of body position on the upper airway of patients with obstructive sleep apnea, Am. J. Respir. Crit. Care Med. 152 (1995) 179–185.

W. Richard, D. Kox, C. den Herder, et al., The role of sleep position in obstructive sleep apnea syndrome, Eur. Arch. Otorhinolaryngol. 263 (2006) 946–950.

H. Saigusa, M. Suzuki, N. Higurashi, K. Kodera, Three-dimensional morphological analyses of positional dependence in patients with obstructive sleep apnea syndrome, Anesthesiology 110 (2009) 885–890.

M.A. Skinner, R.N. Kingshott, D.R. Jones, et al., Elevated posture for the management of obstructive sleep apnea, Sleep Breath 8 (2004) 193–200.

M.A. Skinner, R.N. Kingshott, S. Filsell, D.R. Taylor, Effect of the "tennis ball technique" vs CPAP in the management of position dependent obstructive sleep apnea syndrome, Respirology 13 (2008) 708–715.

T. Soga, S. Nakata, F. Yasuma, et al., Upper airway morphology in patients with obstructive sleep apnea syndrome: effects of lateral positioning, Auris Nasus Larynx 36 (2009) 305–309.

B.A. Soll, K.K. Yeo, J.W. Davis, et al., The effect of posture on Cheyne-Stokes respirations and hemodynamics in patients with heart failure, Sleep 32 (2009) 1499–1506.

I. Szollosi, T. Roebuck, B. Thompson, M.T. Naughton, Lateral sleeping position reduces severity of central sleep apnea/Cheyne-Stokes respiration, Sleep 29 (2006) 1045–1051.

F. Tanaka, H. Nakano, N. Sudo, C. Kubo, Relationship between the body position-specific apnea-hypopnea index and subjective sleepiness, Respiration 78 (2009) 185–190.

J.H. Walsh, K.J. Maddison, P.R. Platt, et al., Influence of head extension, flexion, and rotation on collapsibility of the passive upper airways, Sleep 31 (2008) 1440–1447.

J.H. Walsh, M.S. Leigh, A. Paduch, et al., Effect of body posture on pharyngeal shape and size in adults with and without obstructive sleep apnea, Sleep 31 (2008) 1543–1549.

Chapter 24

Scheduled Sleep Periods as an Adjuvant Treatment for Narcolepsy

Ann E. Rogers
Emory University, Atlanta, GA

PROTOCOL NAME

Scheduled sleep periods as an adjuvant treatment for narcolepsy.

GROSS INDICATION

Scheduled sleep periods are indicated for patients with narcolepsy who are unable to remain awake during the day.

SPECIFIC INDICATION

This intervention is suitable for narcoleptic patients who prefer not to take stimulant medications, and/or those patients whose medications do not completely relieve their excessive daytime sleepiness.

CONTRAINDICATIONS

The treatment is contraindicated in narcoleptic patients with recent increases in excessive daytime sleepiness. Since obstructive sleep apnea is common in patients with narcolepsy, all patients who report an increase in excessive daytime sleepiness need to be evaluated for obstructive sleep apnea.

RATIONALE FOR INTERVENTION

Scheduled sleep periods (naps) and good sleep hygiene have traditionally been recommended for management of excessive daytime sleepiness in narcoleptic patients. However, due to their limited efficacy, naps and good sleep hygiene are no longer recommended as the sole treatments for narcolepsy [1,2].

Behavioral Treatments for Sleep Disorders. DOI: 10.1016/B978-0-12-381522-4.00024-9

STEP BY STEP DESCRIPTION OF PROCEDURES

1. If an established patient continues to complain of daytime sleepiness, evaluate the efficacy of current stimulant therapy. Consider altering the type of stimulant medication, amount of medication, and/or timing of stimulant medication to reduce daytime sleepiness. A nocturnal polysomnogram may be necessary to determine if increased excessive daytime sleepiness is caused by the development of a second sleep disorder, such as obstructive sleep apnea or periodic limb movement disorder.
2. Consider also adherence to and cost of therapy. Narcoleptic patients rarely increase their dosage of stimulant medications and frequently reduce their dosage, often due to fears of becoming addicted to stimulant medications [3]. The costs of medication may also be a factor, with newer medications such as modafinil or armodafinil costing considerably more than older medications such as dexadrine or methylphenidate.
3. If adherence is not an issue and/or patients are unable to tolerate or unwilling to take stimulant medications, have them keep a record of their nocturnal sleep time and when they have difficulties remaining alert during the daytime for at least a week.
4. Use the data obtained from the sleep log to determine placement of the scheduled sleep periods (naps). Naps should be 10 or 15 minutes in duration, and scheduled to precede times when the patient typically has difficulty remaining awake. For example, if the patient typically has trouble staying awake during a 2 pm meeting, a nap could be scheduled at 1:30 or 1:45 pm to increase alertness during the 2 pm meeting.

POSSIBLE MODIFICATIONS/VARIANTS

A single long nap (120 minutes) can be substituted for several short naps. Although the long nap has produced statistically significant increases in alertness on a modified MSLT, mean sleep latencies remained quite low. In addition, all of the alerting effects associated with a 120 minute nap were lost within 3 hours [4].

Regular bedtimes and extended nocturnal sleep periods may also be recommended. Although regular times for arising and retiring may reduce perceived symptom severity, they may have no effect on reducing objectively measured daytime sleepiness [5]. Patients should be cautioned to avoid sleep deprivation; however, extended periods of nocturnal sleep are not necessary, and may further exacerbate the nocturnal sleep disruption that many patients with narcolepsy experience.

PROOF OF CONCEPT/SUPPORTING DATA/EVIDENCE BASE

Although behavioral interventions for the treatment of narcolepsy are very appealing to patients and providers alike, there are limited data supporting their efficacy. In fact, current treatment guidelines [1,2] do not support the use of scheduled sleep periods as the sole method of managing excessive daytime sleepiness in patients with narcolepsy.

Although naps can produce transient increases in alertness, the alerting effects of 15- and 30-minute naps were demonstrated to lose their effectiveness when narcoleptic patients were re-tested 30 minutes after awakening from a nap in one study [6]. Even five short naps per day have been shown to fail to increase performance over a no-nap condition in patients with narcolepsy [7]. One study suggested that a single long nap (120 minutes) may be more effective than several short naps for reducing excessive daytime sleepiness in narcoleptic patients [7].

Although scheduled sleep periods may be useful as an adjuvant to stimulant medications in some patients with narcolepsy, patients who are employed may find it very difficult and/or impossible to take one or two 15-minute naps during their work day, and few employers would tolerate patients taking a 120-minute mid-day nap.

Current practice guidelines [1,2] stress that stimulant medications, rather than scheduled sleep periods, should be prescribed for the relief of excessive daytime sleepiness in patients with narcolepsy.

REFERENCES

[1] S. Keam, M.C. Walker, Therapies for narcolepsy with or without cataplexy; evidence-based review, Curr. Opin. Neurol. 20 (6) (2007) 699–703.

[2] T.I. Morgenthaler, V.K. Kapur, T. Brown, et al., Practice parameters for the treatment of narcolepsy and other hypersomnias of central origin, Sleep 30 (2007) 1705–1711.

[3] A.E. Rogers, C. Cantor, S. Marcus, Compliance with stimulant medications in patients with narcolepsy: measurement with a MEMS trackcap, Sleep (2001).

[4] T. Helmus, L. Rosenthal, C. Bishop, et al., The alerting effects of short and long naps in narcoleptic, sleep-deprived, and alert individuals, Sleep 20 (1997) 251–257.

[5] A.E. Rogers, M.S. Aldrich, X. Lin, A comparison of three different sleep schedules for reducing daytime sleepiness in narcoleptic patients, Sleep 24 (4) (2001) 385–391.

[6] R. Roehrs, F. Zorick, R. Wittig, et al., Alerting effects of naps in patients with narcolepsy, Sleep 9 (1986) 191–194.

[7] J. Mullington, R. Broughton, Scheduled naps in the management of daytime sleepiness in narcolepsy-cataplexy, Sleep 16 (1993) 444–456.

Part III

BSM Protocols for Pediatric Sleep Disorders

Introduction

Brett R. Kuhn

Behavioral Sleep Medicine Services, Children's Sleep Disorders Center, Children's Hospital & Medical Center, Omaha, NE

The majority of sleep disorders are experienced both by children and adults, yet the clinical manifestations, evaluation methods, diagnostic criteria, and treatments differ greatly across these two populations. For example, adults with Sleep-related breathing disorders (SRBD) typically experience excessive daytime sleepiness (EDS), while children may be more likely to present with restless sleep, mouth breathing, and inattention. The etiology of SRBD in children is more often associated with craniofacial abnormalities, neuromuscular disorders, and adenotonsillar hypertrophy than with obesity [1]. In addition, EDS in children may produce "paradoxical" manifestations such as increased activity, aggression, or risk-taking behavior. In children, narcolepsy is not always accompanied by cataplexy, sleep paralysis, or hypnagogic hallucinations in the early stages, making the diagnosis a considerable challenge for some [2,3]. Finally, pediatric "insomnia" differs greatly from what is described in adults, prompting experts to derive a modified definition [4]. Behavioral and pharmacological interventions for pediatric insomnia are clearly distinct from those used in adults [5–7].

Pediatric sleep specialists clearly face unique challenges. They must possess a fundamental knowledge of normal child development in order to accurately evaluate and treat a "moving target" due to rapid physiological and maturational changes in sleep development. For example, EDS can be challenging to assess in early childhood when napping is the norm, and within the context of rapidly decreasing sleep requirements as children age. Culture, family values, and caregiver influences must also be considered, as they play more prominent roles in the initiation, maintenance, and resolution of pediatric sleep disorders compared to their adult counterparts.

Despite these challenges, the field of pediatric sleep medicine has witnessed rapid growth both in professional and public interest. Pediatric sleep clinics and centers are popping up all over the US, and are beginning to show up in other countries. Jobs appear plentiful, and professionals with pediatric expertise are currently in high demand. Students across a variety of disciplines are suddenly expressing interest in careers in pediatric sleep medicine, and there are even a few adult sleep specialists who are "crossing over" to bring their skills to the pediatric arena.

The field of pediatric sleep medicine continues to develop its own professional identity. Students and professionals now have the opportunity to attend child-specific sleep conferences, both in the US and internationally. The past 10 years have witnessed such a proliferation of peer-reviewed journal articles that a separate journal dedicated exclusively to pediatric sleep disorders cannot be far off.

The chapters in this section of the book reflect this growth and represent the current state of the science. Readers will notice that the section contains a number of chapters describing interventions to address the Behavioral Insomnias of Childhood. This emphasis is warranted for two reasons: (1) the large majority of treatment studies, review articles, consensus papers, and practice parameters have focused on this population; and (2) these cases represent the "bread and butter" when it comes to clinical referrals to comprehensive pediatric sleep practices. The section also includes three excellent chapters detailing behavioral treatments for pediatric parasomnias, including sleepwalking and sleep terrors, nocturnal enuresis, and chronic nightmares in adolescents.

Although adenotonsillectomy remains the first-line treatment for childhood OSAs, continuous positive airway pressure (CPAP) is being increasingly called upon as the obesity epidemic impacts more and more children. Tolerance and adherence is the major obstacle to pressure therapies. Readers who make it to the thirty-seventh chapter of this book will be aptly rewarded with a well-written chapter by a leading expert in the development and promotion of CPAP adherence therapies for children. Finally, while there is a solid knowledge-base describing the changing sleep needs and sleep timing associated with puberty. Sleep practitioners sorely lack evidence-based tools to address one of the most rapidly growing public health issues of all: sleep-deprived adolescents. Even the task of identifying an expert to write a chapter on the treatment of adolescent sleep was difficult. Fortunately, two authorities with a wealth of experience working with adolescents stepped up to meet the challenge. The final chapter of this book details the application of motivational interviewing (MI) to help facilitate healthy adolescent sleep behaviors.

I truly believe this talented group of authors succeeded in providing the necessary "how to do it" details that will allow front-line practitioners to positively impact the millions of children and adolescents experiencing disturbed and disordered sleep. It is my hope that the principles and procedures presented in these chapters will also serve as a springboard for future research, especially clinical outcome research designed to develop more effective, "user-friendly" interventions for children, adolescents and their families.

REFERENCES

[1] T.F. Hoban, R.D. Chervin, Pediatric sleep-related breathing disorders and restless legs syndrome: how children are different, Neurologist 11 (2005) 325–337.

[2] S. Kotagal, Narcolepsy in childhood, in: S.H. Sheldon, R. Ferber, M. Kryger (Eds.), Principles and Practice of Pediatric Sleep Medicine, Elsevier Saunders, Philadelphia, PA, 2005, pp. 171–182.

[3] G. Stores, The protean manifestations of childhood narcolepsy and their misinterpretation, Dev. Med. Child Neurol. 48 (2006) 307–310.

[4] J.A. Mindell, G. Emslie, J. Blumer, et al., Pharmacologic management of insomnia in children and adolescents: consensus statement, Pediatrics 117 (2006) e1223–1232.

[5] J.A. Mindell, B. Kuhn, D.S. Lewin, et al., Behavioral treatment of bedtime problems and night wakings in infants and young children, Sleep 29 (2006) 1263–1276.

[6] J.A. Owens, C.L. Rosen, J.A. Mindell, Medication use in the treatment of pediatric insomnia: results of a survey of community-based pediatricians, Pediatrics 111 (2003) e628–635.

[7] C.J. Schnoes, B.R. Kuhn, E. Workman, C. Ellis, Pediatric prescribing practices of Clonidine and other psychopharmacological agents for pediatric sleep disturbances, Clin. Pediatr. (Phila) 45 (2006) 229–238.

Chapter 25

Brief Parent Consultation to Prevent Infant/Toddler Sleep Disturbance

Brian Symon
Kensington Park, Adelaide, South Australia

PROTOCOL NAME

Brief parent consultation to prevent infant/toddler sleep disturbance.

GROSS INDICATION

This intervention is preventative in nature, and targets families with children less than 4 weeks old.

SPECIFIC INDICATION

The intervention is appropriate for any family wishing to help their infant maximize sleep quality and sleep duration.

CONTRAINDICATIONS

There are few families where there is a clear contraindication. Contraindications include:

- major medical problems where very significant medical interventions are required and must take precedence over all other issues (an example might be major cardiac abnormalities);
- weight loss or very poor weight gain, where this has to be the first priority for the family and their carers.

In our experience, some families are not contraindicated but in practice may be less likely to succeed. For example:

- if the parents or mother come from a culture where co-sleeping is the norm or it is her wish;

Behavioral Treatments for Sleep Disorders. DOI: 10.1016/B978-0-12-381522-4.00025-0

- if the parents, have a strong belief in a particular philosophy of care (e.g., "attachment parenting");
- if there has been a previous infant disaster (e.g., SIDS);
- where there has been major technical difficulty in achieving pregnancy or previous miscarriage (precious conception);
- if there is parental dispute (e.g., separation with trauma and distress while the child is weeks or months old);
- if the child has suffered major neurological damage (e.g., severe totally dependent cerebral palsy).

There are families that some may consider to have the status of "contra-indications", or where success might not be anticipated, but where, in practice, we have found outcomes to be good. These include:

- families with low levels of parental education – this is NOT a contraindication;
- families of low socio-economic status;
- where there are modest levels of neurological deficit in the child (e.g., Down syndrome)
- single-parent families.

RATIONALE FOR INTERVENTION

- Up to 46 percent of parents report infant sleep problems [1–5].
- These problems include not sleeping through the night, delay in achieving sleep, and atypical behavior at wakening. These sleep disturbances may have serious negative consequences, including postnatal depression, family breakdown, and child abuse [3,6,7].
- Disturbances may be long-lasting, with one study finding that, based on parental reports, 41 percent of children with sleeping disturbance at 8 months still had difficulties at 3 years [7].
- Studies of sleep achievement show that all individuals, including babies, "learn" to fall asleep with certain external environmental cues [1,8,9].
- Sleep initiation is repeated several times during the night, as all individuals repeatedly awaken for brief periods. However, these awakenings and returns to sleep are often not understood by parents.
- Parents can inadvertently contribute to unwelcome night crying when they rock, hold, pat, or feed their infant to sleep. The child may learn to re-initiate sleep repeatedly by signaling (crying) for the parent to repeat similar behaviors [10].
- Techniques of resolving sleep problems in infants and young children that have shown the best and most persistent results involve behavior modification [4,11,12].
- Given the widespread nature of the problem and the potential for serious consequences, preventing the development of sleep problems is a superior strategy.

- Behavioral interventions have a well-reported efficacy in decreasing sleep disturbance from the time of birth [5,11–13].
- Given the frequency of these problems and their impact upon family life, a simple intervention available from primary care services would be of value.
- The intervention described is time-efficient, highly effective, and cheap to deliver. It can be provided by a trained nurse, and does not increase infant distress as measured by crying times.

In our study [14] the tutorial was provided to families one on one, but there is no reason why it could not be delivered to groups or included in current antenatal programs.

STEP BY STEP DESCRIPTION OF PROCEDURES

The intervention, utilized in the study, consists of a single, 45-minute tutorial delivered by a trained nurse. However, any health professional with an understanding of infant sleep could be trained to deliver the program. The author has many years' experience of working with trained nurses. Patient outcomes are essentially the same for nurse and doctor. In practice, the number of visits varies from as few as one, as studied, to multiple visits spread over weeks or months in some families.

In the RCT described [14], families were recruited immediately after the birth of their child. They were found by reading birth notices in the single local daily newspaper. The birth notice was then cross-referenced with the local telephone book, and if the families could be identified they were rung and offered an opportunity to participate in the study. In the context of assisting families in the community, there are many options for recruitment of families. Self-referral from friends and relatives dominates all others in the author's experience. However, mothers' groups, antenatal classes, Internet fora, referral from other professionals, and lactation classes may all be points of referral.

Families are met by the trained nurse. Both partners are encouraged to attend, and the visit is scheduled to take place by 3 weeks of age if at all possible. The infants are weighed to make sure that the intervention is not being applied to infants who are malnourished. In clinical practice, families attend at varied times and for quite different numbers of visits. Some families will present as early as 36 weeks' gestation. This timing is quite approximate, but is found to be useful in that the parents are receptive and not affected by fatigue and the stresses of a newborn who may or may not be doing well. After birth, families may present at any time. The concept of a "preventative" protocol becomes less applicable as the infant ages, and beyond 12 weeks it is probably worth seeing the consultation as "resolving" a problem.

The 45-minute tutorial contains two elements: background knowledge about infant sleep, and a guide on how to manage the baby at home. In a clinic, this can be considerably expanded upon. When the focus of your work is

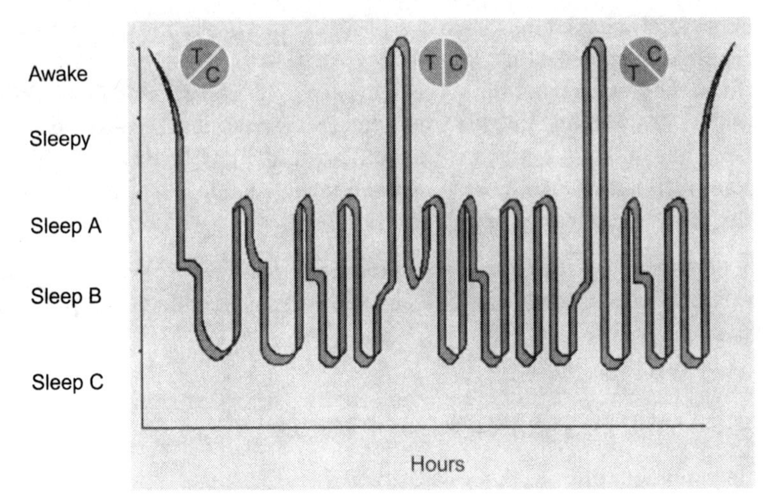

FIGURE 25.1 Multiple sleep cycles.

problem prevention in the first 12 weeks of life, there is an increased number of elements that require the carers' support. Feeding technique, weight gain, maternal nutrition and self confidence, paternal understanding and support of his partner all become relevant to success in achieving high-quality sleep.

Background Knowledge (Part I of the Protocol)

Background knowledge emphasizes six basic points:

1. A block of sleep contains multiple *sleep cycles* (Figure 25.1).
   Teaching about the existence of sleep cycles is critical to the parents' understanding. While well known to those with an interest in the field, it is not a common element of lay knowledge. In neonates, sleep cycles tend to be about 45 minutes long.
2. Sleep achievement is in part *cue dependent*.
   Explaining cues of sleep is again straightforward. Practical examples, such as sleeping with a companion or with a familiar pillow, enhance comprehension. Reverse examples (e.g., the difficulty of sleeping in the back seat of a car) also help to emphasize the role of sleep cues.
3. Cues of sleep are *learned*, can be changed and then relearned.
   Cues of sleep are, in fact, variable. Examples such as learning to sleep with a new partner, moving house to a suburb with new sounds, or buying a new bed are readily understood. It is important to teach that sleep cues can change with time and be easily relearned. As adults we know this to be true from our life experience, but emphasizing the point is important for parental understanding.

4. Sleep achievement is usefully regarded as a *learned skill.*
   By combining points (2) and (3), we now teach that sleep functions as a learned skill. Understanding that both achieving and maintaining sleep are learned skills is critical for all that follows. Fortunately for the care provider, this point is rapidly understood by the mother once we get to the next point.
5. *Fatigue interferes* with the learned skill of sleep achievement.
   If sleep truly functions as a learned skill, then, like all human skills without exception, as we become more sleepy the skill is more difficult to achieve. Every woman who has been a mother rapidly understands this point. Fatigue is virtually a universal experience in mothers. All mothers have had personal experience of being tired to the point that achieving sleep is difficult. In this intervention, we emphasize that newborn infants are exquisitely fatigue sensitive. They rapidly become tired to the point that achieving sleep is difficult. The newborn baby may be only 10–20 minutes overtired before their ability to achieve and maintain sleep is impaired.
6. *Cues of sleep achievement that are parent independent* are the most successful.
   Avoid sleep transitions which involve parental assistance. Allow a child to achieve sleep alone. As sleep achievement is in part cue dependent, and as sleep is cyclical, if sleep achievement is usually parent dependent, then at later sleep achievement events within a block of sleep the child will seek parental cues again.

The point here is to guide parents to allow a child to complete the process of sleep achievement independently as often as possible.

The above six points provide a basic framework whereby a parent can understand sleep in their newborn child.

To simplify and summarize at the end of this part of the tutorial, it is emphasized that sleep is usefully regarded as a learned skill; that, like all skills, if the child becomes tired the ability to perform the skill is impaired; and that parent-independent cues of sleep are most useful.

Advice for Home with a New Baby (Part II of the Protocol)

This advice is most appropriate in the first 3 or 4 weeks of life.

Parents receive advice from numerous sources that often varies greatly. In addition, there is often an overlay of emotive content. It is common for mothers to receive a message that unless they, the mother, look after their child in a particular way, there will be dire consequences for the child's life.

It is important to recognize that the mother is risk averse in the extreme. She has undergone major hormonal readjustments, and may be experiencing a flood of powerful emotions. She needs support, understanding, and practical advice. Guilt is never an ethical or useful strategy for guiding patients. This is even more true in this setting.

This intervention attempts to simplify and perhaps oversimplify the situation, which aids in helping the mother feel that she will succeed and does understand the important issues.

A major starting point is to state that there are only two significant issues: feeding and sleeping. If these are managed successfully, all other issues will generally resolve with minimal effort. This, of course, assumes good health. If the child has a medical problem of significance, this must take pre-eminence.

1. *Feeding and nutrition.*
   - Baby:
     - breast or bottle feed 2–3 to 4–5 hourly on demand;
     - there may be a need for occasional top-up bottles on busy days;
     - try to achieve a weight gain of approximately 30 g per day (note that the range of healthy weight gain varies from 20 to 60 g per day).
   - Mother:

     Note that while breast-feeding, the mother's physiology changes significantly. The lactating mother's energy needs increase by a factor of 50–100 percent. This is a fact rarely taught to families. To assist in maintaining such an energy intake:
     - it is recommended that the mother has three good meals per day, with an aim to increase calorie intake by at least 2000 calories per day
     - drinking and hydration are important; the mother should drink 1–1.5 l of full-cream milk per day in any format that she likes;
     - particularly with a first-born child, it should be possible for the mother to sleep in the afternoon for 30–60 minutes.

     Caring for the mother's well-being is a fundamental part of caring for the child.
2. *Sleep.*
   - In the first 3 weeks or so, life for the newborn is basically feed, sleep, feed, sleep, feed and sleep.
   - Try to achieve 18–21 hours of sleep per day (note that this aim is higher than some other authors in that it deletes the skewing to lower levels caused by children with sleep disturbance in large population studies).
   - Try to keep feeding times fairly short (15–30 minutes is recommended).
   - Avoid over-handling. Excessive handling in the neonatal period is a major cause of infant fatigue, loss of sleep skills, and then poor sleep. The cumulative impact of fatigue disrupting sleep can lead to major sleep disruption.
   - Avoid over-handling by friends and relatives.
   - Let sleeping babies sleep if the weight gain is acceptable. The only exception is to limit continuous daytime sleeps to not longer than about 4 hours.

- Individual sleeping periods should be 2–5 hours for the newborn. These will increase with age. At night particularly they become longer – for example, 6 hours at 6 weeks, 8 hours at 8 weeks, and 12 hours at 12 weeks. Note that the 12-hour sleeps include at least one feed.
- Waking times will be 20–40 minutes in the day, and shorter at night. This time includes all handling, feeding, and changing. Understanding the limits to the child's ability to interact at this age is fundamental in the attempt to avoid overtiredness.
- Minimize cues of sleep that regularly use parental care. When babies are ready to sleep, put them down and let them go to sleep with minimal intervention.

To conclude the information part of the tutorial, a few general points are made:

- Babies will often be very sleepy by the end of the feed, and can go straight down to sleep.
- The bowel is often opened frequently, and if the milk supply is strong in the first month this may be as often as four to eight times per day. (This reassures the parents that such frequent bowel actions are not diarrhoea.)
- If the feeding is going well and the recommended sleep volumes are achieved, the baby may not cry a great deal.
- Despite days where crying is minimal, there will always be some days where the baby has been a little too busy, becomes overtired, and will cry from fatigue even when well fed. In this setting, parents are guided to provide a small amount of additional care. This may include an extra feed to double-check for hunger, minor direct contact and physical reassurance, but parents are given permission to leave the baby to settle independently. In babies of this age (i.e., under 1 month old), parents are guided to leave the baby to cry down for 10–20–30 minutes. As some parents find this distressing, they are given guidance to leave the baby for as long as they feel comfortable, but are warned of the dangers of over-handling, particularly when the baby is tired or overtired.

Parents are then given an opportunity to ask further questions, but in the majority of cases, apart from clarifying one or two points already included in the teaching, they feel adequately informed.

The parents are provided with a printed copy of the tutorial content to take with them. A copy of the information sheet can be found at http://silentnights.org/. In clinical practice, it is found that provision of written material relevant to the consult is helpful.

A simple summary of the first 3 months is useful to the parents, and this can be given at any time:

- *Month 1.* This is a time of feeding, sleeping, and growth. Interactions with the baby are minimized.

- *Month 2*. The month of "awakening". The baby is learning about affection, and will logically put energy into increasing parent contact time. Parents gain here by guiding the baby to sleep independently, and to keep sleep volumes long; 18–21 hours of sleep per day is still normal. This is a time when the parents and the baby begin to share affection and communication. Smiling commences.
- *Month 3*. The month to establish some long-term patterns. Evening bed time is beginning to develop predictability of between 6 and 7 pm. Day-time sleep patterns are establishing. Aim to achieve 12 hours of sleep at night, including one or two feeds, by about 12 weeks. The baby is now developing quite significant social skills, has obvious interest and affection for the family, and an interest in the world around. By 3 months, it is hoped that there will be a fairly predictable pattern of feeding and sleeping around the 24-hour clock. The child usually has developed quite meaningful skills of communication, and has started to vocalize, share affection with a wider range of people and to have a "personality".

After 12 weeks of age, if all is going well the family is encouraged to take complete control of the review process. If they feel confident, they need no further help. If they feel concerned about any issue they are welcome to return, but they take control of the process.

POSSIBLE MODIFICATIONS/VARIANTS

Clinical experience indicates that additional visits can enhance effectiveness. There are other choices for delivering the information to parents. Group sessions can be very helpful, where multiple families share experiences. Website support is very useful in that large amounts of information can be delivered to the reader. Email communication is often requested by families, but is limited by the amount of information that can be written in response to a question. Face-to-face strategies are the most effective.

Enhancements to the single session program could include the following:

- Provision of the information at a visit while the mother is pregnant. In clinical practice, the author attempts to see women at about 36 weeks' gestation. The information given is as above. The difference here is that the woman is still pregnant, often feeling well, and is welcoming of a "plan of action".
- Seeing the family when the baby is about 2–3 weeks old. The family is now facing some of the real issues and dilemmas of having a child at home. The information is as above, and the document given to the family is the same. In practice, the visit often focuses upon the issues of feeding and weight gain. At this visit, it is re-emphasized that life is largely feed and go straight back to sleep.
- Seeing the family when the child is about 4 weeks old. The documentation is the same, but the baby is now beginning to develop periods of wakefulness. These are described as "happy wake times". Weight gain is checked.

Feeding choices that the mother has made are supported when weight gain is good; if weight gain is poor or marginal, a range of strategies is used to ensure adequate nutrition. The author notes that about 75 percent of his patients are breastfeeding at 12 weeks.

- Seeing the family when the child is about 8 weeks old. A new document is introduced called "The perfect night at 12 weeks" (this document can be found at the URL http://silentnights.org/). The "happy wake time" is discussed again. The baby's signals of fatigue are described and emphasized, as is the limited ability to be awake. A timetable for the day is suggested as a "soft plan". The family is guided that this is the general direction, rather than a hard and fast set of times and rules.
- Seeing the family when the child is about 12 weeks old. The same document is used to guide the consultation. The baby is again checked for weight gain and nutrition. Sleep achievements for the baby are checked, and again the family is gently guided in the direction of sleep times described in the above sheet.

PROOF OF CONCEPT/SUPPORTING DATA/EVIDENCE BASE

Parent education/prevention is conceivable the most economical and time-efficient approach to behaviorally based pediatric sleep problems. It is also a highly effective approach. A recent review sponsored by the American Academy of Sleep Medicine concluded that parent education/prevention is one of only two treatment modalities to meet the most stringent criteria for evidence-based practice [15].

The peer-reviewed evidence supporting this particular prevention protocol was published in 2005 [14]. The results of this study are summarized as follows:

- 268 families were studied, with the intervention consultation occurring in the first 2–3 weeks of life. Families were randomized to interventions and controls.
- The intervention was a 45-minute consultation with a trained nurse.
- Data returned recorded 3273 days of sleep diaries, with every 10-minute period coded for sleep, feeding, awake, or crying.
- Total sleep time was 15 hours or more per 24 hours for 62 percent of recorded days in the intervention group, compared with 36 percent in the control group ($P < 0.001$).
- At 6 weeks of age, intervention infants slept a mean 1.3 hours per day more than control infants (95% CI, 0.95–1.65), comprising a mean 0.5 h more night sleep (95% CI, 0.32–0.69) and 0.8 h more daytime sleep (95% CI, 0.56–1.07).
- At 12 weeks, intervention infants slept a mean 1.2 hours per day more (95% CI, 0.94–2.14), comprising 0.64 h more night sleep (95% CI, 0.19–0.89) and 0.58 h more daytime sleep (95% CI, 0.39–1.03).

- There was no significant difference in crying time between the groups.
- At 5-year follow-up there were five divorces in the controls and none in the interventions ($P < 0.02$).

REFERENCES

[1] R. Ferber, Sleep, sleeplessness, and sleep disruptions in infants and young children, Ann. Clin. Res. 17 (1985) 227–234.

[2] K.L. Armstrong, R.A. Quinn, M.R. Dadds, The sleep patterns of normal children, Med. J. Aust. 161 (1994) 202–206.

[3] S.M. Kerr, S.A. Jowett, Sleep problems in pre-school children: a review of the literature, Child Care Health Dev. 20 (1994) 379–391.

[4] P. Ramchandani, L. Wiggs, V. Webb, G. Stores, A systematic review of treatments for settling problems and night waking in young children, Br. Med. J. 320 (2000) 209–213.

[5] H. Hiscock, M. Wake, Randomised controlled trial of behavioural infant sleep intervention to improve infant sleep and maternal mood, Br. Med. J. 324 (2002) 1062.

[6] P. Boyce, J. Stubbs, The importance of postnatal depression, Med. J. Aust. 161 (1994) 471–472.

[7] B. Zuckerman, J. Stevenson, V. Bailey, Sleep problems in early childhood: Continuities, predictive factors, and behavioural correlates, Pediatrics 80 (1987) 664–671.

[8] R. Ferber, Solve Your Child's Sleep Problems, Simon & Schuster, New York, NY, 1985.

[9] W. Richman, A community survey of characteristics of 1–2 year olds with sleep disruptions, Am. Acad. Child Psychiatry 20 (1981) 281–291.

[10] M.C. Johnson, Infant and toddler sleep. A telephone survey of parents in one community, Dev. Behav. Pediatrics 12 (1991) 108–114.

[11] I. James-Roberts, J. Sleep, S. Morris, et al., Use of a behavioural programme in the first 3 months to prevent infant crying and sleeping problems, J. Paediatr. Child Health 37 (2001) 289–297.

[12] A. Wolfson, P. Lacks, A. Futterman, Effects of parent training on infant sleeping patterns, parents' stress, and perceived parental competence, J. Consult. Clin. Psychol. 60 (1992) 41–48.

[13] V.I. Rickert, C.M. Johnson, Reducing nocturnal awakenings and crying episodes in infants and young children. A comparison between scheduled awakenings and systematic ignoring, Pediatrics 81 (1988) 203–211.

[14] B.G. Symon, J.E. Marley, A.J. Martin, E.R. Norman, Effect of a consultation teaching behaviour modification on sleep performance in infants: a randomised controlled trial, Med. J. Aust. 182 (5) (2005) 215–218.

[15] B. Symon, Your Baby, University of Adelaide, Adelaide, 1997.

RECOMMENDED READING

Australian Bureau of Statistics, Information Paper: 1991 Census – Socio-Economic Indexes for Areas, ABS, Canberra, 1993.

R. Barr, M. Kramer, C. Boisjoly, et al., Parental diary of infant cry and fuss behaviour, Arch. Dis. Child 63 (1988) 380–387.

Centers for Disease Control and Prevention. Epi Info, version 6.04a [computer program]. Centers for Disease Control and Prevention, Atlanta, GA, 1996.

S.M. Kerr, S.A. Jowett, L.N. Smith, Preventing sleep problems in infants: A randomised controlled trial, J. Adv. Nur. 24 (1996) 928–942.

K.Y. Liang, S.L. Zeger, Longitudinal data analysis using generalised linear models, Biometrica 73 (1986) 13–22.

J.A. Mindell, B. Kuhn, D.S. Lewin, et al., Behavioral treatment of bedtime problems and night wakings in infants and young children, Sleep 29 (10) (Oct 1 2006) 1263–1276.

S. Pocock, Clinical Trials – A Practical Approach, Pittman Press, Bath, 1983.

SAS Institute, The Gennod Procedure, SAS-STAT Software, Changes and Enhancements Through Release 6.12, SAS Institute, Cary, NC, 1997.

Chapter 26

Unmodified Extinction for Childhood Sleep Disturbance

Robert Didden
Behavioural Science Institute/Department of Special Education, Radboud University, Nijmegen, The Netherlands

Jeff Sigafoos
School of Educational Psychology & Pedagogy, Victoria University of Wellington, Karori, Wellington, New Zealand

Giulio E. Lancioni
Department of Psychology, University of Bari, Bari, Italy

PROTOCOL NAME

Unmodified extinction for childhood sleep disturbance.

GROSS INDICATION

Unmodified extinction is an effective treatment for childhood insomnia. It is effective in reducing inappropriate bedtime behaviors (e.g., crying, repeatedly getting out of bed, and tantrums) that interfere with sleep onset and maintenance. These behaviors are often maintained by reinforcement in the form of parental attention and insufficient limit setting. These child behaviors often occur at bedtime and at waking up at night (night waking) or in the early morning. This treatment may also be effective in case of co-sleeping, whereby child and parent sleep in the same bed.

Although extinction is typically used in young children, it may be used in infants and in older children as well.

SPECIFIC INDICATION

Unmodified extinction is indicated for the treatment of the behavioral insomnias of childhood: limit setting and sleep onset types.

Behavioral Treatments for Sleep Disorders. DOI: 10.1016/B978-0-12-381522-4.00026-2

CONTRAINDICATION

There is no contraindication to the use of unmodified extinction. However, prior to starting an extinction procedure, any somatic, neurological, or other factor that may be responsible for bedtime and night-waking problems should be assessed and ruled out. There are many such factors, such as breathing difficulties, epilepsy, and melatonin synthesis disturbance. For example, a distinction should be made between bedtime resistance and delayed sleep phase disorder, as the latter has a different etiology and treatment (e.g., chronotherapy, melatonin).

The use of extinction in children with anxiety disorders and in parents with mental health problems is at the clinician's discretion. It should be noted that results of several studies indicate that extinction is also effective for sleep problems in infants of depressed and psychological disturbed parents [1].

RATIONALE FOR INTERVENTION

During their development, most children will show some type of inappropriate behavior during bedtime and at night. They may acquire inappropriate sleep onset associations that disrupt the sleep–wake rhythm. From a learning theory point of view, inappropriate behaviors are acquired through operant conditioning – that is, are shaped and maintained by their reinforcing consequences. Disruptive behavior or non-compliance may be negatively reinforced if that behavior results in escape from or avoidance of an unpleasant situation. Children learn that as a result of a tantrum or resistance, they are allowed to stay awake with their parents in the living room, to watch television or to play with their favorite toys. In this example, parents may have difficulties in adequately enforcing bedtime limits because of their past behaviors, which have inadvertently "rewarded" bedtime refusal behaviors. The child's disruptive behavior at bedtime is then strengthened, and he or she will probably exhibit the same behavior at bedtime in the future.

Problematic behaviors may be positively reinforced if they result in the receipt of a pleasant event. Children may learn that they will receive parental attention upon exhibiting disruptive behaviors. For example, parents go to visit a child in his or her bedroom contingent upon the child calling out for parents and/or crying. These behaviors are maintained if they are followed by a strong reinforcer, namely parental attention.

If disruptive behaviors are operants, their frequency may be reduced by removing the reinforcer. Extinction is an effective treatment for such behaviors, and involves terminating the reinforcement contingency that maintains a behavior, which results in a reduction in a behavior's occurrence over time [2]. The extinction approach consists of several procedures: (1) time out from positive reinforcement (e.g., parental attention); (2) planned ignoring (e.g., of attention maintained disruptive behavior); and (3) extinction of escape and avoidance behaviors. Extinction has been show to be effective in reducing childhood disruptive behaviors, such as tantrums and aggressive behavior [3], and feeding problems [4].

In terms of treatment of childhood sleep disturbance, the implication is that withdrawing reinforcement for inappropriate bedtime behaviors will result in elimination of such behaviors, and as a result, improved sleep onset may be facilitated.

STEP BY STEP DESCRIPTION OF PROCEDURES

The objective of extinction it to change the usual strategies by parents for their child's inappropriate bedtime behaviors. Unmodified extinction entails the requirement that reinforcement for inappropriate bedtime behaviors is completely withdrawn. This intervention should always be used in combination with establishing stimulus control over bedtime (i.e., setting a bedtime routine) and reinforcement for appropriate bedtime behaviors (e.g., lying quietly in bed, being compliant with parental requests, going to bed without resistance).

Four steps may be identified during the process of functional assessment and intervention with extinction.

Step 1: Functional Assessment

Before implementing extinction, it is important to conduct some type of functional assessment [5]. The objective of a functional assessment is to identify the operant function of inappropriate child behaviors, and type of reinforcement contingencies (positive, negative) "delivered" by parents and that maintain these behaviors. The therapist should get a detailed picture of the child's behaviors, and parental strategies to deal with such behaviors. Knowledge about the interaction between child and parent may lead to the identification of the operant function, if any, of the child's inappropriate bedtime behavior. If parents are unable to provide detailed information for a functional assessment, it is recommended to ask them to keep a sleep diary during a period of at least 2 weeks. During this period, they should record the time at which the child was put to bed, the number of night-time awakenings, and the type of inappropriate child behaviors. It is also important that parents record their own behavior as a response to their child's behavior. If necessary, both parents may keep a log separately, to identify any differences between parents in their management styles and experiences with the child's inappropriate bedtime behaviors.

Ideally, a functional assessment should result in the identification of the events (i.e., parental behaviors) that elicit and maintain inappropriate bedtime behaviors in the child.

Step 2: Providing General Information about Sleep to Parents

Parents should be informed about typical sleep patterns in children, and that bedtime refusal behaviors and night wakings in children may be part of their development. During the course of development, an appropriate sleep–wake rhythm is acquired through interactions between constitutional child variables (e.g., temperament, activity levels) and aspects of the environment (e.g. parental management style). An appropriate sleep–wake rhythm is, to a large extent, the result of a learning process. Parents should be informed that their child's inappropriate bedtime behaviors are elicited and maintained (i.e., rewarded) by how they manage these behaviors.

Step 3: Bedtime Routine and Reinforcement for Appropriate Bedtime Behaviors

Parents should establish a consistent bedtime routine. The function of establishing stimulus control is that it signals absence of reinforcement and, eventually, falling asleep. Stimulus control is established by implementing a bedtime routine that is more or less fixed (also during the weekend), and limited in duration (15–45 minutes). Parents should be advised to withhold positive and/or negative reinforcement for any sleep-disrupting behaviors during the routine.

From the first night of treatment with unmodified extinction, parents should provide positive reinforcement for appropriate bedtime behaviors (for a sample protocol, see Chapter 31). That is, parents should provide attention/comfort for child behaviors that are incompatible with inappropriate bedtime behaviors and compatible with sleep onset. This may take the form of compliments for remaining in bed, comforting the child when he or she lies quietly in bed, etc. It is necessary that parents know which activities and objects are reinforcing for the child, and that at the same time do not interrupt appropriate sleep onset associations (i.e., falling asleep). Reinforcement should never be given following an incident of inappropriate behavior. In older children, reinforcement for appropriate sleep may be given the next day, and may take the form of compliments and preferred activities and objects. However, the child should be able to associate these reinforcers with his or her appropriate bedtime behaviors displayed during the night before.

Step 4: Unmodified Extinction – Bedtime and Night Wakings

With unmodified extinction, reinforcement of inappropriate sleep behaviors should be completely withdrawn and withheld. Parents refrain from their usual management strategies so as to ensure that the child's inappropriate bedtime behaviors are no longer reinforced (i.e., are extinguished). During extinction, it is critical that both parents agree on and adhere to the same management style when dealing with their child's inappropriate bedtime behavior. Other family members and neighbors should be informed about the possibility of an extinction burst (see below).

Extinction consists of limit-setting and systematic ignoring for settling problems and night waking/early waking. Parents set a bedtime that is appropriate for the child's age, and at a time when the child usually shows signs of sleepiness. A bedtime routine (e.g., bath, bottle, bedtime) should be established that takes between 15 and 45 minutes, depending on the child's age. The child is complimented for compliance to parental requests. However, parents withhold reinforcement for any occurrence of bedtime refusal, which may consist of resistance or non-compliance, repeatedly coming out of bed, crying, or calling out. For example, if a child refuses to stay in bed at bedtime, parents are instructed to return the child back to bed until he or she remains there, and parents must also withhold any actions that could inadvertently reinforce inappropriate behavior – for example, refrain from talking (too much) to the child. While implementing extinction, parents should be aware that it may take many times (e.g., tens of times) before extinction becomes effective (i.e., before the child eventually remains in his or her bed).

Inappropriate child behaviors during the night may take the form of, for example, coming out of bed, crying, calling out, and disturbing parents by entering their bed, and are the result of inappropriate sleep onset associations. The child has learned that after waking up at night, inappropriate behaviors result in some type of parental reinforcement in the form of comfort, feeding, and play activities. Unmodified extinction entails that these parental responses (reinforcers) are completely withheld, and the child's behavior is ignored. No instances of inappropriate child behavior should be followed by reinforcement in order to prevent intermittent reinforcement, which makes the child's behavior more resistant to treatment. That is, if the parent wants to check on the child after, say, three bouts or periods of crying, and comforts the child, this may provide an example of intermittent reinforcement. Such actions by the parent strengthen the disruptive behavior instead of extinguishing it. The child learns that eventually the reinforcer will be provided if the behavior is shown for long enough.

During the first 3–5 nights of intervention, the therapist and parent(s) should have daily contact by phone and/or email in order for the therapist to provide support to the parents, especially when an extinction burst occurs. It is important for the parents to know that their child is safe. The procedure should be adapted or its implementation postponed in case of illness of the child.

It is important to note that extinction does *not* lead to a worsening of the quality of the parent–child relationship; neither does it negatively influence the attachment process [6,7]. Most parents worry about this, and they should be reassured.

Extinction Burst and Spontaneous Recovery

The most important side effect of unmodified extinction is the possible occurrence of a so-called "extinction burst" [8]. That is, the frequency and severity of the child's inappropriate bedtime behaviors may substantially increase during the first nights of the treatment. However, it should be noted that this burst is a sign of the procedure's effectiveness, and not its ineffectiveness.

Parents should be aware that sleep problems may reappear where usual routines are disrupted. This is known as spontaneous recovery, but in reality the recovery is rarely spontaneous [9]. Instead, recovery often appears when there is a change in the environment, such as staying in another bed (e.g., when visiting other people), during holidays or illness, and possibly seasonal changes.

POSSIBLE MODIFICATIONS

No doubt, unmodified extinction is potentially stressful for parents, and therefore it might not be an acceptable treatment option for many. The best known modification of unmodified extinction is graduated extinction (for a description of this procedure, see Chapter 27). Another modification of the unmodified extinction procedure with parental "absence" is unmodified extinction with parental "presence", which involves parents withholding reinforcement while remaining in the child's room at bedtime and at night [10]. It is our experience that parents find unmodified extinction with parental "absence" less stressful than its alternative, whereby parents remain in close proximity to a child who is engaging in crying or tantrums.

PROOF OF CONCEPT/SUPPORTING DATA/EVIDENCE BASE

Several literature reviews have concluded that unmodified extinction for sleep problems in children is a highly effective and 'well-established' treatment approach [11–14]. A quantitative review of intervention studies on bedtime and night-waking problems showed that extinction had an average Cohen's *d* effect size of 1.58, which indicates a large treatment effect [12]. In a review of 52 studies, it was found that extinction has strong support for its effectiveness, and extinction was effective in eliminating bedtime and night-waking problems in 17 out of 19 empirical studies in which young children participated [14].

Unmodified extinction has also been shown to be effective in the treatment of sleep problems in children with various types of developmental disabilities, such as intellectual and/or physical disabilities and autism [13].

It is our clinical experience that if unmodified extinction is implemented consistently, it is highly likely to lead to a substantial reduction or even elimination of a child's sleep problems within several days. Overall, successful treatment with extinction for childhood sleep disturbance may have positive effects on parental well-being and the child's daytime behavior [14,15].

REFERENCES

[1] M. Thunström, A 2.5-year follow-up of infants treated for severe sleep problems, Ambul. Child Health 6 (2008) 225–235.

[2] D. Lerman, B. Iwata, Developing a technology for the use of operant extinction in clinical settings: an examination of basic and applied research, J. Appl. Behav. Anal. 29 (1996) 345–382.

[3] M. O'Reilly, G. Lancioni, I. Taylor, An empirical analysis of two forms of extinction to treat aggression, Res. Dev. Disabil. 20 (1999) 315–325.
[4] C. Piazza, M. Patel, C. Gulotta, et al., On the relative contributions of positive reinforcement and escape extinction in the treatment of food refusal, J. Appl. Behav. Anal. 36 (2003) 309–324.
[5] C. Herzinger, J. Campbell, Comparing functional assessment methodologies: A quantitative synthesis, J. Autism Dev. Disord. 37 (2007) 1430–1445.
[6] K. France, Behavior characteristics and security in sleep-disturbed infants treated with extinction, J. Pediatr. Psychol. 17 (1992) 467–475.
[7] M. Van Ijzendoorn, F. Hubbard, Are infant crying and maternal responsiveness during the first year related to infant–mother attachment at 15 months? Attach. Hum. Dev. 2 (2000) 371–391.
[8] D. Lerman, Prevalence of the extinction burst and its attenuation during treatment, J. Appl. Behav. Anal. 28 (1995) 93–94.
[9] R. Waller, N. Mays, Spontaneous recovery of previously extinguished behavior as an alternative explanation for extinction-related side effects, Behav. Modif. 31 (2007) 569–572.
[10] T. Morgenthaler, J. Owens, C. Alessi, et al., Practice parameters for behavioral treatment of bedtime problems and night wakings in infants and young children: An American Academy of Sleep Medicine report, Sleep 29 (2006) 1277–1281.
[11] J. Mindell, Empirically supported treatments in pediatric psychology: Bedtime refusal and night wakings in young children, J. Pediatr. Psychol. 24 (1999) 465–481.
[12] B. Kuhn, A. Elliott, Treatment efficacy in behavioral pediatric sleep medicine, J. Psychosom. Res. 54 (2003) 587–597.
[13] R. Didden, J. Sigafoos, A review of the nature and treatment of sleep problems in individuals with developmental disabilities, Res. Dev. Disabil. 22 (2001) 255–272.
[14] J. Mindell, B. Kuhn, D. Lewin, et al., Behavioral treatment of bedtime problems and night wakings in infants and young children, Sleep 29 (2006) 1263–1276.
[15] J. Reid, A. Walter, S. O'Leary, Treatment of young children's bedtime refusal and nighttime wakings: a comparison of standard and graduated ignoring procedures, J. Abnorm. Child Psychol. 27 (1999) 5–16.

RECOMMENDED READING

A. Kazdin, Behavior Modification in Applied Settings, sixth ed., Wadsworth Publishers, Florence, KY, 2000.

The Journal of Applied Behavior Analysis regularly publishes studies on the effectiveness of extinction for childhood disruptive behaviors.

Chapter 27

Graduated Extinction: Behavioral Treatment for Bedtime Problems and Night Wakings in Young Children

Lisa J. Meltzer
Sleep Center, Children's Hospital of Philadelphia, Philadelphia, PA
Department of Pediatrics, University of Pennsylvania School of Medicine, Philadelphia, PA

Jodi A. Mindell
Department of Psychology, Saint Joseph's University, Philadelphia, PA
Sleep Center, Children's Hospital of Philadelphia, Philadelphia, PA

PROTOCOL NAME

Graduated extinction: behavioral treatment for bedtime problems and night wakings in young children.

GROSS INDICATION

Bedtime problems and night wakings, typically involving inappropriate sleep associations and/or limit-setting problems, in young children (ages 6 months to 5 years).

SPECIFIC INDICATION

This intervention is indicated for:

- behavioral insomnia of childhood – sleep onset association type;
- behavioral insomnia of childhood – limit-setting type;
- behavioral insomnia of childhood – combined type.

Frequent night wakings are the hallmark symptom of Behavioral Insomnia of Childhood – Sleep Onset Association type (BIC–SOA), typically seen in children older than 6 months. BIC–SOA is caused by negative sleep associations that interfere with falling asleep at bedtime and returning to sleep independently throughout the night. BIC–limit-setting type is typically manifested

Behavioral Treatments for Sleep Disorders. DOI: 10.1016/B978-0-12-381522-4.00027-4

as avoidance of bedtime, frequent requests after lights out, as well as refusal to get into bed, to stay in bed, or to participate in the bedtime routine. Finally, BIC–combined type occurs when a child has features of both SOA and limit-setting subtypes, often with difficulties limit-setting leading to the development of negative sleep associations.

CONTRAINDICATIONS

Potential contraindications include:

- severe anxiety disorder in the child;
- a child with past trauma (e.g., abuse, neglect);
- where prolonged crying is medically contraindicated (e.g., a cardiac condition).

These potential contraindications may not in all cases prevent the use of graduated extinction. Clinical judgment that weighs the benefits of treating the sleep issues versus the possible risks of treatment must be utilized in specific clinical situations.

RATIONALE FOR INTERVENTION

Bedtime problems and night wakings are highly prevalent, with studies indicating that 20–30 percent of young children experience these sleep problems [1]. Such problems can result in significant sleep loss in young children, which can impact all aspects of a child's well-being and daytime functioning [2]. In addition to the impact on the child, these sleep problems also negatively impact families, with sleep problems placing a significant burden on parents (e.g., increased rates of maternal depression) and the parent–child relationship [3,4].

There are several important underlying mechanisms related to sleep that can result in parental complaints of bedtime problems or night wakings in young children. Clinicians must be familiar with these in order to educate parents and provide an effective intervention approach.

Sleep onset associations. Sleep onset associations are conditions that must be present to help a child fall asleep at bedtime, and return to sleep following an arousal. A positive sleep association is one where the child is able to fall asleep without assistance, such as thumb sucking, pacifiers, or a stuffed animal. A negative sleep association is one where another person or circumstance is required to help a child fall asleep, such as nursing, being rocked, or riding in the car.

Night wakings are normal. Night wakings or arousals are a part of normal sleep. At the end of each sleep cycle, a child will have a brief arousal before returning to sleep. A child who has a negative sleep association at bedtime to fall asleep will also likely require this same association during the night to help him or her return to sleep following each of these brief arousals. For example, an infant who is nursed to sleep at bedtime will also need to be nursed back to sleep several times during the night following each normal arousal. Similarly, following a normal arousal a preschooler whose parent lies with him at bedtime will either need a parent to lie with him during the night, or he might move to the parents' bed for the remainder of the night.

Bedtime behavior problems are often difficult to manage. A normal part of early development is for children to test the limits or rules set by their parents. This is how young children explore their environment, and learn the difference between right and wrong. In addition, children are often "rewarded" by additional parental attention when they misbehave. Along with everyone being overtired, which can interfere with emotion regulation on the part of both children and their parents, managing bedtime behavior problems can be challenging for even the most skilled parents. Bedtime problems can be effectively managed with parental consistency in terms of bedtime routines, a set bedtime, and how parents respond to their child's behavior.

Graduated extinction is an effective treatment for bedtime problems and night wakings in young children, and is more acceptable for parents than extinction. Graduated extinction is an empirically supported treatment approach for bedtime problems and night wakings in young children [5,6]. In addition, this approach is often more acceptable to parents than extinction approaches in which parents are to ignore their child for prolonged periods [7]. Because it is less stressful for parents, they are more likely to be consistent in their responses to bedtime problems and/or night wakings, decreasing attrition rates and increasing success.

The traditional application of graduated extinction to bedtime involves parents ignoring bedtime crying and tantrums for a specific period of time, and then briefly checking on their child. The duration between parental checks is determined by the child's age and temperament, as well as how long parents can tolerate their child crying [5]. Either a fixed schedule (e.g., checking every 5 minutes) or a progressive schedule (increasing the time between checks; e.g., 5 minutes, 10 minutes, then 15 minutes) can be instituted. These checking methods are described in Step 5.

Prior to implementing graduated extinction approaches, however, there are several areas that must be addressed to ensure treatment success.

STEP BY STEP DESCRIPTION OF PROCEDURES

Educate Parents about Normal Sleep and Child Development

The first step for a graduated extinction intervention is to educate parents about normal sleep in children, with the understanding that sleep needs change over the first few years of a child's life.

- *Newborns (0–3 months)* generally sleep between 10 and 18 hours a day, but this can be longer for premature infants. There is no clear day–night difference in terms of newborn sleep patterns, with multiple short sleep periods (45 minutes to 4 hours) across a 24-hour span. Around 8–12 weeks, sleep patterns begin to consolidate, with differentiation between day and night and a more predictable sleep–wake schedule.

- *Infants (3–12 months)* have a total sleep time of around 12–13 hours (9–10 hours at night and up to 4 hours obtained during daytime naps), with significant individual variability. Sleep consolidation continues to occur, with the majority of 6-month-olds able to sleep for a prolonged period at night (at least 6–8 hours), and two to three daytime naps.
- *Toddlers (12 months–3 years)* have a total sleep time of 12–14 hours, with approximately 9–12 hours at night, with an additional 2–4 hours of sleep time during naps. Again, there is individual variability in sleep times in toddlers. By 18 months, most toddlers have transitioned from two naps to one nap per day.
- *Preschoolers (3–5 years)* have decreased sleep needs due to the phasing out of daytime naps, with an average of 11–13 hours of sleep per 24 hours. By the age of 5 years, only 25 percent of children continue to nap during the day.

Along with sleep need, it is important for parents to understand that night wakings are normal, and that a negative sleep onset association (e.g., nursing an infant to sleep, lying with a child to help him or her fall asleep) can contribute to the development and maintenance of night wakings.

Cognitive reasoning is another developmental change in young children that can interfere with sleep onset. As children develop reasoning skills, they can quickly learn how to delay bedtime by making multiple requests for parental attention, which can contribute to and perpetuate bedtime problems. Parents need to understand that it is normal for their child to "test the limits" at bedtime, and that parents must set consistent limits to ensure treatment success.

Establish a Sleep Schedule and a Bedtime Routine

Prior to instituting any intervention, a therapist needs to ensure that a child is falling asleep at a consistent and age-appropriate time (generally by 7:30 pm for infants, and 7:30–8:30 pm for toddlers/preschoolers). The child's circadian rhythm also needs to be considered when selecting an appropriate and consistent bedtime. For example, if a child typically falls asleep around 9 pm but is put to bed at 7 pm, this will result in prolonged bedtime resistance, increased difficulties for the child in falling asleep, and decreased parent tolerance of recommended interventions. In this case it is better to set the bedtime to 9 pm and gradually fade earlier (i.e., advance bedtime by 15 minutes every 3–4 nights). Although an early bedtime is recommended here, and research has found that a bedtime earlier than 9 pm results in more sleep and fewer sleep difficulties [8], individual bedtimes will need to be set in consideration of a specific family's values and schedule, and in relation to cultural differences.

It is also important to have a consistent wake time in the morning and nap times during the day. Sleep schedules in young children should not differ on weekdays and weekends.

Recent research indicates that a consistent bedtime routine can reduce bedtime resistance and improve sleep consolidation [9]. A bedtime routine should consist of three or four soothing activities that occur on a nightly basis (e.g., bath, books, prayers, bed) for a total of 30–40 minutes. An ideal bedtime routine is one that moves progressively toward the child's sleeping environment. For most families, it will be important to institute these two steps (i.e., consistent bedtime routine and sleep schedule) prior to continuing with a graduated extinction treatment.

Stabilize Parent Behaviors and Sleep Location at Bedtime and during the Night

Frequently, parents are inconsistent in their parenting behaviors at bedtime and how they respond through the night. For example, one night a parent may lie down with a child, and the next night refuse. Prior to making changes, it is important first to stabilize parental behavior, providing children with a consistent response every night. Further, children should be falling asleep at bedtime in their own room. Often this involves the institution of a negative sleep association (e.g., lying with the child in the child's room at bedtime). However, based on principles of partial reinforcement schedules, it is more important to have a consistent baseline behavior that can then be modified.

The same is true for night wakings, with parents immediately responding to a child's night waking rather than reinforcing prolonged crying. For example, if a parent is eventually going to bring a child into their bed, they should do so immediately following the first waking, rather than making their child "cry it out" for the first two wakings, and then bringing the child to the parents' bed following the third waking. Prior to the initiation of graduated extinction, it is recommended that all family members obtain as much sleep as possible. The stabilization of parental behaviors should allow for this additional sleep.

Select a Global or Targeted Approach

During the development of a treatment plan, it is best first to articulate the final goal. The steps to get to this goal will require negotiation with the parent, and are based on the child's temperament and parent tolerance. In addition, some parents are ready to tackle all sleep issues, while others prefer to make one change at a time.

The first decision in designing a treatment plan is to determine whether to take a global approach and focus on both bedtime and night wakings, or to take a more specific approach of making changes only at bedtime, while having parents quickly and consistently respond to their child during the night. Research indicates that changes made only at bedtime (i.e., child learning to fall asleep independently) generalize to night wakings within about 2 weeks, and this targeted approach is often the approach that is more acceptable to parents. This approach also decreases sleep loss in both the child and his or her parents. This is important, as sleep loss can contribute to increased night wakings and difficulties settling at bedtime, as well as parental frustration and exhaustion.

Implementing the Graduated Extinction Intervention

Once the bedtime routine, bedtime, and parental behaviors have been consistently followed for 1–2 weeks, the next step is gradually to remove the negative sleep onset association (e.g., nursing, parent lying next to child). The actual steps vary by the negative sleep onset association, and are outlined below. Each step is followed for at least 3 nights, but more typically for 4–7 nights until the behavior has stabilized.

Infants Who Are Nursed to Sleep

Step 1. Move nursing to an earlier part of the routine, and then rock the child to sleep without nursing.

Step 2. At the completion of the bedtime routine, the parent should place infant in the crib awake and leave the room, returning to check on the child for a brief period, maintaining minimal contact and interaction. Parents can check on a consistent schedule (e.g., every 3 minutes) or at increasing intervals (e.g., 3 minutes, 5 minutes, 10 minutes). No research has indicated the efficacy of one approach over the other.

The above approach is also applicable for children who are bottle-fed, with the exception that Step 1 would be to taper the bottle by one ounce per night until the bottle is no longer part of the falling asleep routine. The family should then move to Step 2.

For parents who are less tolerant of their child's crying, a progressive withdrawal of the parent involvement may be indicated. For example, following Step 1 above, the following would be implemented for an infant sleeping in a crib:

- Place infant in crib awake and provide no physical contact, yet parent is present next to crib until child is asleep.
- Place infant in crib awake, and parent then moves half the distance from the crib to the bedroom door, remaining present until the child is asleep.
- Place infant in crib awake, and parent remains present in the doorway until the child is asleep.
- Place infant in crib awake, and parent leaves the room, checking on the child as described in Step 2 above.

Another variation combines the two above approaches and involves having the parent take progressively longer breaks but continuing to be present while the child falls asleep. For example, the parent leaves the room for 2 minutes, and then returns and remains until the child is asleep. The next night the parent leaves the room for 3 minutes and then returns and remains until the child is asleep. Although this may seem that the crying is being reinforced by the child's protests, it is effective in exposing children to increasing periods of not having their parent present. With an increasing length of time that the parent is out of the bedroom, the end goal is for the child to fall asleep without the parent present. The parent's return cannot be contingent upon the child's cries, but rather be previously specified (e.g., "I have to go turn on the dishwasher, I'll be right back").

The determination of which approach to use with a specific child should be based on how likely the parent is to be consistent and follow through, as well as how the child responds when the parent checks on him or her. For example, a parental check may provide comfort to some children, while for other children a parental check will only make them more upset. Similarly, some parents can tolerate their child's crying while others prefer minimal crying, thus the former would do better with the checking approach while the latter would do better with the gradual removal of parental presence approach.

Young Children Who Fall Asleep with Parent Lying Down with Child, or Fall Asleep in Parents' Bed

A similar approach to above can be implemented when the situation involves a parent lying down with a child in his or her bed until asleep.

Step 1. The parent sits on the bed with the child, or on the floor next to the bed, and remains until child is asleep.
Step 2. The parent sits half the distance to the bedroom door, and remains until the child is asleep.
Step 3. The parent sits in the doorway and remains until the child is asleep.
Step 4. The parent sits in the hall outside the child's room (outside the child's line of vision) and remains until the child is asleep, providing brief verbal responses if needed (e.g., "I'm here, go to sleep").
Step 5. The parent takes breaks that increase in length until the child is consistently falling asleep without the parent present in the hallway.

Problem-Solve Barriers to Treatment Adherence

Once the treatment plan has been developed, it is important to problem-solve with parents all the potential obstacles, to ensure treatment adherence and increase the likelihood of treatment success. For example, a discussion of differing parenting styles and mutual agreement to the treatment plan is critical in two-parent households. Another common concern is the potential disturbance of close neighbors or other children in the household during the implementation of the intervention. It is important to discuss how parents respond in cases where the child is prone to vomit or have other extreme behavioral responses when upset.

Education about the usual course of treatment is also important. Parents should be informed that often the behavior gets worse before it gets better; thus, the second night of a graduated extinction approach often results in prolonged crying. Extinction bursts are also common, and thus parents need to be prepared for a return of bedtime struggles and night wakings days to weeks following significant improvement.

Educate Parents about Potential Pitfalls to Ongoing Treatment Success

Once treatment has been successfully implemented and the child's sleep is significantly improved, a discussion of potential pitfalls can help mediate future setbacks. For example, it is expected that illness and disruption to the child's schedule (e.g., vacations, birth of another child) will result in sleep disruption. Future developmental milestones and other transitions (e.g., discontinuing pacifier use, moving to a bed from a crib, etc.) can also result in the return of sleep issues. A focus on maintaining night-time rules and parental consistency typically prevents the development of ongoing sleep issues.

POSSIBLE MODIFICATIONS/VARIANTS

See above for general recommendations.

In specific circumstances – for example, for children with developmental delays, psychiatric disturbances, or medical disorders – a more gradual approach may be appropriate and more acceptable to parents. Behavioral approaches in these populations should be the first line of treatment, with the understanding that it may take longer than in typically developing and healthy populations.

PROOF OF CONCEPT/EVIDENCE BASE

Behavioral intervention, including graduated extinction, for bedtime problems and night wakings in young children is well documented and empirically supported. Such empirical basis has resulted in previous reviews supporting the efficacy of this behavioral intervention [10,11] and more recently, the publication of practice parameters by the American Academy of Sleep Medicine [6]. For graduated extinction, specifically, the companion review of the literature [5] to the standards of practice found 14 studies involving 748 participants had been conducted on the efficacy of graduated extinction, with an additional 9 studies utilizing similar behavioral principles but variations of graduated extinction (e.g., gradual removal of parental presence). These studies provided empirical support for the efficacy of graduated extinction and its variants. In addition, behavioral interventions were recommended and found to be effective in improving secondary outcomes (child's daytime functioning, parental well-being) in children with bedtime problems and night wakings.

REFERENCES

[1] J.A. Owens, Epidemiology of sleep disorders during childhood, in: S.H. Sheldon, R. Ferber, M.H. Kryger (Eds.), Principles and Practices of Pediatric Sleep Medicine, Elsevier Saunders, Philadelphia, PA, 2005, pp. 27–33.

[2] J.E. Bates, R.J. Viken, D.B. Alexander, et al., Sleep and adjustment in preschool children: Sleep diary reports by mothers relate to behavior reports by teachers, Child Dev. 73 (1) (2002) 62–74.

[3] P. Lam, H. Hiscock, M. Wake, Outcomes of infant sleep problems: A longitudinal study of sleep, behavior, and maternal well-being, J. Pediatr. 111 (3) (2003) 203–207.

[4] J.K. Bayer, H. Hiscock, A. Hampton, M. Wake, Sleep problems in young infants and maternal mental and physical health, J. Paediatr. Child Health 43 (1–2) (2007) 66–73.

[5] J.A. Mindell, B.R. Kuhn, D.S. Lewin, et al., Behavioral treatment of bedtime problems and night wakings in infants and young children, Sleep 29 (10) (2006) 1263–1276.

[6] T.I. Morgenthaler, J. Owens, C. Alessi, et al., Practice parameters for behavioral treatment of bedtime problems and night wakings in infants and young children: An American Academy of Sleep Medicine report, Sleep 29 (10) (2006) 1277–1281.

[7] V.I. Rickert, C.M. Johnson, Reducing nocturnal awakening and crying episodes in infants and young children: a comparison between scheduled awakenings and systematic ignoring, Pediatrics 81 (2) (1988) 203–212.

[8] J.A. Mindell, L.J. Meltzer, M.A. Carskadon, R.D. Chervin, Developmental aspects of sleep hygiene: findings from the 2004 National Sleep Foundation Sleep in America Poll, Sleep Med. 10 (7) (2009) 771–779.

[9] J.A. Mindell, L. Telofski, B. Wiegand, E.S. Kurtz, A nightly bedtime routine: Impact on sleep in young children and maternal mood, Sleep 32 (5) (2009) 599–606.

[10] B.R. Kuhn, A.J. Elliott, Treatment efficacy in behavioral pediatric sleep medicine, J. Psychosom. Res. 54 (6) (2003) 587–597.

[11] J.A. Mindell, Empirically supported treatments in pediatric psychology: Bedtime refusal and night wakings in young children, J. Pediatr. Psychol. 24 (6) (1999) 465–481.

RECOMMENDED READING

K.G. France, J.M.T. Henderson, S.M. Hudson, Fact, act, and tact: A three-stage approach to treating the sleep problems of infants and young children, Child Adolesc. Psychiatr. Clin. N. Am. 5 (3) (1996) 581–599.

H. Hiscock, J. Bayer, L. Gold, A. Hampton, et al., Improving infant sleep and maternal mental health: A cluster randomised trial, Arch. Dis. Child 92 (11) (2007) 952–958.

J.A. Mindell, B.R. Kuhn, D.S. Lewin, et al., Behavioral treatment of bedtime problems and night wakings in infants and young children, Sleep 29 (10) (2006) 1263–1276.

J.A. Mindell, J.A. Owens, A Clinical Guide to Pediatric Sleep: Diagnosis and Management of Sleep Problems, second ed., Lippincott, Williams, & Wilkins, Philadelphia, PA, 2009.

T.I. Morgenthaler, J. Owens, C. Alessi, et al., Practice parameters for behavioral treatment of bedtime problems and night wakings in infants and young children: An American Academy of Sleep Medicine report, Sleep 29 (10) (2006) 1277–1281.

Chapter 28

Extinction with Parental Presence

Karyn G. France
Health Sciences Centre, University of Canterbury, Christchurch, New Zealand

PROTOCOL NAME

Extinction with parental presence.

GROSS INDICATION

This intervention is indicated for settling and night waking problems in infants between 6 and 24 months of age. Infants of this age often present with sleep disturbance, including an inability to fall asleep at night without intense parental involvement, resulting in the infant being placed in the cot already asleep or with the parent present. This means the infant lacks the skills to self-settle and forms inappropriate sleep associations (such as parental contact and feeding) rather than appropriate cues (such as internal feelings of tiredness, and the crib or bed). Consequently when the infant inevitably awakens during the night, the same associations are required for sleep reinitiation. This results in awakenings each night requiring the parent to be present.

Parents accept that infants require intervention throughout the night until they are able to sustain a longer period of sleep without feeding. Unfortunately, if inappropriate associations are formed the young child may continue with sleep onset and night waking problems indefinitely. These kinds of persistent sleep problems in infants and young children are associated with a number of adverse developmental sequelae [1].

SPECIFIC INDICATION

This approach requires that the infant still sleeps in a crib or other setting where he or she is confined, although it can be modified for older preschoolers sleeping in a bed. It is particularly suitable for parents who are anxious about leaving the infant, for infants experiencing developmentally typical separation anxiety, and for infants who have developed fear of the crib as a result of prior extinction programs carried out unsuccessfully.

Behavioral Treatments for Sleep Disorders. DOI: 10.1016/B978-0-12-381522-4.00028-6

CONTRAINDICATIONS

This is a precise technique which requires that parents adhere exactly to the protocol. Parents need the ability to understand and adhere to the program, which does require a change in household routines for at least a week. Some parents with high anxiety or depression may find this technique too stressful. It requires that the baby is able to sleep in the same place for several weeks, and that the parent sleep in the same place as the baby for at least 1 week.

This program should not be undertaken when the child is unwell. It is contraindicated in children with chronic conditions which make it unwise to allow the child to cry – for example, asthma, hernia, or epilepsy.

Medical explanations for the sleep problems should be ruled out, as should severe family dysfunction which might compromise the correct use of the program or should itself be the focus of intervention.

RATIONALE FOR INTERVENTION

The rationale for this intervention draws on both learning theory and attachment theory. Social learning theory explanations of infant sleep problems describe the parents and child as caught in the kind of escape conditioning (coercion trap) described originally by Patterson [2]. The parents and child are both negatively reinforced for maintaining the conditions under which the infant learned to fall asleep. Specifically, these conditions are being out of the crib at sleep onset, with the parent present and interacting intensively with the child. These conditions are created at bedtime and re-established after each awakening.

The successful removal of reinforcement for signaling upon settling and awakening will eventually lead to decreases in resistance to settling, and in the frequency and duration of night awakenings. However, the initial stages of removing this reinforcement through extinction lead to a Post Extinction Response Burst (PERB), which is an increase in responding after the reinforcement has been withdrawn.

The PERB is evidenced as an increase in crying and duration of awakening in the first few nights of an extinction program. This distress in infants and accompanying distress in parents has been of concern, and has led to the development of modifications of extinction, most notably gradual programs such as controlled crying or fading. Unfortunately, learning theory would predict that such approaches would lead to less robust changes than an unmodified program. Intermittent parental intervention would impede progress and provide many more opportunities for relapse [3].

The extinction with parental presence program overcomes these difficulties. The parent's presence is constant and non-contingent, hence it does not act as a reinforcer. Consequently, the extinction protocol is kept intact. The parent's presence acts to decrease anxiety and consequently distress on the first few nights of the program. Once the crib, rather than the parent, has become the discriminative stimulus for sleep onset, removal of the parent from the room is less likely to stimulate distress.

This explanation is consistent with attachment theory, which acknowledges anxiety experienced by both parent and child on separation [4]. Continued parental presence relieves this infant anxiety until the infant learns to settle in the presence of new, more appropriate sleep-related stimuli. The new responses create a behavior trap whereby the infant replaces the previous responses (waking and crying) with new ones (settling in the presence of the crib), which finally obviates the need for anxiety reduction, because the infant no longer experiences being alone in the crib as an unfamiliar, distressing situation.

STEP BY STEP DESCRIPTION OF PROCEDURES

There are multiple steps in this intervention:

1. Assess suitability of the family
2. Record the sleep problem
3. Introduce the intervention
4. Choose a starting night
5. Set up the room
6. Bedtime and early evening
7. Parent's bedtime
8. Morning
9. Troubleshooting/fears
10. Monitoring and support
11. Transition out of the room
12. Maintaining progress and follow-up.

Assess Suitability of the Family

Prior to deciding on treatment, a full description of the presenting problem and parents' responses to it should be obtained. This should include a description of a typical night, parents' expectations for improved sleep, duration of the problem and precipitating events if present, as well as parents' attempts to solve the problem now and in the past. In addition, a developmental and medical history should be obtained, paying attention not only to infant development but also to the parent–child relationship and stressors on the family which may exacerbate the sleep problems through environmental disruption or parental behavior. The suitability of the child's sleeping arrangements should also be established.

Important considerations are: whether parents' expectations for their child are developmentally appropriate; parents' knowledge about sleep and the role they may play in it; the extent of previous, unsuccessful attempts at intervention; the presence of medical problems which may make intervention unwise; and parental anxiety, depression, or attachment problems which may make intervention difficult or inappropriate. Previous unsuccessful attempts to remedy the sleep problem may have made the child more resistant to extinction. They may also have led to other problems, such as conditioned fear of the crib. Nonetheless, the nature of this program makes it an excellent choice in these situations.

Record the Sleep Problem

The use of a diary to record the sleep problem is of benefit. It enables the therapist to ascertain exactly what happens in response to night waking and settling problems, and gives the parents and therapist a ready source of information about their infants' improvement over the course of the intervention. The diary should cover, for each night, the time the infant is placed in bed; whether he or she is awake or asleep; the time taken to settle to sleep; any parental interventions or periods out of the cot during settling; the number, time and duration of night awakenings; details of parental responses to night awakening; and, finally, the time awake in the morning.

Introduce the Intervention

It is important that parents are committed to following a sleep program through to its conclusion. If not, and the parents repeatedly stop and start this or other programs, the sleep problem may deteriorate and the child may develop unwanted side effects, such as fear of the crib or conditioned vomiting. It is important therefore to refrain from persuading parents to follow this or any other program. Ensure they are fully informed of what is involved prior to making their decision.

This intervention involves one parent's presence in the infant's room whenever the child is awake, and for the duration of the parent's own sleep. It is an extinction program in that although the parent is present, he or she does not interact with the child during the night unless the child is ill or in danger.

Parents can be informed that this program is gentler than unmodified extinction. It is gentler because the infant is aware of the parent's presence in the room, so separation anxiety is reduced. Consequently, there is less likelihood of the infant experiencing a severe PERB [3]. Parents can also be informed that there is evidence that it resolves the sleep problem more effectively than other modifications of extinction [3]. On the other hand, parents also need to be aware that they need to stay in the room with the child while he or she is awake and learning to settle. This means they will need to listen to a certain amount of crying.

Parents are given a rationale in order to acquaint them with what they need to do, what to expect, and how the program works. Parents are told that it is usual for everyone to wake occasionally during the night, and that we learn to simply go back to sleep. Young children may be prevented from learning to go back to sleep if their parents are present every time they need to resume sleeping. Parents can be informed that, while they likely have a role in maintaining their child's sleep disturbance, in most cases sleep problems are multi-causal.

The need to remove reinforcing responses to the child when he or she is settling to sleep or awakens during the night is explained. The PERB is explained with use of a simple diagram showing the PERB and spontaneous recoveries [5]. These points, where parents are most vulnerable to abandoning the program, are identified, as is the risk of exacerbating the sleep problem, making it harder to change in the future, should they choose to do so.

Parents are then asked to plan how they might fit this program into their and their child's routine along the following dimensions.

Choose a Starting Night

The most disruption to the household routine will occur during the first 3 nights, so parents are advised to begin the program at a time when there will be minimum impact – on the Friday of a weekend, for example. Parents should also be advised to begin the program at a time when they are likely to have a settled routine for the next month. Beginning when a family holiday is planned in the next few weeks would not be appropriate.

Set up the Room

The program requires the child to be sleeping in the room where he or she will continue to sleep once the program is over, and requires one parent to move in and sleep in another bed in that room for the first week of the program. There is no reason why the program cannot be followed in the parent's bedroom, so long as that is the room where the child will continue to sleep. It can also be followed if the child shares a room with another child, so long as the other child is moved from the room for the first week of the program.

Bedtime and Early Evening

Decide, together with the parents, on a suitable bedtime for the child. This is usually between 7.30 and 8.30 pm, and will vary within this time depending on family routines such as parents' working hours. Negotiate a routine which will signal to the child that it is bedtime. This should not be drawn out. An example might be to change into pajamas, finish a bottle in the living room, and have a song. The child should be placed in the crib awake at bedtime, then the parent bids goodnight and lies in the second bed.

The parent feigns sleep and does not respond to the child while the child is settling to sleep. On the first night of the program there can be considerable crying during the settling period, but, if the child is aware of the parent in the room, there is likely to be less crying than on other programs [3]. If the child appears not to see the parent in the room, the parent can clear his or her throat and increase the light level a little.

Once the child has settled to sleep for the first time, the parent can leave the room and continue with usual evening activities, returning to feign sleep in the second bed, without interacting with the child, as soon as the child has a night waking. The parent can again leave the room once the child has settled back to sleep.

Parent's Bedtime

The parent repeats the process until his or her own bedtime. At that point the parent settles to sleep in the second bed in the child's room, again feigning sleep when the child wakes.

Morning

Children undergoing a sleep program, and who are settling earlier in the evening than they are used to, may awaken earlier in the morning once their sleep begins to consolidate. This is temporary, and the child will sleep for a longer stretch so long as the parent does not allow the child up increasingly early for the day. For this reason, an earliest "up time" is decided with the parent prior to the program. This is usually 6 am, unless the parents rise earlier themselves. Any waking prior to that is treated as a night waking, and waking after that period is treated as rising time. Parents are advised to make rising a clear contrast to night-time – for example, by taking the child to a light and active area of the house rather than to the parent's bed, where he or she may fall asleep again. Parents can relax this practice during the maintenance phase.

Troubleshooting/Fears

Prior to the program, allow the parents to express their fears and the possible challenges they may face in carrying out the program. Parents often express a fear that a lack of response to the child may be damaging to the parent–child relationship. They may also fear that the child will get out of the crib, hurt him- or herself, or become ill.

There is evidence that there is in fact an improvement in the parent–child relationship after a sleep program [6]. The other problems are practical, and can be planned for. An additional mattress can be placed on the floor for an active child who might get out of the crib. If there is danger (e.g., the child gets in a difficult position) this should be remedied, but with minimal response to the child. In the case of illness, the program should be stopped until the child is well again. The program can be resumed at that point. If the child has repeated illness, such as chronic ear infections, then a program is not likely to be effective until this problem has been remedied.

Monitoring and Support

Parents require considerable support during sleep programs, and it is advisable to make contact with the parent on a daily basis. A 24-hour number to call at the beginning is also a good idea, if feasible. There is a risk that parents may deviate from the program if they do not have this support, and that may lead to an increased risk of conditioned fear of the crib, and a sleep problem which becomes increasingly intractable.

Transition Out of the Room

If the program is carried out correctly, an improvement in the child's sleep will be visible in the recordings by the fourth night of the program, and distinct improvement attained by the end of the first week. After that period, the aim is to consolidate progress and accustom the child to sleeping in his or her own bed without the parent being present.

On the eighth night of the program, the parent resumes sleeping in his or her own bed. Difficulty settling and night waking are not attended to, and are likely to be of much shorter duration. We have found that infants cope with this transition with little perturbation, but, in a very small number of cases, if there is an increase in crying consequent to the move then the parent can move back for a few more nights and successfully withdraw again after that.

Maintaining Progress and Follow-up

After the daily contact of the first week, parents should be contacted about twice weekly for the next 3 weeks. Diaries should continue to be completed. After the fourth week, provided progress continues, the family is moved to the maintenance phase. The maintenance phase can be sustained indefinitely, and is similar to the practice of parents whose children are good sleepers. The parent responds to the child whenever there is sustained crying in the child's room. The parent checks for reasons and remedies them quietly, leaving the child to settle back to sleep once the reason has been addressed. If there is no reason for the crying, the parent responds minimally and leaves the room. Should difficulty settling and night crying increase again, in the absence of illness, the program can be resumed. It is likely this can occur without the parent returning to the room, and if dealt with promptly, marked improvement is likely within a few nights.

After maintenance has been successfully implemented for 2 weeks, then regular contact can be terminated and the parents make contact only if they need further advice. Sleep problems may resume, particularly after a disruption such as an illness or a holiday, and parents may need to return to the program briefly after these events. The clinician may wish to check in after a few weeks to ensure that progress has been maintained.

POSSIBLE MODIFICATIONS/VARIANTS

This program can be used with older preschoolers, and has been dubbed "camping out" in some quarters. Rewards should be added for children with sufficient language (usually over 2 years of age). When the child is in a bed, unconfined, the program needs to be modified. The parent sits in a chair rather than lying in a bed, as the child will need to be returned to bed repeatedly – in fact, every time the child gets up, until he or she eventually settles. The parent needs to return the child to bed gently but firmly, without further interaction. The parent can then leave the room or sleep in a second bed, depending on the time of the night.

It is wise to allow a preschool child to visit the bathroom during the night. This should be accomplished quietly, and with minimum interaction.

PROOF OF CONCEPT/SUPPORTING DATA/EVIDENCE BASE

There has been research into the efficacy of this program in the form of group and single-case evaluations [3,7]. These have demonstrated that extinction with parental presence leads to improvements in a number of sleep-related variables. Further, unpublished data from both these studies indicate that there is significantly less crying on the first night of the program compared with unmodified extinction and the minimal checking programs. The resolution of the sleep problem is better than the more gradual minimal checking program.

Further support for the program comes from its theoretical base. It is critical to understand the definition of extinction when considering modifications to sleep programs which are intended to make them more gentle. Extinction calls for the complete discontinuation of reinforcement. In contrast, most modifications to sleep programs allow the withdrawal of parental attention to be spaced out, or truncated. This risks converting from an extinction paradigm to one of intermittent reinforcement, with attendant difficulties.

Extinction with parental presence, in contrast, manages to retain the extinction paradigm intact. Reinforcing consequences are discontinued by decreasing parental intervention to sub-reinforcing intensity. Parental intervention is maintained at that level without the intermittent interaction with the child which characterizes the other modified programs. Meanwhile, non-contingent parental presence relieves infant anxiety until the infant learns to settle in the presence of new, more appropriate sleep-related stimuli.

The result is a program which retains the effectiveness of an extinction paradigm while decreasing infant anxiety evidenced by a marked decrease in crying compared with both unmodified and more gradual extinction programs.

REFERENCES

[1] J.A. Mindell, B. Kuhn, D.S. Lewin, et al., Behavioral treatment of bedtime problems and night wakings in infants and young children, Sleep 29 (10) (2006) 1263–1276.

[2] G.R. Patterson, Coercive Family Process, Castalia Pub Co., Eugene, OR, 1982.
[3] K.G. France, N.M. Blampied, Modifications of systematic ignoring in the management of infant sleep disturbance: Efficacy and infant distress, Child Fam. Behav. Ther. 27 (2005) 1–16.
[4] J. Bowlby, Attachment and Loss, vol. 2, Separation, Anxiety and Anger, Basic Books, New York, NY, 1973.
[5] K.G. France, J.M.T. Henderson, S.M. Hudson, Fact, act and tact: A three-stage approach to treating the sleep problems of infants and young children, Child Adolesc. Psychiatr. Clin. N. Am. 5 (1996) 581–599.
[6] K.G. France, Behavior characteristics and security in sleep disturbed infants treated with extinction, J. Pediatr. Psychol. 17 (1992) 467–475.
[7] A. Sadeh, Assessment of intervention for infant night waking: parental reports and activity-based home monitoring, J. Consult. Clin. Psychol. 62 (1994) 63–68.

RECOMMENDED READINGS

K.G. France, N.M. Blampied, Infant sleep disturbance: Description of a problem behaviour process, Sleep Med. Rev. 3 (1999) 365–380.
K.G. France, N.M. Blampied, Modifications of systematic ignoring in the management of infant sleep disturbance: Efficacy and infant distress, Child Fam. Behav. Ther. 27 (2005) 1–16.
K.G. France, J.M.T. Henderson, S.M. Hudson, Fact, act and tact: A three-stage approach to treating the sleep problems of infants and young children, Child Adolesc. Psychiatr. Clin. N. Am. 5 (1996) 581–599.
J.A. Mindell, B. Kuhn, D.S. Lewin, et al., Behavioral treatment of bedtime problems and night wakings in infants and young children, Sleep 29 (10) (2006) 1263–1276.
A. Sadeh, Assessment of intervention for infant night waking: Parental reports and activity-based home monitoring, J. Consult. Clin. Psychol. 62 (1994) 63–68.

Chapter 29

Bedtime Fading with Response Cost for Children with Multiple Sleep Problems

Tiffany Kodak
Department of Pediatrics, Center for Autism Spectrum Disorders, Munroe-Meyer Institute, University of Nebraska Medical Center, Omaha, NE

Cathleen C. Piazza
Munroe-Meyer Institute and Department of Pediatrics, University of Nebraska Medical Center, Omaha, NE

PROTOCOL NAME

Bedtime fading with response cost for children with multiple sleep problems.

GROSS INDICATION

Bedtime fading with response cost is indicated for children with or without a developmental disability between the ages of 3 and 18 years. Sleep disturbances are relatively common in children, and may persist and become increasingly problematic if left untreated. In fact, sleep problems may persist for 3 years or more in 84 percent of individuals who initially show symptoms of sleep disturbance [1]. In a survey of typically developing children, approximately 20–30 percent of 1- to 4-year-olds displayed sleep problems [2]. By contrast, the prevalence of sleep disturbance in individuals diagnosed with a developmental disability may be as high as 88 percent [3]. Thus, children with developmental disabilities may be more likely to display sleep disturbance. Sleep problems in children diagnosed with a developmental disability may be especially problematic, because these individuals may be more likely to engage in problem behavior (e.g., disruptive or self-injurious behavior) at bedtime or during night wakings. Parents may need to monitor their child during night wakings, especially if the child engages in problem behavior during this period of time. Consequently, sleep problems may affect the whole family, and parents may feel irritable during the day due to chronic sleep deprivation [4].

Behavioral Treatments for Sleep Disorders. DOI: 10.1016/B978-0-12-381522-4.00029-8

SPECIFIC INDICATION

Bedtime fading is indicated for children with multiple sleep problems (e.g., night wakings, daytime sleep, delayed sleep onset), and/or children with the following diagnoses from the American Academy of Sleep Medicine [5]:

- Behavioral insomnia of childhood – sleep onset association type
- Behavioral insomnia of childhood – limit-setting type
- Behavioral insomnia of childhood – combined type
- Circadian rhythm sleep disorder, delayed sleep phase type
- Circadian rhythm sleep disorder, irregular sleep–wake type.

CONTRAINDICATIONS

Prior to implementing any treatment for sleep disturbances, parents should consult with a physician to determine if any biologically based disorders may be impacting the child's sleep.

RATIONALE FOR INTERVENTION

A variety of treatment procedures for sleep disturbance have been described in the literature, although few of these studies have evaluated treatments for children with multiple sleep disturbances (e.g., waking at night, waking early, difficulty falling asleep, bedtime tantrums). Many of the behavioral treatments that have been evaluated with children exhibiting sleep disturbances are designed to treat one type of sleep disturbance (e.g., bedtime tantrums) [6]. Unfortunately, many children that exhibit signs of sleep disturbance display more than one type of sleep problem (e.g., bedtime tantrums, waking at night, and waking early). Bedtime fading with response cost is one treatment procedure that has an advantage over other behavioral treatments for sleep disturbance because it is effective in treating multiple sleep problems simultaneously. Thus, bedtime fading with response cost is recommended when individuals present with multiple sleep problems that will be targeted during treatment.

A number of components of bedtime fading with response cost may increase the efficacy of treatment. For example, treatment capitalizes on the biological components of sleep. The initial steps in treatment involve placing the child in bed later than his or her typical onset of sleep. As a result, the child may fall asleep quickly upon being placed in bed. In addition, eliminating daytime sleeping (except for scheduled naps for children under the age of 4 years) may result in the child being sleepier near the scheduled bedtime. Finally, establishing a set pattern of sleep and wake cycles may facilitate the regulation of the body's circadian rhythm. Bedtime fading with response cost may also be preferable to other forms of treatment that require parents to implement treatment procedures during the middle of the night, when they are sleepy and may have difficulty following through with certain consequences.

The operant mechanisms responsible for the effectiveness of treatment may be related to enhanced stimulus control and manipulation of establishing operations, although no studies have directly examined these mechanisms. Removing the child from the bed when sleep onset does not occur within 15 minutes (i.e., response cost) and only allowing the child to lie in bed when sleep is highly likely allows bedtime stimuli (e.g., dark room, lying in bed) to be paired with sleepiness and sleep-related behaviors. Therefore, sleep-related behavior may come under the stimulus control of bedtime stimuli, which may result in a rapid onset of sleep when placed in bed, and allow the child to rapidly fall back to sleep during night wakings. In addition, restricting sleep during waking hours or removing the child from bed if sleep onset does not occur within 15 minutes may establish a motivating operation for sleep-related behavior. It has been noted that bedtime fading with response cost closely approximates a combination of two treatments – sleep restriction therapy and stimulus control therapy – shown to be highly efficacious in the treatment of adult insomnia [7].

STEP BY STEP DESCRIPTION OF PROCEDURES

Bedtime fading requires parents to implement treatment at the onset of bedtime. That is, parents place the child in bed at the scheduled bedtime, and observe the child for 15 minutes after they place him or her in bed. If the child is asleep, the parents are able to go to sleep as well. If the child is awake, the parents remove the child from the bed, but allow the child to engage in regular night-time activities (e.g., playing with toys, watching television). Therefore, parents do not have to restrict the child's access to activities if the child is required to stay awake until the next scheduled bedtime. In addition, parents are not required to change the consequences typically provided during night waking. For example, if parents allow the child to co-sleep (i.e., the child sleeps in the same bed as the parents) following night wakings prior to treatment, the child would still be permitted to co-sleep once treatment is initiated. This may prevent tantrums that could occur in the middle of the night if the child is suddenly not permitted to sleep in the same bed as the parents.

The first step of bedtime fading with response cost involves the collection of baseline data. Parents record whether the child is asleep or awake every 30 minutes throughout the day, with the exception of night-time hours, when the parents and child are asleep. However, parents do collect data on the occurrence and duration of any night wakings. When the baseline data are stable, the mean onset of sleep time is calculated by taking thc time that the child fell asleep each night and dividing by the number of nights included in the data sample. For example, if data were collected for 5 days, and the child fell asleep at 11:00 pm, 11:30 pm, midnight, 11:30 pm, and 11:30 pm, the mean onset of sleep during baseline would be 11:30 p.m. (i.e., the sum of each sleep time divided by 5). After the mean time of sleep onset is calculated, 30 minutes is added to this time to determine the initial bedtime during treatment.

Thus, the first night of treatment would involve a bedtime of midnight (i.e., 11:30 pm + 30 minutes). Data on the duration of daytime sleeping are also recorded in baseline. Prior to treatment implementation, the parents should decide on a specific goal for bedtime and morning waking (e.g., 8:00 pm to 7:00 am). This schedule should be based on parents' preference as well as developmental recommendations for the total number of hours of sleep per day based on the child's age (see Appendix 29.1).

Once the initial bedtime is determined from analysis of the baseline data, the parents are required to keep the child awake until this scheduled time. The child can engage in his or her typical night-time activities during treatment. Thus, if the child watches television and plays with toys for 1 hour prior to bedtime, the child is permitted to engage in these same activities once treatment is initiated. We recommend that the parents maintain a consistent bedtime routine prior to and following the initiation of treatment. During treatment, the child is placed in bed at the scheduled bedtime, and parents are permitted to interact with their child in the same manner as they did prior to treatment. That is, parents do not have to change their response to the child's behavior during bedtime. If the parents sat in the room with their child for 5 minutes after placing the child in bed prior to treatment, parents are permitted to continue to sit in the room with the child when treatment is initiated. When 15 minutes have elapsed after the scheduled bedtime, the parents check to see if the child is asleep. If it is unclear whether the child is asleep in bed, parents can stand within 1 ft of the child's bed and whisper their child's name. If the child does not engage in a motor or vocal response (i.e., does not look up or say anything in response to their name), this is taken as an indication that the child is asleep. If the child is not asleep, or responds to their name, the child is removed from the bed and required to stay awake for 1 hour past the scheduled bedtime. Removing the child from the bed if he or she is not asleep within 15 minutes of the scheduled bedtime is the response cost component of treatment. Thus, if the child is placed in bed at 11:30 pm and is awake at 11:45 pm, the child is removed from the bed and kept awake until 12:30 am (a response cost of 1 hour). At 12:30 am, the child is placed in bed and observed after 15 minutes. The 1-hour response cost is implemented until the child is observed to be asleep within 15 minutes of being placed in bed.

Upon night wakings, the parent records the time the child woke up and when the child went back to sleep. The child is permitted to engage in the activities he or she was permitted to do during night-time waking prior to treatment. However, parents should prompt the child, at 30-minute intervals, to go to bed. A morning wake-up time is determined prior to treatment, and the child is not permitted to sleep past the scheduled time. Outside of scheduled nap times (depending on developmental guidelines for daytime naps), the child is not permitted to sleep during the day. If developmental guidelines indicate that nap times are appropriate for the child's age, parents should schedule naps for certain times of the day and only allow the child to nap during these scheduled times. For example, if it is developmentally appropriate for the child to take two 1-hour naps, the parents should schedule these naps at specific times (e.g., midday–1:00 pm and 4:00–5:00 pm), and not permit the child to fall asleep outside of the scheduled nap times. Fading the bedtime schedule consists of adjusting the bedtime based on the time of sleep onset from the previous night. For example, if the child fell asleep within 15 minutes of the scheduled bedtime, the bedtime is made 30 minutes earlier the next night. If the child did not fall a sleep within 15 minutes of the scheduled bedtime, the bedtime is made 30 minutes later for the next night.

POSSIBLE MODIFICATIONS/VARIANTS

The procedure for determining the child's bedtime at the onset of treatment has varied in the literature. The amount of time added to the mean time of onset of sleep calculated during baseline has been reported as either 30 minutes or 1 hour. The recent literature on bedtime fading with response cost has added 30 minutes to the mean sleep onset time [8,9], although one of the initial studies on bedtime fading with response cost added 1 hour [10]. Thus, one potential modification to the description above involves adding 1 hour to the mean time of sleep onset calculated from baseline data. That is, if the mean time of sleep onset is 11:30 pm, adding 1 hour would involve an initial bedtime of 12:30 am at the onset of treatment.

A second variation in the procedure for bedtime fading with response cost involves the method for fading the bedtime. Although the recommendation above involves fading by 30-minute intervals, depending on the time of sleep onset from the previous night, research has also shown that fading by 15-minute intervals may be effective [11]. In addition, Piazza and colleagues adjusted the bedtime following two consecutive nights with sleep onset within 15 minutes of placement in bed. This differs from the recommendation above, which describes fading the bedtime each day if the child falls asleep within 15 minutes of being placed in bed. There may be a benefit to using a somewhat less stringent criterion for fading. First, the child's behavior may take more than 1 day to adjust to a new scheduled sleep time. By fading too rapidly, parents may become frustrated by having to increase the bedtime the day after they were able to decrease bedtime. Parents also may have difficulty keeping track of the target bedtime if the schedule is adjusted each day. Parents may prefer to provide their child with an extra day to respond to treatment before making another adjustment in the schedule. Alternatively, parents may prefer the rapid fading of the schedule because of exhaustion. The initial bedtime is scheduled at a time when the child is likely to have a rapid onset of sleep, and parents may find it difficult to keep their child awake prior to the scheduled bedtime. Furthermore, parents may be sleepy if the initial scheduled bedtime is relatively late at night. Parents may be eager to decrease the bedtime schedule to avoid having to stay up late and/or keep their child awake.

An additional modification to the fading procedure was discussed by Piazza and Fisher [10]. The authors suggested fading the bedtime by 15 minutes once the child reaches a plateau in fading. If the child is not making progress toward reaching the treatment goal (i.e., the final bedtime), parents could consider fading by 15 minutes instead of 30 minutes. Thus, the bedtime could be increased or decreased by 15 minutes each day, depending on the child's time of sleep onset.

A third modification to bedtime fading involves the amount of time the child is required to stay awake when the response cost component of treatment is implemented. In the procedures described above, the child is required to get out of bed and stay awake for an additional hour past the initial scheduled bedtime if the onset of sleep does not occur within 15 minutes of being placed in bed. One alternative, evaluated by Ashbaugh and Peck [8], involved a response cost interval of 30 minutes. Although treatment including a shorter duration of response cost was effective, the procedure was only evaluated with one participant, and the results should be interpreted with caution.

A final modification to bedtime fading with response cost involves eliminating the response cost component from treatment. Piazza and Fisher [11] evaluated bedtime fading without response cost with two children. Results indicated that appropriate sleep (sleeping only during scheduled sleep times) increased and inappropriate sleep (sleeping during unscheduled sleep times) decreased. Thus, the procedure may also be effective in the absence of the response cost component of treatment, although it remains unclear to what extent response cost improves the effectiveness of treatment.

PROOF OF CONCEPT/SUPPORTING DATA/EVIDENCE BASE

A number of studies have evaluated bedtime fading with typically developing children and children with developmental disabilities. Although the majority of the literature on bedtime fading was conducted with individuals diagnosed with developmental disabilities, two studies have evaluated this procedure with typically developing children. For example, Ashbaugh and Peck [8] evaluated bedtime fading with a 2-year-old girl with no developmental or behavioral impairments. In addition, one participant in a study by Piazza and Fisher [11] was of normal intelligence and diagnosed with ADHD. Additional research is required to evaluate bedtime fading with more typically developing children.

Bedtime fading is an effective treatment procedure for reducing multiple sleep problems. That is, bedtime fading may increase the percentage of appropriate sleep (i.e., sleeping during scheduled sleep time periods) [9–11], decrease the percentage of inappropriate or disturbed sleep [8,10], decrease waking multiple times per night [10], and decrease co-sleeping (i.e., sleeping in the parent's bed) [10]. Bedtime fading is more effective than simply scheduling a specific bedtime [9], and results may be maintained for at least 1 year [8,10]. Parents have also reported satisfaction with treatment outcomes, and reported that children who previously refused to go to bed prior to treatment actually requested to go to bed following treatment [10].

REFERENCES

[1] S. Kataria, M.S. Swanson, G.E. Trevathan, Persistence of sleep disturbances in preschool children, J. Pediatr. 110 (1987) 642–646.
[2] B. Lozoff, A.W. Wolf, N.S. Davis, Sleep problems seen in pediatric practice, Pediatrics 75 (1985) 477–483.
[3] C.C. Piazza, W.W. Fisher, S.W. Kahng, A descriptive study of sleep patterns in children with mental retardation and severe behavior disorders, Dev. Med. Child Neurol. 38 (1996) 335–344.
[4] P.C. Friman, C.C. Piazza, Behavioral pediatrics: A logical point of entry into pediatric medicine for applied behavior analysts, in: W.W. Fisher, C.C. Piazza, H.S. Roane (Eds.), Handbook of Applied Behavior Analysis, Guilford Publications, Inc., New York, NY, in press.
[5] American Academy of Sleep Medicine, International Classification of Sleep Disorders, second ed., AASM, Westchester IL, 2005.
[6] L.A. Adams, V.I. Rickert, Reducing bedtime tantrums: Comparison between positive routines and graduated extinction, Pediatrics 84 (1989) 756–761.
[7] B.R. Kuhn, A.J. Elliott, Treatment efficacy in behavioral pediatric sleep medicine, J. Psychosom. Res. 5 (2003) 587–597.
[8] R. Ashbaugh, S.M. Peck, Treatment of sleep problems in a toddler: A replication of the faded bedtime with response cost protocol, J. Appl. Behav. Anal. 31 (1998) 127–129.
[9] C.C. Piazza, W.W. Fisher, M. Sherer, Treatment of multiple sleep problems in children with developmental disabilities: Faded bedtime with response cost versus bedtime scheduling, Dev. Med. Child Neurol. 39 (1997) 414–418.
[10] C.C. Piazza, W. Fisher, A faded bedtime with response cost protocol for treatment of multiple sleep problems in children, J. Appl. Behav. Anal. 24 (1991) 129–140.
[11] C.C. Piazza, W.W. Fisher, Bedtime fading in the treatment of pediatric insomnia, J. Behav. Ther. Exp. Psychiatry 22 (1991) 53–56.
[12] T. Kodak, C.C. Piazza, Assessment and behavioral treatment of feeding and sleeping disorders in children with autism spectrum disorders, Child Adolesc. Psychiatr. Clin. N. Am. 17 (2008) 887–906.
[13] G.J. Cohen (Ed.), American Academy of Pediatrics Guide to Your Child's Sleep, Villard, New York, NY, 1999.

APPENDIX 29.1

A number of treatment procedures have been evaluated with individuals with sleep problems [12]. However, bedtime fading is one treatment procedure that may address multiple sleep problems. Prior to treatment implementation, parents may wish to read additional information regarding treatment procedures and any limitations to treatment. Any of the references provided in the text of the chapter may be obtained to learn additional details about bedtime fading with response cost. The study conducted by Piazza and Fisher [10] provides a comprehensive review of the literature, a thorough description of the procedures for bedtime fading with response cost, and a section on procedural modifications. The article can be obtained online at: http://www.pubmedcentral.nih.gov/picrender.fcgi?artid=1279554&blobtype=pdf.

Developmental guidelines for sleep for children may be obtained from a number of sources. One group providing developmental sleep guidelines is the National Sleep Foundation. These guidelines can be obtained online at: http://www.sleepfoundation.org/site/c.huIXKjM0IxF/b.2419295/k.5AAB/Childrens_Sleep_Habits.htm. *The American Academy of Pediatrics Guide to Your Child's Sleep* [13] provides some guidelines regarding how much sleep children need at different ages. The guidelines listed below reflect total sleep hours in a 24-hour period. Thus, naptimes will need to be taken into account when adding up the child's total hours of sleep.

Birth–6 months	16–20 hours
6 months–12 months	14–15 hours
Ages 1–3	10–13 hours
Ages 3–10	10–12 hours
Ages 11–12	10 hours
Teenagers	9 hours

Chapter 30

The Bedtime Pass

Connie J. Schnoes
Father Flanagan's Boys' Home, Boys Town, NE

NAME OF PROTOCOL

The bedtime pass.

GROSS INDICATION

The *bedtime pass* is a viable and effective strategy to employ for children who present with bedtime struggles or bedtime refusal. Bedtime difficulties typically include resistance to going to bed and falling asleep. Such behaviors are reinforced or sustained by delaying bedtime, and maintaining contact with caregivers.

SPECIFIC INDICATION

The pass is an appropriate intervention or strategy for children who are able to initiate sleep independently in their own beds or rooms [1–3]. The skill of independent sleep initiation consists of:

- ability to fall asleep alone and
- ability to fall asleep in the dark and
- ability to fall asleep in the quiet and
- ability to fall asleep in own bed.

Some children exhibit independent sleep onset skills, but resist remaining in bed or falling asleep for an extended period of time. Bedtime refusal includes resisting getting ready for bed and engaging in the bedtime routine, and/or calling out from bed or coming out of the bedroom after bedtime or upon awakening during the night. These children have the skill to fall asleep on their own, but they demonstrate insufficient motivation to do so.

The bedtime pass is recommended for children who present with behavioral insomnia of childhood – limit-setting type [4]. Diagnostic criteria include:

- the individual has difficulty initiating or maintaining sleep
- the individual stalls or refuses to go to bed at an appropriate time, or refuses to return to bed following a night-time awakening

Behavioral Treatments for Sleep Disorders. DOI: 10.1016/B978-0-12-381522-4.00030-4

- the caregiver demonstrates insufficient or inappropriate limit-setting to establish appropriate sleeping behavior in the child.

CONTRAINDICATIONS

The bedtime pass is not appropriate for children who:

- do not fall asleep on their own in their own beds;
- require parental presence;
- only fall sleep with a TV, radio or specific music playing, while feeding, etc.;
- exhibit a behavioral insomnia of childhood – sleep onset association type;
- exhibit fear of the dark;
- exhibit parasomnias (e.g., sleep walking, sleep talking, night terrors);
- present with breathing-related sleep disorders;
- present with nightmares;
- exhibit narcolepsy.

RATIONALE FOR INTERVENTION

Pediatric sleep problems warrant intervention for several significant reasons:

- Problems with sleep onset and frequent night awakenings are one of the most common childhood concerns expressed by parents
- Approximately 20–40 percent of children and adolescents experience some type of sleep disorder during their lifetime [5,6]
- Untreated pediatric sleep disorders persist over time [7]
- Sleep disorders can have a negative impact on development, emotion, and behavior [8,9].

Behavioral insomnia of childhood – limit-setting type is characterized by the child stalling or refusing to go to bed or follow appropriate bedtime regimens. The child's resistance usually occurs at the start of bedtime, but can also occur during awakenings in the middle of the night. The disruptive bedtime behavior and resulting delayed sleep onset may lead to sleep deprivation. Bedtime resistance often presents as calling out or coming out of the bedroom repeatedly. However, these children ultimately fall asleep independently [4].

The bedtime pass is an extinction-based behavioral protocol. The child is allowed one escape from bedtime (the bedtime pass), and all subsequent bedtime resistance is ignored (extinction). Bedtime signals the end of the child's active participation in the day. Bedtime is functionally equivalent to time out from positive reinforcement including attention, possessions, and movement. That is, children end their active participation with people, toys, play, entertainment, etc., once they go to bed. Disruptive behavior at bedtime may serve to escape the experience of time out from positive reinforcement. The bedtime pass provides the child with an acceptable escape strategy to employ at his or her discretion. The pass functions as a single opportunity to escape this end of active participation. It also assures children that they have one opportunity to have their needs (a drink, potty, hug) met after being put to bed. Extinction is employed when the child engages in bedtime-resistant or disruptive behavior after he or she has used his or her pass to have a request met after bedtime.

The effect of the bedtime pass is a reduction in the number of times a child calls or comes out of his or her bedroom. When the child falls asleep before using the pass, calling or coming out behavior is reduced to zero. One potential reason the child may fall asleep before using the pass is a desire to save the pass for something he or she really wants or needs. In younger children, a desire to keep their bedtime pass object may contribute to their falling asleep before exchanging it to have a want or need met. Whether the child is saving the pass for something important or is reluctant to give up the pass, the child experiences going to bed and falling asleep readily. Thus, bedtime resistance is reduced if not eliminated.

STEP BY STEP DESCRIPTION OF PROCEDURES

Prior to implementing the bedtime pass, it is important for clinicians to ensure the child falls asleep independently in his or her own bed, in a quiet dark room. This step is conducted to confirm the child exhibits behavioral insomnia of childhood – limit-setting type. Once it is determined that the bedtime pass is an appropriate intervention, the child is encouraged and/or assisted to select or make an object to be designated as a bedtime pass. The object can be a stuffed animal (not the child's transitional object), a fancy ticket or card that fits under the child's pillow, etc. A string of beads is not recommended due to safety concerns. Once an object is selected for the pass, how the pass works is explained to the child. The child is informed that the pass is "worth" one opportunity to come out or call out of the bedroom after bedtime, and that if he or she chooses to come or call out of the bedroom, the bedtime pass must be turned over to the parent immediately. Finally, the child is also told that once the pass has been used, he or she cannot come out or call out from the bedroom again, and that if the child does call out or come out, the parents will not talk to him or her.

At bedtime, the child is placed in bed with the bedtime pass tucked in with the child or placed under the pillow, depending on the object used. The parent reminds the child that if he or she needs or wants anything, the bedtime pass can be used one time. After that, the child will have to stay in bed and go to sleep. The first time the child calls or comes out of the room, the parent attends to the child's want or need readily. Once the need or want is addressed, the parent reminds the child that he or she must give the parent the bedtime pass. Once the pass is in the parent's possession, the child is placed back in bed and reminded that there are no more opportunities to call or come out of the bedroom. If the child calls out, the parents ignore the child's attempts to interact. If the child comes out of the bedroom, the parent returns the child to bed with minimal interaction – that is, the parent does not remind the child, reprimand the child, etc. The parent simply, gently and silently, returns the child to bed. Parents respond in this manner until the child falls asleep.

In the morning, it is not necessary or encouraged that parents discuss their child's use of the bedtime pass the night before. Verbal interaction regarding the pass occurs at bedtime. A summary of the implementation procedures is as follows:

1. Select/make a bedtime pass
2. Explain the pass is good for one call out or coming out of the bedroom after bedtime
3. Immediately respond to the child's request/need
4. Collect the pass from the child
5. Ignore all subsequent attempts to call or come out from the bedroom by the child.

As the child consistently goes to bed and falls asleep readily, and the disruptive behavior decreases, the bedtime pass is gradually faded from use. Possible fading procedures include the following:

- Parents decrease the amount of verbal interaction specific to the pass when they put their child to bed. Verbal interaction may transition over time from the full explanation about how the pass works, to a simple review of the procedure, to a brief statement acknowledging the presence of the pass.
- As the child is tucked into bed, the parent, without drawing verbal attention to the pass, simply insures it is present (under the pillow, on the night stand, etc.).
- Parents may alternate between making sure the pass is present (verbally or non-verbally) and no attention to the pass night to night, and gradually decreasing the frequency of ensuring its presence.

POSSIBLE MODIFICATIONS/VARIANTS

One variation to this procedure is to identify with the child an incentive (e.g., special breakfast, toy, coin) to be earned by not using the pass and simply remaining in bed at bedtime. If this modification is included, parents provide the incentive or inform the child that he or she earned the incentive upon getting up in the morning.

Pairing the bedtime pass with sleep restriction therapy (SRT) and a consistent bedtime routine may facilitate a more rapid treatment response. SRT involves restricting the child's time in bed (at night and during naps) to facilitate ready sleep onset. SRT increases the likelihood the child will fall asleep readily upon being put to bed [10]. The bedtime schedule is established based on the child's actual time of sleep onset. This information is readily obtained from a completed sleep diary. Pairing SRT with bedtime fading serves to establish ready sleep onset, and a bedtime schedule that results in increased total sleep time. Bedtime fading involves gradually adjusting the bedtime schedule once the child is falling asleep readily (within 15 minutes of bedtime) [11]. For more information on SRT see Schnoes & Reimers [12].

PROOF OF CONCEPT/SUPPORTING DATA/EVIDENCE BASE

Research indicates the pass is highly effective in reducing bedtime resistance for typically developing toddlers and school-age children [1–3]. The bedtime pass has also been rated as highly acceptable by parents [2,3]. Bedtime resistance was defined as calling/crying out or leaving the bedroom across studies. The first published research on the bedtime pass revealed positive effects for both a 3-year-old boy and a 10-year-old boy [2]. The results of the study revealed that the mean number of nightly episodes of bedtime resistance were 4.6 for the 3-year-old and 2.3 for the 10-year-old during baseline. During the intervention phase, the bedtime pass was effective in eliminating crying out and leaving the room for both children without an extinction burst. These gains were maintained at 1-week follow-up. The data indicated that the children frequently fell asleep and did not utilize their passes.

A multiple baseline design study supported the efficacy of the bedtime pass for four 3-year-old Caucasian males [1]. Mean rates of bedtime resistance ranged from 0.8 to 5.4 episodes during baseline across the four children. During the intervention phase, mean rates of bedtime resistance ranged from 0 to 0.75 episodes per night across the four children. Freeman [1] also conducted an initial component analysis examining the use of the pass alone and the pass plus extinction. The data revealed decreased rates of bedtime resistance when the pass was used alone. When the pass was used in combination with extinction, bedtime resistance was eliminated. Another finding of this study was a reduction in the rates of resistance without an extinction burst.

Moore and colleagues [3] randomly assigned 19 male and female children, aged 3 to 6 years, to the bedtime pass condition or a monitoring control group. Compared to children in the monitoring control condition, children in the bedtime pass condition exhibited statistically significantly less bedtime resistance and time to quiet. The results revealed virtually no change in rates of leaving the bedroom, crying/calling out, and time to quiet for the children in the monitoring control group from baseline to post-test. Children in the bedtime pass condition demonstrated reductions in bedtime resistance and time to quiet from baseline to post-test with gains maintained at 3-month follow-up. Mean rates for the children assigned to the bedtime pass condition were as follows: leaving the bedroom 1.6 (baseline), <0.5 (post-test), and 0.4 (follow-up); crying out 2.4 (baseline), 0.6 (post-test), and 0.1 (follow-up); and time to quiet 43 minutes (baseline), 25 minutes (post-test), and 0.1 minutes (follow-up). Data also revealed the absence of an extinction burst with the implementation of the bedtime pass.

REFERENCES

[1] K.A. Freeman, Treating bedtime resistance with bedtime pass: A systematic replication and component analysis with 3-year olds, J. Appl. Behav. Anal. 3 (2006) 423–428.

[2] P.C. Friman, K.E. Hoff, C. Schnoes, et al., The bedtime pass: An approach to bedtime crying and leaving the room, Arch. Pediatr. Adolesc. Med. 153 (1999) 1027–1029.

[3] B.A. Moore, P.C. Friman, A.E. Fruzzetti, K. MacAleese, Evaluating the bedtime pass program for child resistance to bedtime – a randomized, controlled trial, J. Pediatr. Psychol. 32 (2007) 283–287.

[4] American Academy of Sleep Medicine, International Classification of Sleep Disorders, second ed., AASM, Westchester IL, 2005.

[5] L.J. Meltzer, Mindell J.A. Sleep, sleep disorders in children and adolescents, Pediatr. Clin. N. Am. 29 (2006) 1059–1076.

[6] J.A. Mindell, B. Kuhn, D.S. Lewin, et al., Behavioral treatment of bedtime problems and night wakings in infants and young children, Sleep 29 (2006) 1263–1276.

[7] S. Kateria, M. Swanson, C. Trevarthin, Persistence of sleep disturbances in preschool children, J. Pediatr. 110 (1987) 642–646.

[8] D.W. Beebe, D. Gozal, Obstructive sleep apnea and the prefrontal cortex. Towards a comprehensive model linking nocturnal upper airway obstruction to daytime cognitive and behavioral deficits, J. Sleep Res. 11 (2002) 1–16.

[9] J.A. Mindell, J.A.A. Owens, Clinical Guide to Pediatric Sleep: Diagnosis and Management of Sleep Problems, Lippincott, Williams & Wilkins, Philadelphia, PA, 2003.

[10] A.J. Spielman, P. Saskin, M.J. Thorpy, Treatment of chronic insomnia by restriction of time in bed, Sleep 10 (1) (1987) 45–56.

[11] C.C. Piazza, W. Fisher, A faded bedtime with response cost protocol for treatment of multiple sleep problems in children, J. App. Behav. Anal. 24 (1991) 129–140.

[12] C.J. Schnoes, T.M. Reimers, Assessment and treatment of child and adolescent sleep disorders, in: D McKay, E.A. Storch (Eds.), Cognitive-Behavior Therapy for Children: Treating Complex and Refractory Cases., Springer, New York, NY, 2009, pp. 293–324.

RECOMMENDED READING

K.A. Freeman, Treating bedtime resistance with bedtime pass: A systematic replication and component analysis with 3-year olds, J. Appl. Behav. Anal. 3 (2006) 423–428.

P.C. Friman, Good Night, Sweet Dreams, I Love You: Now Get into Bed and Go to Sleep, BT Press, Boys Town, NE, 2005.

P.C. Friman, K.E. Hoff, C. Schnoes, et al., The bedtime pass: An approach to bedtime crying and leaving the room, Arch. Pediatr. Adolesc. Med. 153 (1999) 1027–1029.

B.A. Moore, P.C. Friman, A.E. Fruzzetti, K. MacAleese, Evaluating the bedtime pass program for child resistance to bedtime – a randomized, controlled trial, J. Pediatr. Psychol. 32 (2007) 283–287.

Chapter 31

The Excuse-Me Drill: A Behavioral Protocol to Promote Independent Sleep Initiation Skills and Reduce Bedtime Problems in Young Children

Brett R. Kuhn
Munroe-Meyer Institute Department of Pediatric Psychology, University of Nebraska Medical Center, Children's Sleep Disorders Center, Omaha, NE

PROTOCOL NAME

The "excuse-me drill": a behavioral protocol to promote independent sleep initiation skills and reduce bedtime problems in young children.

GROSS INDICATION

The Excuse-Me Drill (EMD) is designed to reduce bedtime problems and frequent night-time awakenings in young children. The procedure combines the complementary forces of extinction and reinforcement to teach young children the key skill of independent sleep initiation. The protocol relies heavily on parents' most salient reinforcer, their own presence and attention, to address problematic child behaviors such as bedtime tantrums, frequent requests ("curtain calls"), and coming out of the bedroom.

SPECIFIC INDICATION

The EMD is not limited to any particular population or age range; however, it is most appropriate for:

1. Children with the following diagnoses from the latest edition of the International Classification of Sleep Disorders (ICSD) [1]:
   - Behavioral insomnia of childhood – sleep onset association type
   - Behavioral insomnia of childhood – limit-setting type
   - Behavioral insomnia of childhood – combined type.

Behavioral Treatments for Sleep Disorders. DOI: 10.1016/B978-0-12-381522-4.00031-6

2. Children near the ages 2–6 years who have transitioned, or are in the process of transitioning, from the crib to their own bed.
3. Children whose problem behavior is largely maintained by the reinforcing properties of parental presence and parental attention, or who misbehave in order to escape/avoid separation from parents at bedtime.
4. Parents who indicate a preference to teach their child to become a solitary sleeper, as opposed to parents who prefer to practice routine co-sleeping.

CONTRAINDICATIONS

- Fragile medical conditions (parent or child) that might prevent or interfere with initiating any effort to change habits, behavior, or living situation.
- An inappropriate or inconsistent sleep schedule during which the child is placed in bed at times when he or she is not sleepy.
- Severe child anxiety, especially separation anxiety (including fear of being alone). Before targeting independent sleep skills at bedtime, therapists are encouraged to consider first addressing separation anxiety during the day using empirically supported treatments (e.g., cognitive-behavioral therapy incorporating graduated exposure) [2].
- Sleep-related problem behaviors that are not maintained by the reinforcing properties of parental presence and/or attention.
- Certain children who for various reasons do not find parental presence or social attention to be reinforcing (e.g., neurobehavioral deficits, autism, history of environmental deprivation in early childhood).
- Poor timing. This could involve a number of things, such as upcoming travel, stress and unrest, or disruptions to the typical family schedule (e.g., illness, birth of a new child).
- Parental disagreement regarding treatment goals (e.g., solitary sleeping arrangements vs routine co-sleeping) or disagreement on the appropriateness of the EMD protocol itself.

The conditions above do not represent an exhaustive list of potential contraindications, nor do they represent absolute contraindications. As with any case, sound clinical judgment should be used to weigh the potential risks and benefits of treating the child's sleep disturbance, including the long-term risks of choosing not to treat.

RATIONALE FOR INTERVENTION

- Although young children display a variety of sleep problems (e. g., parasomnias, sleep apnea, disrupted schedule), the predominant presentation consists of an extrinsic dyssomnia involving difficulty settling and frequent night-time awakenings. These two symptoms often coexist, and treatments targeting one symptom frequently generalize to the other. This can be explained by the fact that the process of initiating sleep takes place not just

at bedtime, but also following brief night-time awakenings that are part of a child's normal sleep cycle [3,4].
- Parent sleep practices during sleep initiation (e.g., whether the child is placed into bed awake or already asleep) most strongly predict which young children are described as "good" or "poor" sleepers [5–7].
- Even after children develop the ability to self-sooth and initiate sleep independently, the transition from the crib to a bed presents a formidable challenge for many families. Taking down the crib means that parents no longer have their "toddler containment device", placing increased pressure on their ability to set and enforce effective behavioral limits.
- Bedtime problems during this stage include frequent requests of the parent, crying, tantrums, and leaving the bedroom. Most of these behaviors function to secure parental presence and attention, to delay going to bed, or to avoid separation from the parent. Disruptive bedtime behavior often results in delayed sleep onset and sleep deprivation for both child and parent.

Nearly all treatments for young children with sleep disturbance are designed to specifically target independent sleep initiation skills. Besides prevention and parent education, extinction-based treatments have the strongest research support [8]. There are, however several inherent problems with the use of extinction (EXT):

1. EXT is difficult to execute. In many cases, success relies largely on parents' ability to effectively ignore a child's disruptive bedtime behavior for long periods of time. Parents can easily fall into the trap of selectively reinforcing more severe occurrences, inadvertently strengthening the child's behavior and making it more resistant to intervention.
2. There are several undesirable side effects associated with EXT, including the extinction burst (a temporary increase in frequency, duration, or magnitude of the target behavior), extinction-induced emotional outbursts or aggression, and spontaneous recovery [9].
3. EXT is widely reported in the sleep literature to be viewed poorly by parents. This view is consistent with the treatment acceptability literature indicating that parents prefer positive interventions (e.g., praise, reinforcement vs punishment) designed to increase adaptive child behavior (vs decrease problem behavior) [10].
4. While EXT is highly effective in reducing behaviors (e.g., crying, tantrums) that interfere with sleep initiation, it does nothing to teach or reinforce appropriate child "pre-sleep" behaviors. In other words, EXT eliminates reinforcement for problem bedtime behavior, but the procedure does nothing to teach children what TO DO (e.g., remain in bed quietly until they fall asleep).
5. Both basic and applied research indicates that adding a reinforcement component (especially a "rich schedule" of reinforcement) to EXT produces more rapid and effective results, and reduces the likelihood of undesirable side effects [11,12]. Consequently, implementing EXT as the sole intervention component is rarely recommended [13].

In summary, the EMD protocol enhances the effectiveness of EXT by adding a differential reinforcement schedule to teach young children adaptive behaviors during the pre-sleep period. The reinforcement schedule starts out rich in order to help young children establish newly acquired behaviors, and is gradually thinned to a partial reinforcement schedule to maintain these behaviors over time [14]. Our experience after using this protocol for nearly 15 years in a pediatric sleep clinic suggests that the EMD protocol effectively eliminates problem behaviors that interfere with sleep initiation, reinforces appropriate pre-sleep behaviors to facilitate quicker sleep initiation, and ensures that children learn to fall asleep independently without requiring parental presence.

STEP BY STEP DESCRIPTION OF PROCEDURES

Like most good behavioral interventions, the EMD is best when delivered within the context of other sound clinical procedures (detailed below). Although the intervention presented in this chapter is standardized and prescriptive, successful outcomes rely on obtaining a skilled, comprehensive assessment that identifies behavioral function and informs an *individualized* treatment plan [15]:

1. Teach the child to fall asleep in the desired habitual sleep environment
2. Select an appropriate "start night"
3. Temporarily delay bedtime and manage the sleep schedule
4. Begin the excuse-me drill
5. Create a back-up plan for leaving the bedroom.

Teach the Child to Fall Asleep in the Desired Habitual Sleep Environment

A child's habitual sleep environment, including where and with whom the child sleeps, may vary greatly depending on family values, preferences, economic status, parenting style, and cultural beliefs. Children with behavioral sleep disturbances, however, tend to experience gross inconsistencies in their sleep environment as parents tend to respond to child misbehavior by altering this environment. Once children are sound asleep and can no longer put up resistance, many parents relocate them to their own bed for (hopefully) the remainder of the night. Upon awakening normally in the middle of the night, children find themselves in a "foreign land" where they have virtually no experience initiating sleep – much less independently. Therefore, the first step in this treatment protocol simply involves providing children with multiple opportunities to initiate sleep in their desired habitual sleep location (often their own bed and bedroom). Parents are encouraged to place their child in bed drowsy but still awake. For the first week or two, parents may continue to provide any other familiar sleep associations (e.g., rocking, singing, back rub, lying next to them in bed) to facilitate quick and cooperative sleep onset.

This recommendation is typically delivered as the family's first homework assignment toward the end of the first appointment following the presentation of the clinical impressions. In our experience, 5–10 percent of children respond to this treatment component alone, obviating the need for further intervention.

Recommendation: *For now, Richie should be required to fall asleep in his own bed and bedroom each and every time (e.g., bedtime, following night-time awakenings, naps). Mrs Cunningham may continue to remain with Richie in his room until he falls asleep. If Richie wakes up in the night to cry out, or enters the parent's bedroom, Mrs Cunningham will immediately re-enter Richie's bedroom (or return him to his bedroom), and remain with him until he falls asleep again. The short-term goal is to help Richie become more comfortable and accustomed to falling asleep in his own bed and bedroom.*

Families with children who already initiate sleep consistently in the desired sleep environment may skip this step and begin with the next treatment component. The following three steps are typically installed together during the second clinic appointment, given that the first step was accomplished successfully.

Select an Appropriate "Start Night"

Discussing the best time to begin the EMD is best accomplished during a clinic visit, as long as all of the active "players" are present. Delaying the protocol may be warranted in the event of upcoming travel or disruptions to the family schedule (visitors, illness, birth of new child). In many cases, families choose to implement the EMD on a night (often Friday night) when both parents will be home and they have the weekend ahead of them.

Temporarily Delay Bedtime and Manage the Sleep Schedule

In order to increase homeostatic sleep drive, parents are instructed to temporarily delay the child's bedtime beginning the first night they implement the EMD. The objective of this step is to increase the likelihood of quick sleep onset and decrease the duration of bedtime resistance. The new bedtime can be chosen by calculating the child's average sleep onset (clock time) based on parents' report of the most recent three or four nights (or by obtaining a pre-treatment sleep diary). Readers may recognize this treatment component as a variation of Piazza's bedtime fading protocol (see Chapter 29 of this book), with the exception that 30 minutes is not added to the average sleep onset time to prevent younger children from becoming over-tired and fussy/irritable. Once the child is routinely falling asleep independently within 20–30 minutes of being placed in bed, bedtime is gradually faded earlier (about 15 minutes every couple of nights) until the original bedtime (or parents' bedtime goal) is reached.

Delaying the bedtime increases the risk of circadian drift; therefore, parents are asked to tightly maintain usual morning wake-times and nap-times. This recommendation prevents the child from "making-up" lost sleep following the introduction of a later bedtime and novel behavioral protocol, ensuring that one bad night does not become two, three, or thirty.

Recommendation: *It is extremely important to keep the morning wake time and daytime naps constant (same as pre-treatment) so Joanie does not "make up" for lost sleep following a difficult night. This will increase the likelihood that she will fall asleep more quickly the next evening. Please communicate this recommendation to daycare staff in charge of napping. During planned awake times, Joanie should be kept awake by engaging her in outdoor activities, games, sensory stimulation, or exercise to prevent her from drifting off to sleep. An action plan should be made to keep Joanie awake during high-risk situations like watching a movie or a long car ride.*

The Excuse-Me Drill (EMD)

Now that the child is falling asleep easily in his or her habitual sleep environment (usually with the help of parental presence), the clinician introduces the "parent-ectomy." Specifically, parents are taught to strategically deliver frequent but brief "bursts" of social attention when the child displays appropriate (e.g., sleep-compatible) bedtime behavior. Clinicians may wish first to provide a description of the underlying process (or function) driving the child's behavior before recommending and demonstrating the EMD, for example:

A sleep-friendly environment tends to be devoid of stimulation. Young children, however, often find this type of environment unpleasant and may work to avoid it, much like a time-out. Consequently, the bedtime routine or bedroom environment itself may trigger child misbehavior, much like a long, boring car ride, or when a parent becomes preoccupied on the phone. Children quickly realize that remaining quietly in bed is simply not an effective strategy to recruit their parents' presence or attention. Instead, they learn to exit the bedroom or to engage in behaviors uniquely crafted to recruit parents into their bedroom. During these "curtain calls", children often make frequent requests for extra drinks, hugs, kisses, or they suddenly become interested in learning how clouds are formed. After delivering the child's sixteenth glass of water in a single night, most parents figure out that it's not thirst that the child is trying to quench.

The beauty of the EMD protocol is that it relies on parent behaviors that are already known to be reinforcing to the child. By simply reversing the contingency, parents deliver these social reinforcers in response to appropriate rather than inappropriate in-bed behaviors. Upon completing the normal bedtime routine, the parent places the child in bed and says, "Excuse me, I need to go ... [insert reason] ..., but I will be right back to check on you." On the first trip, the parent barely crosses the threshold of the bedroom and (before the child has the opportunity to misbehave) quickly returns to the child to provide physical presence, attention, a calm touch, and labeled verbal praise for "being a big girl" and "staying quietly in your bed." All aspects of the reinforcement schedule, including the duration of visits, the reward "value" of parent behavior during visits, and the distance/duration away from the bedroom during excuse-me trips, start on a thick schedule but are gradually faded over subsequent nights as the child develops increased behavioral mastery.

Recommendation: *Please run the "excuse-me" drill at bedtime. Provide attention freely and frequently to reinforce Ralph whenever he is practicing "sleep compatible" behaviors. Upon putting him in bed and turning off the lights, you might say, "Excuse me, I need to ... I'll be right back." You can then leave Ralph's bedroom, but return quickly (i.e., after no longer than a few seconds) to praise Ralph for lying quietly. Continue regularly to walk into his bedroom to provide attention, physical presence, a calm touch, and verbal praise whenever he is (a) quiet, (b) lying down in bed, and (c) calm. These brief visits can be gradually delayed from every few seconds to a maximum of every 15 minutes. Make sure you are out of the room when Ralph falls asleep so he learns to do so independently of your presence. Inappropriate behaviors (e.g., demanding, calling out from the bedroom) are, of course, to be ignored. Politely presented special requests (e.g., for a drink or extra hug) may be fulfilled at your discretion, but only when Ralph makes the request during a "strategic attention" visit earned by practicing appropriate bedtime behavior.*

The clinician can demonstrate the essential concepts of the EMD during an office visit. Once rapport is established with the child, the clinician politely says to the child: "Please show me how you can be a big girl and sit nicely in this chair." With parents observing, the clinician prompts the child into a chair (representing the bed) and provides enthusiastic labeled praise for sitting nicely. The clinician gradually moves across the room and out the door for a couple of seconds before returning to deliver another round of attention and labeled praise ("I love how you are sitting quietly in the chair, keeping your arms and legs still"). The office "drill" can be repeated two to three times, with the clinician closing the office door and remaining in the hallway for increasing intervals (typically from 30 seconds to 1 minute, depending upon the child's age and attention span), before returning to praise the child.

Create a Back-up Plan for Leaving the Bedroom

The effectiveness of even carefully crafted reinforcement programs may be limited without the inclusion of EXT as a part of the treatment package [9,13]. Implementing EXT for problem bedtime behavior, however, becomes a major challenge when children exit the bedroom to enter the living area. This behavior is not uncommon during the introduction of the EMD, before the child has come into contact with the new reinforcement contingency. If the child comes out of the bedroom, the parent immediately returns him or her to the bedroom, saying briefly "it is bedtime" or "get back in bed," while minimizing eye contact and attention. Upon returning the child to the bedroom, he or she is given one warning: "If you come out of the bedroom again I will have to close your door." Before securing children in a room, parents first must make sure to prepare the room by removing breakable items or furniture (mirrors, unsecured dressers) that might result in harm to the child during a tantrum or destructive behavior. If parents are not comfortable closing and securing the child's bedroom door, other options may be used to secure the child in the room, such as installing a mesh security gate at the threshold of the bedroom. Once secured, the parent remains quietly in the hallway, ignoring inappropriate behavior, until the child demonstrates self-calming skills. Upon 3–5 seconds of quiet behavior, the parent immediately opens the door or removes the gate, enters the room, and if necessary places the child back in bed. The EMD is re-initiated, and this cycle is repeated until the child falls asleep independently.

POSSIBLE MODIFICATIONS/VARIANTS

Clinicians are *encouraged* to modify and derive creative alterations to this protocol in order to account for differences in clinical presentation and individual treatment goals. Sample modifications that may be employed include the following:

- For children with high-rate disruptive behavior, it may be advisable to first address child compliance through an empirically based behavioral parent training program such as Parent–Child Interaction Therapy [16].
- If considerable child resistance with the EMD is anticipated at bedtime, the procedure can be practiced first during the day using short homework sessions. The session would not terminate with child sleep initiation; rather, following a set number of successful repetitions. Tangible rewards can be added for successful homework completion.
- To start with, parents and clinicians can decide whether to implement the EMD during bedtime only or throughout the entire night (e.g., sleep re-initiation). With overwhelmed or sleep-deprived families, clinicians may advise parents to initially focus just on bedtime skills until improvement is noted. If needed, parents can later institute the EMD to promote independent sleep initiation following night-time awakenings, and finally during naptimes. The introduction of EMD across conditions could be paired with a signal (stimulus) to make it clear to the child the EMD is now in place.

  Recommendation: *For now, please handle middle-of-the-night awakenings as you normally have in the past and simply document them on the sleep diary. If needed, we will directly address these awakenings once Arthur is falling to sleep quickly and independently at bedtime.*

- Consider combining the EMD with other effective interventions (e.g., the Sleep Fairy book [17]). Delayed delivery of tangibles rarely competes with the immediacy and saliency of parental presence and co-sleeping. However, using tangibles concurrently with the EMD, or introducing tangibles as children develop increased independent sleep skills, may help overcome road-blocks and maintain long-term progress. Incorporating the bedtime pass (see Chapter 30 of this book) with the EMD can be extremely helpful for older children with anxiety or separation issues.

- In addition to targeting independent sleep skills and problematic bedtime behavior, the EMD can be helpful in reducing or eliminating undesirable co-sleeping for parents who prefer solitary sleeping arrangements. The EMD can also be incorporated into graduated exposure trials for children with mild night-time anxiety, by fading parental presence and reinforcing coping skills and brave bedtime behavior.

Finally, clinicians must be prepared to help parents identify common pitfalls that interfere with the success of the EMD. Although not an exhaustive list by any means, some of these problems may include:

- Failure to monitor and maintain a consistent sleep–wake schedule during the early phases of the EMD;
- Parents who are reluctant to make *any* changes once they experience success, such as fading the bedtime earlier to ensure the child is obtaining sufficient sleep;
- Failure to eliminate long-distance interactions with the child (communicating with the child from the living room);
- Fading parent checks too quickly and falling back into the previous habit of responding to misbehavior;
- Running the EMD but failing to ensure the parent is out of the bedroom when the child initiates sleep.

PROOF OF CONCEPT/SUPPORTING DATA/EVIDENCE BASE

At this time there are no controlled, large group studies demonstrating the efficacy of the EMD with sleep-disturbed children. The EMD has been described in a couple of uncontrolled, small "n" conference presentations [18,19], and it is currently being evaluated in two pilot studies. Anecdotally, the EMD has been used extensively (within the context of other clinical procedures described in this chapter) in a pediatric sleep clinic for nearly 15 years, generally with positive outcomes and widespread parent approval. Empirically based clinicians may derive more comfort, however, in knowing that the EMD simply represents the clinical application of proven, fundamental principles of behavior. Numerous intervention studies have used various forms of reinforcement and EXT to effectively address commonly occurring as well as novel behavior problems in both children and adults. There is solid evidence that problem behavior responds more readily, with fewer side effects, when EXT and reinforcement are combined, versus using either as the sole intervention component (see, for example, Petscher and Bailey [12], Lerman and Iwata [13], Grow et al. [20] and Waters et al. [21]).

REFERENCES

[1] American Academy of Sleep Medicine (AASM), The International Classification of Sleep Disorders, Diagnostic and Coding Manual, second ed., American Academy of Sleep Medicine, Westchester, IL, 2005.

[2] W.K. Silverman, A. Dick-Niederhauser, Separation anxiety disorder, in: T.L. Morris, J.S. March, (Eds.), Anxiety Disorders in Children and Adolescents, second ed., Guilford Press, New York, NY, 2004, pp. 164–188.

[3] T.F. Anders, M.A. Keener, Developmental course of nighttime sleep–wake patterns in full-term and premature infants during the first year of life: I, Sleep 8 (1985) 173–192.

[4] M.M. Burnham, B.L. Goodlin-Jones, E.E. Gaylor, T.F. Anders, Nighttime sleep–wake patterns and self-soothing from birth to one year of age: a longitudinal intervention study, J. Child Psychol. Psychiatry 43 (2002) 713–725.

[5] W. Anuntaseree, L. Mo-Suwan, P. Vasiknanonte, S. Kuasirikul, A. Ma-A. Lee, C. Choprapawan, Night waking in Thai infants at 3 months of age: Association between parental practices and infant sleep, Sleep Med. 9 (2008) 564–571.

[6] D. Fehlings, Frequent night awakenings in infants and preschool children referred to a sleep disorders clinic: the role of non-adaptive sleep associations, Child Health Care 30 (2001) 43–55.

[7] B.L. Goodlin-Jones, M.M. Burnham, E.E. Gaylor, T.F. Anders, Night waking, sleep–wake organization, and self-soothing in the first year of life, J. Dev. Behav. Pediatr. 22 (2001) 226–233.

[8] J.A. Mindell, B. Kuhn, D.S. Lewin, L.J. Meltzer, A. Sadeh, Behavioral treatment of bedtime problems and night wakings in infants and young children, Sleep 29 (2006) 1263–1276.

[9] B.A. Iwata, G.M. Pace, G.E. Cowdery, R.G. Miltenberger, What makes extinction work? An analysis of procedural form and function, J. Appl. Behav. Anal. 27 (1994) 131–144.

[10] T.M. Reimers, D. Wacker, L.J. Cooper, Evaluation of the acceptability of treatments for children's behavioral difficulties: Ratings by parents receiving services in an outpatient clinic, Child Fam. Behav. Ther. 13 (1991) 53–71.

[11] D.C. Lerman, B.A. Iwata, M.D. Wallace, Side effects of extinction: prevalence of bursting and aggression during the treatment of self-injurious behavior, J. Appl. Behav. Anal. 32 (1999) 1–8.

[12] E.S. Petscher, J.S. Bailey, Comparing main and collateral effects of extinction and differential reinforcement of alternative behavior, Behav. Modif. 32 (2008) 468–488.

[13] D.C. Lerman, B.A. Iwata, Developing a technology for the use of operant extinction in clinical settings: an examination of basic and applied research, J. Appl. Behav. Anal. 29 (1996) 345–382 discussion 383–385.

[14] B.F. Skinner, The Behavior of Organisms, Appleton-Century-Crofts, New York, NY, 1938.

[15] B.R. Kuhn, Sleep disorders, in: M. Hersen, J.C. Thomas (Eds.), Handbook of Clinical Interviewing with Children, Sage Publications, New York, NY, 2007, pp. 420–447.

[16] C.B. McNeil, T.L. Hembree-Kigin, (Eds.), Parent–Child Interaction Therapy, second ed., Springer, New York, NY, 2010.

[17] R.V. Burke, B.R. Kuhn, J.L. Peterson, Brief report: A "storybook" ending to children's bedtime problems – the use of a rewarding social story to reduce bedtime resistance and frequent night waking, J. Pediatr. Psychol. 29 (2004) 389–396.

[18] C.T. Yancey, B.R. Kuhn, My child won't sleep!!: Using the excuse-me drill to increase bedtime compliance and self-initiated sleep onset, presented at: Annual Munroe-Meyer Interdisciplinary Poster Session; 2006, April; Omaha, NE.

[19] B.R. Kuhn, M.T. Floress, T.C. Newcomb, Strategic attention for children's sleep-compatible behaviors: Treatment outcome and acceptability of the "excuse-me drill", presented at: Association for Behavioral and Cognitive Therapies. Orlando, FL, Nov., 2008.

[20] L.L. Grow, M.E. Kelley, H.S. Roane, M.A. Shillingsburg, Utility of extinction-induced response variability for the selection of mands, J. Appl. Behav. Anal. 41 (2008) 15–24.

[21] M.B. Waters, D.C. Lerman, A.N. Hovanetz, Separate and combined effects of visual schedules and extinction plus differential reinforcement on problem behavior occasioned by transitions, J. Appl. Behav. Anal. 42 (2009) 309–313.

RECOMMENDED READING

J. Bailey, M. Burch, How to Think Like a Behavior Analyst, Lawrence Erlbaum, Mahwah, NJ, 2006.

K.G. France, N.M. Blampied, Infant sleep disturbance: description of a problem behaviour process, Sleep. Med. Rev. 3 (1999) 265–280.

J.A. Mindell, J.A. Owens, A Clinical Guide to Pediatric Sleep: Diagnosis and Management of Sleep Problems, second ed., Lippincott Williams & Wilkins, Philadelphia, PA, 2010.

The Journal of Applied Behavior Analysis routinely publishes studies on the clinical application of fundamental principles of behavior-change.

Chapter 32

Day Correction of Pediatric Bedtime Problems

Edward R. Christophersen
University of Missouri at Kansas City School of Medicine and Staff Psychologist, Children's Mercy Hospital and Clinics, Kansas, MO

Kathryn Harnett McConahay
Pediatric Associates, Kansas City, MO

PROTOCOL NAME

Day correction of pediatric bedtime resistance.

GROSS INDICATION

Although ignoring tantrums/fussing is perhaps the most effective procedure for children who resist going to bed, many parents report that they "cannot stand to ignore the pleas of their children at bedtime". Day correction of bedtime problems encourages parents to begin ignoring their child's inappropriate behavior earlier in the day, when presumably the parents have more stamina or willpower, and can experience success with the procedure under less trying circumstances than bedtime.

SPECIFIC INDICATION

In order for children to be able to fall asleep on their own, either at bedtime or after a night waking, they must be able to calm themselves enough that they are able to fall asleep. The day correction of bedtime problems procedures facilitates the acquisition of these self-calming procedures during the day, when many more opportunities exist for such learning to occur under much better conditions.

CONTRAINDICATIONS

We have encountered parents in our clinic who are absolutely adverse to hearing their child exhibit distress of any kind. In those cases where a child lacks good self-quieting skills, procedures such as ignoring and its many variations

Behavioral Treatments for Sleep Disorders. DOI: 10.1016/B978-0-12-381522-4.00032-8

may be doomed to fail since they require that the child exhibits a skill that is either not in his or her repertoire, or that may be present but is not evidenced in the presence of a parent.

RATIONALE FOR INTERVENTION

One of the most common concerns that parents of young children have is that they cannot get their children to bed at night, or their children wake up in the middle of the night and cannot get back to sleep by themselves. The vast majority of the time, these problems stem from the fact that such children do not have self-quieting skills. Self-quieting skills refer to children's ability to quiet themselves when they begin to get upset about something. Most of the time, children with bedtime problems have had help or assistance from their parents in quieting at bedtime. This help may consist of nursing the child to sleep, rocking the child to sleep, lying down with the child, or allowing the child to drift off to sleep in the parents' bed. The day correction method targets critical skills that are needed by young children during the day and night. Once children have developed self-quieting skills during the day, and have had at least 1 week to practice these skills, they can usually learn to self-quiet at night within 3–4 nights [1].

Building self-quieting skills appears to be crucial in an infant's development, because the skills teach a baby to adapt to his environment. As Brazelton (p. xi) said, "the job for parents is to learn the fine line between when to intervene and when to leave the baby alone to find his own competent behavioral pattern of self-calming." [2]. The beauty of the day correction procedures [1] is that we are able to demonstrate them during an office visit, and observe both the parent and the child's reaction to them. If, after the office demonstration, it is apparent that the parent(s) will not be able to follow through with the procedures, then one of many alternatives can be offered to the parent(s), such as the other bedtime protocols described in this book.

STEP BY STEP DESCRIPTION OF PROCEDURES

Encouraging the Development of Self-Calming Skills

Although the disciplinary procedure referred to as "time-out" has been around for almost 50 years, many parents have found that, in their words, "it doesn't work". One reason that we believe that it doesn't work is that parents are using time-out to coerce or force their children to stop engaging in behavior that the parents don't like or don't want to see continued. The reason that many children "misbehave" is that they don't have the skills for dealing with situations that they don't like; they don't have the skills for self-quieting, or, as it applies to adults, "coping skills". We sometimes see this referred to as "anger control skills", and these children are often said to have "bad tempers", to be "strong willed", or to be "difficult children". Many parents, with the best of intentions, will put a great deal of effort into trying to convince their children, using lecturing, explanations, and reasoning, into behaving differently. When this fails, they move into what we refer to as their "coercive mode" – that is, they are going to get the child to behave the way they want the child to behave, no matter what it takes. This often leads to direct confrontations that are unpleasant for both parent and child, and usually accomplish nothing beneficial. And, during this process, the parents are unwittingly making the situation worse by modeling coercive behavior for their child.

In order to educate parents about the importance of shifting their focus from coercion to teaching, we are now recommending that parents begin giving their children the opportunity to learn "self-quieting skills". There are several major components to teaching these skills:

1. Reduce nagging, lecturing, threatening, and warnings as much as possible – preferably eliminate them completely.
2. Provide the child with a great deal of brief, non-verbal, physical contact – usually, we recommend 100 brief physical touches a day in addition to normal caregiving activities. These touches are not meant to be rewards; rather, they are meant to let the child know, non-verbally, that he or she is loved. The reason for insisting that such contact be "non-verbal" is our experience that talking to children when they are engaged in a task often disrupts them enough that they never complete the task.
3. Use brief, non-emotional "chill-outs". This is usually in the form of "chill-out interrupting". For example, if the parents have been providing the child with a lot of brief, non-verbal physical contact when the child wasn't bothering them, then when the child does interrupt the parent, all the parent needs to say is "chill out interrupting". Then, it's extremely important that the parent ignores the child until he or she is quiet, or has regained his or her composure. During these "chill-outs", the parent should refrain from all warnings, nagging, and reminders of what the child did or did not do. Basically, the parent should strive to completely ignore the child during a chill-out, until the child has calmed down. During the chill-out period, the child does not exist. No eye contact. For chill-out to end, the child must calm him- or herself down or gain control for 2–3 seconds, or turn 18 years old – whichever comes first. The child may call his or her parents names, strike them, or have a tantrum on the floor, but until the child calms down he or she does not exist. At first this will not be easy for most parents to do; that's why we typically demonstrate these procedures during an office visit. Most parents have never seen the "other side of a tantrum". After most children do self-calm, they are typically quite pleasant and cooperative, even cuddly. But because so many parents give in to tantrums, either by giving their child what the child wants or assisting the child in calming down, they never get to see how their child behaves after self-calming.

While the parent is ignoring the child, the child (1) needs to be able to see his or her parent, (2) see that the parent is not upset, and (3) see what the child is missing out on. When demonstrating these procedures during an office visit, we will engage the parent in a conversation of mutual interest that has nothing to do with the child's behavior, often having to do with the parent's vocation, vacation, or something remarkable going on in their lives.

Remember, we are giving the child multiple opportunities to learn self-control – a skill that will be used throughout life. After the child gains control, or calms down for just 2–3 seconds, we prompt the parent to resume time-in. We remind the parent that there is no need to remind the child what he or she did prior to the chill-out, or to discuss the chill-out. Even if it takes an individual child a couple of days or a week to learn how to calm him- or herself down, having this skill can help to make the household a much more pleasant place to live. Over time, the child's time to chill-out should gradually be extended from the original 2–3 seconds up to about 30 seconds. This process typically takes place over a period of a week or two.

POSSIBLE MODIFICATIONS/VARIANTS

When we see children who present with temper tantrums, and we have taken reasonable efforts to rule out developmental delays and reactive attachment disorder, we often elect to demonstrate for parents how to effectively NOT respond to temper tantrums – or, as it is often called in the literature, ignore the tantrum. This typically involves waiting (usually a short time) for something to happen that the child reacts to with a tantrum, then instructing the parents to ignore the tantrum while we filibuster by talking to the parents to distract them while they are attempting to ignore their child's fussing. Predictably, the children engage in the behaviors that have worked for them at home to get their parent to re-engage with them, allowing us to see, firsthand, what parental behaviors have been maintaining the tantrums at home. Christophersen (2003), available from the American Psychological Association, is a videotape/DVD demonstration of these procedures [3]. In this videotape, the author demonstrates with a young mother the process of ignoring her toddler's protests during a tantrum until he self-calms and then she is immediately prompted to pay attention to him again. Such a process provides the parents with the confidence that the procedures will work as described because they have seen them work. A crucial part of this demonstration is that the child almost always calms down and starts to engage in some play behavior, whereupon we prompt the parent to resume paying attention to the child; this allows us to point out that there is "no residual effect". Not only are the children not mad at their parents for ignoring them; they are typically more affectionate than they were prior to the tantrum. Often, this is the first time the parents have seen the child stop a tantrum by him- or herself, and, more importantly, the first time they have seen that the tantrum did not harm their child. This can be empowering to parents who believed all along that their child wasn't capable of stopping his or her own tantrum. We have used this office demonstration with a wide variety of populations, including children referred for management of general behavior problems secondary to being born with cardiac problems (e.g., transposition of the great vessels) that mandated, at least until surgery had successfully corrected their congenital condition, that parents attend to their every whim so that they did not cry unnecessarily. In these situations, our experience has been that the tantrums are always brief, probably owing to the child's getting exhausted very quickly and thereby losing the drive to continue with the tantrum.

In addition to working to encourage the development of self-calming skills during the day, we incorporate some pretty standard procedures from the sleep literature, including:

1. Instruct parents to wake the child up at about the same time every morning. Be sure that the parent gets the child up while he or she is still playing quietly, instead of waiting until the child is crying.
2. The child should be put to bed at about the same time every night, alone, awake, and tired.
3. Parents should ensure the child has his or her meals at about the same time every day.
4. Parents should ensure that the child gets vigorous exercise every day.
5. Encourage parents to use time-out during the day for most misbehavior. Time-out should not be over until the child has self-quieted. Make sure that the parents are not avoiding any opportunities to use time-out. Every time-out helps with self-quieting skills.
6. Encourage parents to adopt a bedtime routine for the last 30 minutes before bedtime that is quieting to the child, and to follow a similar routine every night. It's best to not vary from the routine until good bedtime habits are well established.
7. Parents should use time-in during the day whenever their child is engaged in an activity that they consider acceptable.
8. Instruct parents to place several soft toys in their child's bed that can ultimately be used as "transition objects".
9. If parents do feel the need to check their child during the night, suggest that they refrain from talking to the child or turning on the light, and refrain from picking the child up or tucking the child in again.

When children who are referred for sleep issues present with significant behavior problems, a clinical decision must be made, based upon adequate assessment of the sleep issues as well as the behavioral issues, about the role that the sleep issues play. In many instances, addressing the sleep issues first can help with the resolution of the behavioral issues, and in some cases working on the behavioral issues first can help with the resolution of the sleep issues.

PROOF OF CONCEPT/SUPPORTING DATA/EVIDENCE BASE

Edwards and Christophersen [4] reviewed some of the published studies on ignoring as a treatment procedure, pointing out that although extinction was the most effective procedure in the behavioral treatment literature, many parents reported that they could not do it or chose to not do it. Edwards [5] was the first to provided reliable preliminary data (using time-lapse videotape recordings [6]) to suggest that parents can be instructed to encourage the development of sleep-onset skills by setting occasions for their child to learn self-quieting skills during the day. Similarly, Harnett [7], using a multiple baseline design across six young children, showed a rapid decrease in the amount of child protest and parental attention to the child at bedtime. The six children averaged protests during 48 percent of the intervals during baseline (with a range from 0 to 76 percent). The next condition, Extinction with Clinician Assistance, decreased these percentages to a mean of 30 percent. Subsequent Parent Implementation without Clinical Assistance, over the next 4 days increased this slightly to an average of 32 percent. In the follow-up condition, child protests continued at a low rate of 21 percent with a range from 0 to 24 percent. These findings were maintained at 1-month follow-up for five of the six families. Social validation measures showed that parents were very satisfied with all components of the treatment package, and would recommend this intervention to a friend with a similar problem.

ACKNOWLEDGMENT

Preparation of this protocol was supported, in part, by a grant from the Katherine B. Richardson Associates Fund, Children's Mercy Hospitals and Clinics.

REFERENCES

[1] E.R. Christophersen, Beyond Discipline: Parenting that Lasts a Lifetime, second ed., Overland Press, Shawnee Mission, KS, 1998.

[2] T.B. Brazelton, Foreword, in Sammons WA, The Self-Calmed Baby: A Revolutionary New Approach to Parenting Your Infant, Little Brown & Co., Boston, MA, 1989.

[3] E.R. Christophersen, Parenting Young Children, Part of the Relationships. APA Psychotherapy Video Series, APA, Washington, DC, 2003.

[4] K.J. Edwards, E.R. Christophersen, Automated data acquisition through time-lapse videotape recording, J. Appl. Behav. Anal. 26 (1993) 503–504.

[5] K.J. Edwards, The use of brief time-outs during the day to reduce bedtime struggles, Diss. Abstr. Int. 54 (1993) 2181.

[6] K.J. Edwards, E.R. Christophersen, Treating common sleep problems of young children, J. Dev. Behav. Pediatr. 15 (1994) 207–213.

[7] K.J. Harnett, An analysis of daytime and bedtime interventions for sleep-onset problems, Diss. Abstr. Int. (1994) 53.

RECOMMENDED READING

E.R. Christophersen, S.L. Mortweet, Treatments that Work with Children: Empirically Supported Strategies for Managing Childhood Problems, APA Books, Washington, DC, 2001.

E.R. Christophersen, S.L. Mortweet, Parenting that Works: Building Skills that Last a Lifetime, APA Books, Washington, DC, 2003 (translated into Italian, Korean, and Icelandic).

J.A. Mindell, J.A. Owens, A Clinical Guide to Pediatric Sleep: Diagnosis and Management of Sleep Problems, Lippincott, Williams & Wilkins, Philadelphia, PA, 2003.

S.L. Mortweet, E.R. Christophersen, Coping skills for the angry/impatient/clamorous child: a home and office practicum, Contemp. Pediatr. 21 (2004) 43–55.

Chapter 33

Graduated Exposure Games to Reduce Children's Fear of the Dark

William L. Mikulas
Department of Psychology, University of West Florida, Pensacola, FL

PROTOCOL NAME

Graduated exposure games to reduce children's fear of the dark.

GROSS INDICATION

This intervention is indicated for children with fear of the dark.

SPECIFIC INDICATION

The games are particularly useful for darkness fear in children approximately 4–10 years old. This fear may manifest in many ways, including statements about being afraid, crying at night-time, clinging to parents in dark situations, trembling when in or approaching dark situations, having tantrums at bedtime, refusing to sleep in a bedroom alone, insisting on a parent staying in room until the child is asleep, insisting on lights being on, having restless nights, and frightened calling out to parents.

CONTRAINDICATIONS

Fear of the dark needs to be assessed within the context of other behavior problems and the dynamics of the family. Other behaviors may need to be treated first or in conjunction, including:

- stress that accentuates fears;
- resistance to going to bed;
- attention-seeking and related reinforcement;
- sleep disorders;
- night terrors.

Behavioral Treatments for Sleep Disorders. DOI: 10.1016/B978-0-12-381522-4.00033-X

RATIONALE FOR INTERVENTION

Fear of the dark is the most common fear in children aged 4–7 years. It is often confounded with going to bed, time to get to sleep, calling to parents, and/or getting into the parents' bed. These often lead to child–parent problems and family stress. Parents' frustration and anger may lead to other problems, including child abuse [1].

Exposure therapy is now a well-established successful behavioral therapy for anxiety disorders, particularly simple and/or social fears [2–4]. The reduction of affect is due to respondent conditioning, but, in addition, "exposure therapy" usually includes operant and modeling components. We have explicitly dealt with all these components in our games, instructions to the parents, and storybook (discussed below).

The proposed treatment is carried out by the parents in the home, which generally makes the treatment more effective and much less expensive than treatment by a professional in a clinic. The treatment program is also a powerful way to teach parents basic behavioral parenting skills that they can apply in many situations. This includes the use of reinforcement, shaping, modeling, and games. The treatment is brief and fun (which is very important with children), as opposed, for example, to desensitization components of progressive muscle relaxation and imagined scenes, which many children find difficult and boring.

The intervention can potentially catch the fear early when it is easier to treat, because parents might wait longer until the fear-related problems get worse before considering professional therapy. The children learn basic self-control skills they can apply in many situations, and this, coupled with their self-mastery of the fear of the dark, is a powerful way to increase their overall self-concept, self-esteem, self-efficacy, and internal locus of control [5].

STEP BY STEP DESCRIPTION OF PROCEDURES

The exposure consists of a sequence of games, most of which involve gradually spending more and more time in the dark. Since parents coordinate and perhaps model these games, the first step is instructing the parents. We use written instructions, but it could also be done in person, individually or in a group. Instructions and education include the nature of fear of the dark, rationale for the treatment, and general related advice, such as avoiding scary movies and television, particularly before bedtime. Behavioral instructions include the use of reinforcement (e.g., praise, smiles, hugs, tangible reinforcers), the logic of shaping (e.g., gradually increasing time in the dark), and how to adapt the materials to the child's needs and interests. Weekly phone calls at a preset time and/or e-mails between parent and professional are important to stay in contact, answer questions, and provide support. In some cases, parents are instructed in how to keep various types of records related to the program. This might be done for research, to demonstrate change, to check on the children's and parents' progress, and/or to encourage and monitor shaping. One measure is based on the child's approach/avoidance to dark situations that are fearful to that child – for example, how close will a child come to going into a dark room, or how long will the child stay in the dark room before needing to come out? This could be coupled with the child's self-report of fear on a five-point scale.

Great individual differences in the specifics and intensity of fear of the dark require that parents adapt choice and frequency of games to their children. Shaping is continually emphasized. Ask if the child thinks he or she can play the game. Encourage, but do not force. If the child is not ready, break the game into smaller steps or skip the game. As a general rule, stay with the game as long as the child is interested and progressing. Move on when the child is ready, but freely return to previous games.

Next is the sequence of games that we have used. Obviously, the games could be modified or replaced for children of different ages, interests, or cultures. The games should generally be played in order, but the child does not have to master one before going on to the next.

- *Blindfold game.* The blindfolded child tries to find large pieces of furniture or an easily placed toy in his room. Parents are instructed in shaping (gradually making the toy harder to find) and reinforcement (e.g., hugs and praise).
- *Puppet game.* The child learns to relax by tensing and relaxing muscles in the order of arms, hands, legs, and neck. The image is one of a marionette who tenses up when strings are pulled and then relaxes when the strings are released.
- *Toy-in-the-room game.* The child goes into a dark room to get a toy from a designated place. Shaping and reinforcement are again emphasized, as in the blindfold game.
- *Animal friends game.* In a dark room, the child guesses the animal who would make the animal sound that a parent makes from another room. It is suggested that parents begin with easily identified sounds and not make scary sounds. Shaping is accomplished by lengthening the time the child lies in the dark waiting for the next sound.
- *Animals-on-the-wall game.* Parents are shown how to make hand shadows of a goose, dog, bird, and camel. In the child's darkened bedroom, parent and child make various shadows on the wall in the beam of a flashlight. Scary shadows are discouraged.
- *Toy-in-the-dark-game.* This is similar to the toy-in-the-room game, except the child is not told where in the dark room the toy will be. Shaping and reinforcement are again stressed.
- *Flip-the-switch game.* When a parent yells "Go!" from an adjacent room, the child in the bedroom gets up from the floor, turns off light, and goes to lie in bed before the parent arrives to turn light back on. Shaping includes how long the child stays in the dark until the light goes back on.

- *Find-the-noisy-box game*. The game begins in a totally dark house, with the child lying in his or her bed. A parent in another room shakes a cereal box. The child finds the parent by going through the dark house turning on light switches. Shaping occurs through increasing the difficulty of finding the parent, and lengthening the time the parent waits before shaking the box.
- *Puppet game*. This relaxation exercise is now expanded to include arms, legs, face, forehead, neck and shoulder, stomach, and toes.

POSSIBLE MODIFICATIONS/VARIATIONS

For the purpose of this chapter the games are presented as a separate and effective treatment, but in our complete program the games are embedded in a storybook called *Uncle Lightfoot* (see "Recommended Reading", below). The story tells of Michael, a young boy with a fear of the dark, who goes to visit his "Uncle" Lightfoot, an Indian living in the country. Throughout the fun adventures of the story, Lightfoot plays various related games with Michael – the games described above. Through the games, Michael overcomes his fear and is proud of his new skills. Children greatly enjoy the story, and almost always want to have it re-read to them.

Michael is a coping model who overcomes his fears, is pleased with his accomplishments, and is rewarded by others. Thus, a modeling component to reduce fears is added to the exposure-based games. Most of the children who hear the story want to play the games that Michael played. In addition, seeing where the games lead in a positive context can help reduce resistance that some fearful children or parents may have about exposure treatments. Relative to shaping and use of hierarchies, as the story progresses situations are more and more potentially anxiety-producing, and they become more difficult and involve more encounters with the dark. The book and games have gone through many revisions, based on research and feedback from parents.

Instructions to parents include use of the book and games. The book should be read at night, as much or little as is appropriate and desired. One approach is to allow the child to play the games immediately as the story is being read to the child. Another approach is to read the book through several times before playing any of the games. Choice of approach may include such factors as severity of the fear and individual child preferences.

PROOF OF CONCEPT/SUPPORTING DATA

Research on earlier versions of the materials found them to be effective, fun, and inexpensive [6,7]. There were many very dramatic cases of behavior change. Combining all subjects, there were statistically significant changes due to the treatments – changes that were significantly different than for control subjects, such as a parental attention control group. Research by others on earlier versions of the materials found the book plus games to be significantly effective, with improvement slightly increased at a 12-month follow-up [8].

REFERENCES

[1] B. Johnson, H. Moore, Injured children and their parents, Children 15 (1968) 147–152.
[2] D.H. Barlow, L.B. Allen, M.L. Choate, Toward a unified treatment for emotional disorders, Behav. Ther. 35 (2004) 205–230.
[3] R.J. McNally, Mechanisms of exposure therapy: How neuroscience can improve psychological treatments for anxiety disorders, Clin. Psychol. Rev. 27 (2007) 750–759.
[4] B.A. Thyer, M. Baum, L.D. Reid, Exposure techniques in the reduction of fear: a comparative review of the procedure in animals and humans, Adv. Behav. Res. Ther. 10 (1988) 105–127.
[5] W.L. Mikulas, The Integrative Helper: Convergence of Eastern and Western Traditions., Wadsworth, Pacific Grove, CA, 2002.
[6] W.L. Mikulas, M.F. Coffman, Home-based treatment of children's fear of the dark, in: CE Schaefer, JM Briesmeister (Eds.), Handbook of Parent Training, Wiley, New York, 1989, pp. 179–202.
[7] W.L. Mikulas, M.F. Coffmann, D. Dayton, et al., Behavioral bibliotherapy and games for treating fear of the dark, Child Fam. Behav. Ther. 7 (1985) 1–7.
[8] I. Santacruz, F.J. Mendez, J. Sanchez-Meca, Play therapy applied by parents for children with darkness phobia: comparison of two programmes, Child Fam. Behav. Ther. 28 (2006) 19–35.

RECOMMENDED READING

M.F. Coffman (2009). Uncle Lightfoot: Overcoming Fear of the Dark. footpathpress@yahoo.com.

Chapter 34

Scheduled Awakenings: A Behavioral Protocol for Treating Sleepwalking and Sleep Terrors in Children

Kelly Byars
Divisions of Pulmonary Medicine and Behavioral Medicine/Clinical Psychology, Cincinnati Children's Hospital Medical Center, Cincinnati, OH

PROTOCOL NAME

Scheduled awakenings: a behavioral protocol for treating sleepwalking and sleep terrors in children.

GROSS INDICATION

Scheduled Awakenings (SA) has demonstrated efficacy for treating young children with chronic and severe sleepwalking (SW) and sleep terrors (ST) [1–5].

SPECIFIC INDICATION

Most cases of SW and ST are benign, self-limited, and resolve spontaneously without the need for a targeted intervention such as SA [6–7]. SA is most appropriate when the following indications are present.

1. Patient has undergone a comprehensive clinical sleep evaluation confirming diagnosis [7].
2. Non-rapid eye movement (NREM) parasomnia is evidenced by the following:
   - ambulation or terror episode (crying/loud screaming in conjunction with autonomic nervous system and behavioral symptoms of extreme fear) occurs during sleep [8]
   - evidence of altered state of consciousness (e.g., difficult to arouse; mental confusion if awakened; complete or partial amnesia for episode, dangerous or potentially dangerous behaviors) [8].

Behavioral Treatments for Sleep Disorders. DOI: 10.1016/B978-0-12-381522-4.00034-1

3. Symptoms are chronic (persistence >3 months) [3,9].
4. Frequency of SW or ST episodes is severe (episodes occur almost nightly, or at least multiple times per week) [3,9].
5. SW or ST episodes occur at a highly predictable time each night [6,10].
6. Parent or primary caregiver present in the home is fully aware of the demands of the treatment protocol and is willing to implement the protocol consistently over a treatment interval of at least 1–4 weeks.

CONTRAINDICATIONS

There are no published data specifically stating when SA is contraindicated for treating SW or ST. However, in clinical settings it is likely that the intervention would not be appropriate or effective, and/or would be quite difficult to implement, in the following circumstances:

- when the patient has underlying primary sleep disorder (e.g., obstructive sleep apnea, periodic limb movement disorder);
- when episodes are infrequent (less than weekly);
- when the timing of events is unpredictable;
- when episodes could be easily managed using standard management practices (see Table 34.1) [6,7,11];
- when sleep deprivation is a significant clinical issue, and targeted intervention to increase total sleep time takes precedence over intervening specifically to treat SW or ST [4,5,10];
- when parent or primary caregiver is unable or unwilling to implement the protocol.

RATIONALE FOR INTERVENTION

There are three primary hypotheses regarding the underlying mechanism for scheduled awakenings in reducing or eliminating SW and ST. First, it has been proposed that repeated scheduled awakenings alter the child's sleep cycle in such a way that the altered underlying electrophysiology of partial arousal is either prevented or interrupted, and results in remission of the disturbing behavioral features of these events [1,2,4]. However, this proposed mechanism does not explain why partial arousal events do not return once SA is discontinued. Those in favor of this hypothesis have suggested that possibly the pathophysiology of NREM parasomnias is somehow corrected by repetitive awakening, and thus maintained even after SA is terminated.

An alternative hypothesis suggests that the repetition of scheduled awakenings conditions the patient to spontaneously arouse (i.e., self-arousal) just prior to a parasomnia episode and thus avoids the event altogether despite the abnormal physiology [1]. A third possible mechanism has been proposed based on the increased susceptibility for partial arousal parasomnias in sleep-deprived

TABLE 34.1 Standard Management Practices for Uncomplicated Sleepwalking and Sleep Terrors [10,11,14]

Educate and reassure the child and family about sleepwalking and sleep terrors
- Common in children
- Benign condition
- Not suggestive of psychological disturbance
- Do not lead to psychological harm

Safety precautions to consider
- Lock all outside doors and windows
- Heavy curtains at windows
- Install security systems to signal if child attempts to leave home
- Install motion alarms/bells on bedroom door to signal if child leaves bedroom
- Discourage child from sleeping on top bunk
- Consider moving mattress to floor
- Remove any obstructions from bedroom or objects on floor that might cause injury (e.g., toys on floor)

Sleep hygiene practices to promote optimal sleep and prevent/reduce likelihood of partial arousal events
- Age-appropriate sleep schedule to promote adequate sleep
- Consistent timing of sleep–wake cycle
- Minimize parental intervention during events as this may lead to increased agitation or prolonged episode
- Discuss potential triggers/exacerbating conditions (e.g., sleep deprivation, sleep in unfamiliar surroundings, illness)
- Attempt to avoid/minimize triggers/exacerbating conditions

individuals during rebound slow-wave sleep [4,5]. Two similar intervention studies documented unexpected and unexplained increases in the total sleep time of patients treated with scheduled awakenings. Based on this unanticipated finding, it was suggested that the efficacy of SA may simply have been due to increased total sleep time and a related reduction in the density of slow-wave sleep [4,5].

STEP BY STEP DESCRIPTION OF PROCEDURES

To date there has been limited published guidance regarding implementation of the procedures that constitute SA [12,13]. Integration of data from the published protocols [1–5] yields the following specific procedural variables that vary considerably across studies: (1) length of baseline assessment, (2) timing of awakenings, (3) method and duration of waking, (4) duration of treatment, and (5) rate of treatment tapering [12,13]. The implementation of SA generally follows three phases of treatment (see Table 34.2). While it is possible that a particular version of the treatment protocol has greater clinical utility, the current published literature does not definitively support one variation over the

TABLE 34.2 Treatment (Tx) Phases of Scheduled Awakenings Protocol

Phase of Treatment	Specific Focus of Tx
I. Baseline monitoring/Tx planning	Clinical assessment, training in sleep monitoring, sleep diary assessment, develop treatment plan
II. Active Tx	Implement Tx, continue sleep diary assessment, adjust Tx as clinically indicated
III. Tx tapering/termination	Continue sleep diary assessment, decrease frequency of Tx based on frequency of events

other. In order to best guide clinicians interested in using SA to treat SW and ST, the step by step procedures delineated below are a synthesis of all of the published studies. In clinical practice, it is advised that the treating clinician work with the caregiver implementing the treatment to establish concrete steps for implementation that are realistic for the family. This is best achieved by sitting down with the family before treatment is initiated and discussing the treatment plan. The clinician should assess whether or not the caregiver is comfortable with the plan, and confident he or she can implement the protocol.

Baseline Monitoring/Treatment Planning

It is important to note that typically children do not present to a clinician with a formal diagnosis, but with a clinical complaint or problem [7]. Thus it is critical that a child be formally evaluated before treatment is initiated. Detailed discussion of the assessment procedures required for making a clinical diagnosis of partial arousal parasomnia are beyond the scope of this chapter. In brief, the formal sleep evaluation should include a comprehensive sleep history [7], and polysomnography or EEG if nocturnal seizures are suspected. Ruling out an underlying primary sleep disorder (e.g., obstructive sleep apnea, periodic limb movement disorder) is essential. There are resources available that can guide the reader regarding the clinical assessment of sleep disorders [7,11,14,15]. Once a clinical diagnosis of SW or ST is confirmed, a detailed baseline assessment is required before implementing treatment.

Observing and documenting the timing and frequency of partial arousal events is critical to the success of SA. Thus, a parent or caregiver must closely monitor and document the child's sleep using a sleep diary (see Table 34.3). The sleep diary should be maintained on consecutive nights during a designated baseline period. Ideally, the baseline assessment should be completed in no less than 2 weeks.

Once the baseline sleep diary has been completed, the clinician and family should review the data together. If (as delineated in specific indications above) the partial arousal episodes are frequent (i.e., almost nightly) and occur

TABLE 34.3 Sleep Diary for Use with Scheduled Awakenings Protocol

Name: ______________________________

	Sunday	Monday	Tuesday	Wednesday	Thursday	Friday	Saturday
Date:							
1. Time child put to bed							
2. Time child fell asleep							
3. Time episode began							
4. Duration of episode							
5. Description of child behavior during episode							
6. Description of parent responses to child during episode							
7. Wake up time							
8. Nap timing and duration (minutes)							

at a very predictable time each night, then the following steps should be followed for developing a treatment plan and instructing the caregiver regarding implementation:

1. Use the sleep diary to determine the typical time of onset for partial arousal episodes.
2. Use the sleep diary to calculate the average latency from the time the child falls asleep until the time of onset of partial arousal episodes.
3. Use the two data points above to discern the pattern of onset of partial arousal events and to determine the optimal timing for scheduled awakenings.
4. Awaken the child 15–30 minutes prior to the estimated onset time for the partial arousal episode.
5. Continue to keep a sleep diary throughout treatment so that treatment progress can be monitored.

6. Waking the child can be accomplished by light touching or verbal prompting.
7. Once aroused (evidenced by verbalization and/or eyes opening), allow the child to return to sleep.
8. Continue SA every night during the first week of treatment.
9. If no episodes occur during the first week of treatment, begin treatment fading (see discussion of treatment fading below).
10. If the child has any episodes during the first week of treatment, continue nightly scheduled awakenings during the second week of treatment and subsequent weeks until the child goes for an entire week without any episodes, and then begin treatment fading (see discussion of treatment fading below).

Active Treatment

Although the above procedures appear very straightforward, the actual implementation may prove challenging in some cases. Treatment challenges should be anticipated and discussed prior to recommending this treatment so that families are aware of treatment demands, and so that problems can be effectively managed when they occur. Research reports and anecdotal evidence suggest that parents may find the intervention difficult to implement, particularly if the intervention is applied at a time after the parent has already gone to sleep. This being the case, families may be eager to terminate the intervention as soon as they perceive improvement. Because there is no definitive length of treatment supported in the literature, treatment duration is managed based on the child's response to treatment. It is recommended that clinicians advise parents to view treatment in weekly increments, and that decisions regarding modifying or terminating treatment should be made on a week-to-week basis. Because treatment response can be very quick, weekly consultation between family and clinician during treatment is recommended.

There may be situations when the scheduled awakening triggers a partial arousal episode or results in the child becoming fully alert and remaining awake for a prolonged period. If this occurs on several consecutive nights, then the timing of the scheduled awakening should be advanced (i.e., moved earlier) by 15 minutes. Advancing the scheduled awakening time in a similar manner is also recommended if the child has a partial arousal episode before the scheduled awakening time. Delaying (i.e., moving later) the scheduled awakening time may be necessary in situations when partial arousal episodes do not resolve but occur at a later time during the night after treatment has been implemented.

Treatment Fading/Termination

There are no definitive guidelines for fading treatment based on the current empirical base. Of the five published treatment studies, only two dictated a fading schedule which was routinely accelerated by families (i.e., parents terminated therapy earlier than recommended). It is recommended that the treating clinician works closely with the family to dictate a fading schedule that is clinically appropriate and practical for the family to accomplish. An example of a fading schedule that is systematic and predictable is to start treatment fading after 7 consecutive nights without SW or ST, slowly reducing the number of scheduled awakenings per week by skipping a night during the week (complete awakenings on 6 out of 7 nights). During subsequent weeks, skip additional nights (1 per week – 5 of 7 nights, 4 of 7 nights, etc.) until scheduled awakenings have completely faded out [4]. Once scheduled awakenings have been completely discontinued, the treatment is completed. In the event that SW or ST reoccurs in the future, the protocol can be reinstituted.

POSSIBLE MODIFICATIONS/VARIANTS

A protocol using the same name ("scheduled awakenings") [16–19] has demonstrated efficacy for treating problematic night wakings in infants, toddlers, and preschoolers [12–13]. The protocol requires close monitoring of nocturnal awakenings. After a clear pattern of awakenings has been established, scheduled awakenings are implemented 15–30 minutes prior to the time that nocturnal awakenings are predicted to occur. After the child is awakened, parents are instructed to attend to the child's perceived needs (e.g., rocking, patting, feeding) until sleep is reinitiated. The time of the scheduled awakening is gradually delayed (i.e., moved later) so that continuous uninterrupted sleep is increased and frequency of spontaneous awakenings is reduced. SA is discontinued when the child is sleeping through the night.

PROOF OF CONCEPT/SUPPORTING DATA/EVIDENCE BASE

The efficacy of SA as a treatment for SW and ST has been demonstrated in young children (3–12 years of age) with parasomnias that were classified as severe (almost nightly occurrence) and chronic (persisting greater than 3 months). The evidence is limited to five published studies [1–5]. The first published reports were uncontrolled case reports that reported elimination of SW [2] and ST [1] after brief use (1 week or less) of SA. In each of these case reports, treated children had no reoccurrence of parasomnia at 1-year follow-up. More recently, three multiple baseline studies demonstrate the efficacy of SA for eliminating SW [3] and significantly reducing ST [4,5]. In each of these studies, parasomnias were eliminated or significantly reduced over long-term follow-up (6–12 months post-treatment). Based on established guidelines for rating psychological treatments using the weight of empirical evidence, SA is classified as a "*promising treatment*" for SW and ST [12].

REFERENCES

[1] B. Lask, Novel and non-toxic treatment for night terrors, Br. Med. J. 297 (1988) 6648.

[2] J.D. Tobin, Treatment of somnambulism with anticipatory awakening, J. Pediatr. 122 (1993) 426–427.

[3] N.C. Frank, A. Spirito, L. Stark, J. Owens-Stively, The use of scheduled awakenings to eliminate childhood sleepwalking, J. Pediatr. Psychol. 22 (1997) 345–353.

[4] V.M. Durand, J.A. Mindell, Behavioral intervention for childhood sleep terrors, Behav. Ther. 30 (1999) 705–715.

[5] V.M. Durand, Treating sleep terrors in children with autism, J. Posit. Behav. Interv. 4 (2002) 66–72.

[6] T. Mason, A.I. Pack, Pediatric parasomnias, Sleep 30 (2007) 141–151.

[7] G.M. Rosen, D.P. Kohen, M.W. Mahowald, Parasomnias, in: M.L. Perlis, K.L. Lichstein, (Eds.), Treating Sleep Disorders: Principles and Practice of Behavioral Sleep Medicine, John Wiley & Sons, Hoboken, NJ, 2003, pp. 393–414.

[8] The International Classification of Sleep Disorders, Diagnostic and Coding Manual, second ed., American Academy of Sleep Medicine, Westchester, IL, 2006.

[9] International Classification of Sleep Disorders, Diagnostic and Coding Manual, American Sleep Disorders Association, Rochester, MN, 1990.

[10] V.M. Durand, Sleep Better! A Guide to Improving the Sleep for Children with Special Needs, Paul H. Brookes, New York, NY, 1998.

[11] J.A. Mindell, J.A. Owens, A Clinical Guide to Pediatric Sleep: Diagnosis and Management of Sleep Problems, Lippincott Williams & Wilkins, Philadelphia, PA, 2003. 42–54.

[12] B.R. Kuhn, A.J. Elliot, Treatment efficacy in behavioral pediatric sleep medicine, J. Psychosom. Res. 54 (2003) 587–597.

[13] B.R. Kuhn, D. Weidinger, Interventions for infant and toddler sleep disturbance: a review, Child Family Behav. Ther. 22 (2000) 33–50.

[14] R. Ferber, Assessment of sleep disorders in the child, in: R. Ferber, M. Kryger, (Eds.), Principles and Practice of Sleep Medicine in the Child, W. B. Saunders Company, Philadelphia, PA, 1995, pp. 45–53.

[15] A. Sadeh, Clinical assessment of pediatric sleep disorders, in: M.L. Perlis, K.L. Lichstein, (Eds.), Treating Sleep Disorders: Principles and Practice of Behavioral Sleep Medicine, John Wiley & Sons, Hoboken, NJ, 2003, pp. 344–364.

[16] R.J. McGarr, M.F. Hovell, In search of the sand man: shaping an infant to sleep, Educ. Treat. Children 3 (1980) 173–182.

[17] C.M. Johnson, S. Bradley-Johnson, J.M. Stack, Decreasing the frequency of infants' nocturnal crying with the use of scheduled awakenings, Fam. Pract. Res. J. 1 (1981) 98–104.

[18] C.M. Johnson, M. Lerner, Amelioration of infant sleep disturbances: II. Effects of scheduled awakenings by compliant parents, Infant Ment. Health J. 6 (1985) 21–30.

[19] V.I. Rickert, C.M. Johnson, Reducing nocturnal awakening and crying episodes in infants and young children: a comparison between scheduled awakenings and systematic ignoring, Pediatrics 81 (1988) 203–212.

RECOMMENDED READING

V.M. Durand, Sleep Better! A Guide to Improving the Sleep for Children with Special Needs, Paul H. Brookes, New York, NY, 1998.

J.A. Mindell, Sleeping Through the Night: How Infants, Toddlers, and Their Parents Can Get a Good Night's Sleep, Harper Collins Publishers, New York, NY, 2005.

J.A. Mindell, J.A. Owens, A Clinical Guide to Pediatric Sleep: Diagnosis and Management of Sleep Problems, second ed., Lippincott Williams & Wilkins, Philadelphia, 2010.

Chapter 35

Imagery Rehearsal Therapy for Adolescents

Barry Krakow
Sleep & Human Health Institute, Maimonides Sleep Arts & Sciences, Ltd, Albuquerque, NM

PROTOCOL NAME

Imagery rehearsal therapy for adolescents.

GROSS INDICATION

Imagery Rehearsal Therapy (IRT) is indicated for treatment of chronic nightmares in adolescents, and for potential treatment of acute nightmares in adolescents. IRT is useful for various types of disturbing dreams, not necessarily those classically defined as nightmares, which nosologically include an awakening with a feeling of fear or anxiety. Repeatedly in research studies, it is clear that not all patients, adults or adolescents, awaken from their nightmares, which has thus promoted the term "bad dreams" or "disturbing dreams" for this subset. While there is some evidence that bad dreams and nightmares might reflect a difference in severity, we have found that IRT works well on both categories.

SPECIFIC INDICATION

There is reason to believe that chronic nightmares appear to be driven by a conditioning process – that is, they appear to function as a learned behavior, and IRT may be best suited for nightmares stemming from this process. However, this view is predicated on the fact that among trauma survivors who perceive their traumatic experiences as the sole precipitating cause or perpetuating influence on the problem there is less interest or willingness to attempt IRT, whereas among those who might report they are "tired of having nightmares" we see greater interest in attempting IRT. There are insufficient data to know whether the above information is simply an explanation of who will or who won't respond to IRT, or just who will or who won't attempt the use of IRT.

Among adolescents, the same dichotomous thinking holds as well. Most adolescents seeking treatment for nightmares suffer from other psychiatric

Behavioral Treatments for Sleep Disorders. DOI: 10.1016/B978-0-12-381522-4.00035-3

conditions, usually anxiety, depression, or PTSD. They may perceive nightmares as part of the psychiatric condition or they may be "tired of having nightmares", and wonder whether something else (e.g., IRT) can help them. Moreover, because adolescents are closer to childhood than adults, they tend to resonate with instructions regarding the use of imagery in the mind's eye, perhaps because they are not so far removed from the time when their imagination may have been used more regularly for make-believe and other fantasies common in younger children.

While there are few (perhaps only one) controlled studies on IRT in adolescents, there are increasing anecdotal reports of its use in children and adolescents, and increasing interest in nightmares in the same populations. From social networking, it is clear that parents have used the IRT technique in children as early as 18 months of age, so it is likely more studies and reports will be forthcoming on the use of IRT in a broad range of children and adolescent age groups.

CONTRAINDICATIONS

There is clear evidence that any imagery technique can lead to overstimulation in susceptible individuals – for example, PTSD patients. Thus, in PTSD patients with extremely severe nightmares as well as daytime imagery dysfunction in the form of flashbacks, daymares, or traumatic memories, caution is strongly advised when considering an IRT program of therapy. Other contraindications would include individuals who report a complete inability to access their imagery system. There is no evidence that IRT works for other parasomnias such as sleep terrors, REM behavior disorder, or hypnagogic hallucinations.

Among adolescents the same caveats hold, although, again because adolescents may be more in tune than adults with the concept and application of imagery, it is conceivable that more severe adolescent nightmare patients can be coached through an IRT program with a reasonable likelihood of success. However, it cannot be repeated often enough that the clinician must determine whether the co-morbid diagnosis (most often PTSD) is so severe that it must be the primary focus of therapy well before considering nightmare treatment.

RATIONALE FOR INTERVENTION

Nightmares are commonly viewed in children and adolescents as a maturational process that is unlikely to require treatment [1]. Scant attention is given to nightmares and nightmare treatments (for children or adolescents) in the medical, psychiatric, and psychological literature, not to mention the clinical setting [2]. Because of the conventional wisdom that nightmares in children and adolescents decrease with time, a nightmare disorder at this age is more likely diagnosed subsequent to severe psychosocial stress such as the death of a caregiver, divorce, sexual/physical abuse, or neglect [3]. Notwithstanding these views, there is a small body of research that indicates nightmares occur frequently in childhood and adolescence [4–7]. One study surveying a random sample of adolescents (mean age 17 years) demonstrated a prevalence of 6.8 percent for frequent nightmares [8]. Another study of 11- to 14-year-olds yielded a prevalence of 20 percent, although it did not employ random sampling methods [9]. This is consistent with a meta-analysis that indicates nightmare prevalence in children and adolescents is fairly high; rates ranged from a peak in early childhood of 42.2 percent at age 2.5 years, followed by a progressive descent toward adolescence with a final prevalence of 7.3 percent at age 16 years [10].

For nightmare chronicity in adults, 42 percent reported an onset before the age of 15 years and slightly more than one-half of adult chronic nightmare sufferers developed their problem before the age of 20 years. Thus, a substantial number of adolescents appear to suffer from chronic nightmares, and for many it appears likely that the problem persists into adulthood [10]. Morbidity associated with nightmares and related sleep disturbances in adolescence is not inconsequential. Manni and colleagues [11] divided a large sample of 17-year-old adolescents into two groups: poor sleepers (non-restorative sleep quality), and those who reported restorative sleep quality. They noted that nearly 50 percent of those in the poor-sleep group suffered from frequent nightmares, and of 15 dependent variables relating to sleep factors, nightmares attained the highest odds ratio at 62.1 (confidence interval 95%, 58.0–64.4) in their logistic regression model for predicting poor sleep.

Nightmares may also represent a specific marker for a history of sexual trauma in abused children and adolescents [12].

Despite this potentially high prevalence of nightmares and their impact on sleep, there has been only one controlled treatment study (non-randomized), to our knowledge, assessing nightmare treatment in children or adolescents [13]. Halliday [14] lists several case reports that present individual patients treated with a variety of techniques, such as desensitization, play therapy, storyline alterations, extinction, or "face and conquer" (lucidity). Handler [15] successfully treated an 11-year-old with a combination of implosive therapy and a relationship approach. Cavior and Deutsch [16] used systematic desensitization to effectively treat a 16-year-old inmate for his recurrent nightmare. Palace and Johnston [17] utilized the dream reorganization approach on a 10-year-old boy with recurrent, traumatic nightmares, and Pellicer [18] utilized eye-movement desensitization and reprocessing for the treatment of nightmares in a 10-year-old. In the largest study on the treatment of nightmares in children and adolescents, Wile [19] describes the "auto-suggested dreams" approach that he used on 25 children and adolescents who had suffered from nightmares for various periods of time, ranging from a few days to a few months. The technique centered on the simple instruction: "Think about what you would like to dream about tonight". The children tended to have improvement within a few weeks to a few months. Follow-up ranged from a few months to 5 years (median 1 year), with no relapses [19].

Based on adult literature and treatment paradigms for PTSD, it would not be surprising to see future development of exposure-based treatments for nightmares in adolescents. In our work with adolescents, however, we have observed in one controlled study, and anecdotally in the clinical environment, that IRT has efficacy and effectiveness, and IRT is not primarily an exposure-based treatment, albeit the very process of discussing nightmares no doubt can be considered some degree of exposure [20].

IRT operates on the premise that nightmares may be a learned behavior. In some manner, a child or adolescent who initially responds to a daytime stressor with anxiety or fear and then disturbing dreams the same night or that week may be developing a "circuit" that works on the premise: "bad things = bad dreams". One could argue that such a circuit clearly exists in that conventional wisdom and dream research frequently describe nightmares as a place to process adverse daytime experiences. The question arises then as to why the "circuit" continues to operate if someone has successfully processed the daytime experiences. PTSD patients with successful treatment of their PTSD may still report residual nightmares, which is a counterintuitive fact, given that the expectation is that when PTSD is treated effectively, say with exposure therapy, then surely nightmares (a symptom of PTSD) ought to disappear [21].

This persistence of nightmares in the face of other psychiatric interventions is one of the main issues that led our research teams to begin speculating on whether nightmares should be more accurately conceptualized as an independent or co-morbid sleep disorder in most cases of nightmare disorder [21]. From this vantage point, the question continuously arises as to why these nightmares stick, which has led to theories about disturbing dreams as a learned behavior.

IRT is a therapy that specifically works to empower the patient to engage or re-engage their natural human imagery system and create new images for rehearsal, which we assume influence nocturnal images in some fashion to interrupt the nightmare cycle. How this process unfolds and whether what we are describing is valid are matters for future research.

STEP BY STEP DESCRIPTION OF PROCEDURES

An IRT program can be offered in three major steps:

1. Facts about nightmares
2. Practicing pleasant imagery
3. Imagery rehearsal treatment of nightmares.

Facts About Nightmares

The first step explores common questions chronic nightmare sufferers ask about their disturbing dreams, and includes discussion about how nightmares can affect one's sleep. Discussion points focus on linking nightmares to untoward effects on sleep, which then helps the patient to appreciate that nightmares are "independent", and can be directly treated. Remarkably, the majority of nightmare sufferers do not automatically assume nightmares are bad for their sleep. They tend to view nightmares as a mental health thing that's occurring during sleep, but they may not be clear that it actually worsens sleep. We usually discuss:

- the linkage of nightmares to sleep problems;
- fear of nightmares provoking sleep onset insomnia;
- fear of returning to sleep post-nightmare provoking sleep maintenance insomnia;
- that nightmares appear to fragment sleep and thus degrade sleep quality.

This first part of the program can also begin to raise questions about the cause of nightmares:

- What is the initial cause of nightmares?
- Why do nightmares persist in some people?
- What might it mean if nightmares have not responded to treatment with medications or psychotherapy?
- Is it possible to imagine that we have more control over nightmares than we might have thought possible?

Practicing Pleasant Imagery

The second step gives each participant the opportunity to attempt visualization exercises to assess his or her ability to create images and to monitor for unpleasant images. Seven simple behavioral techniques (thought stopping, breathing, grounding, talking, writing, acknowledging, and choosing) are taught, to cope with unpleasant images that might occur during any practice of pleasant imagery. This part of the program focuses on teaching the adolescent to engage or re-engage with his or her natural imagery system (for more details, imagery is discussed at length in *Sound Sleep, Sound Mind*, see Recommended reading, below). Key points raised include the following:

- Imagery is a natural component of the human brain.
- Imagery is accessed repeatedly throughout the day to solve problems – for example, remembering driving instructions, locating something misplaced, knowing what's in the fridge before you go to eat it, and so on.
- The capacity to actively engage one's imagery system may take different forms, but it is most reliably understood as "active daydreaming" or "guided daydreaming".
- Imagery exercises are not meant to be intense efforts yielding meditative or hypnotic-like states; they may or may not be comfortable, but it is best to evoke pleasant images when re-engaging the system.

- The goal is to help the individual realize that imagery is a naturally occurring form of "thinking" in the human mind, which is somewhat akin to the dream state because of its use of visual imagery and because images provide broader brushstrokes of what's on your mind compared with verbal thoughts (self-talking).
- Last, with practice of pleasant imagery, it becomes clear that the human mind can influence some of the images that emerge in the mind's eye; therefore, if such images can be influenced in the waking state, might not such influence extend to the sleep state?

Imagery Rehearsal Treatment of Nightmares

The final step teaches the three-step process of selecting a nightmare, changing it with the instruction "change it anyway you wish", and then rehearsing the new set of images (identified as a "new dream") in the waking state. With the imagery rehearsal technique, participants are taught to write down the material for learning purposes, but they are encouraged to continue using the process mentally. If individuals believe that writing down the old nightmare and new dream is helpful to the process, then they are encouraged to continue in that manner. Participants are instructed to practice the technique (with the sole emphasis on rehearsing new dreams, not nightmares) for at least a month on a daily basis, 5–20 minutes per day, and to do so in the context of working with no more than two "new dreams" each week regardless of how many nightmares they experienced. In practice, this instruction seems to be followed about 50 percent of the time, in that one prior study showed that the average use of IRT post-treatment was every other day for the first month. We recommend follow-up at 4 and 12 weeks post-treatment to review progress, and the use of an outcomes questionnaire facilitates this process.

Notes on the Application of IRT

Pearls we have learned in the application of the IRT steps include the following:

1. Strongly discourage a patient who wants to select his or her worst, most vivid, most trauma replay-like nightmare on the first attempt at IRT. Such dreams may set the stage for failure, by overwhelming the patient with what amounts to unplanned desensitization. The goal is to learn a process called, "changing a nightmare to a new dream and then rehearsing the new dream".
2. If at all feasible, avoid suggestions to the patient regarding the instructions "change the nightmare anyway you wish". It's the patient's nightmare and it's the patient's mind; he or she has the ability to intuit some ideas on how to change it, and it's not at all inconceivable that one empowering

component of IRT is that it encourages the patient to shoulder the responsibility for designing the changes. It is as if the patient is taking charge at this moment, which may be a trigger to enhance self-efficacy.

3. In light of the above, we almost never offer example(s) to patients on what a changed dream might look like until they have attempted the process and reported on how it evolved for them. Later, in group format, for example, we'll discuss "new dreams" among the patients, which gives them a chance to see that some changed the beginning, the middle, or end. Some change a few words, a few images, or just one thing. Some changed nothing at all, but they decided to feel differently about the dream content. Giving the patient a wide berth appears to have utility.
4. Tailor the three steps of the program to the patient. An adolescent with severe PTSD will likely need to spend meaningful time on all three steps to digest the material in order to embrace, or at least acknowledge, a new perspective on nightmares. However, some adolescents may need fewer of these coaching components because their imagery systems are already somewhat engaged or fairly well developed in ways that can more easily acquire and apply the three-step instructions for IRT, perhaps in just one session.

POSSIBLE MODIFICATIONS/VARIANTS

There are numerous variants of IRT, across all age groups, although most work has been done in adults. The major variations include the following:

1. *Group vs Individual Treatment.* There is a number of studies describing the use of IRT as a group treatment or individually, suggesting equivalency, but there are more randomized controlled trials (RCTs) using groups.
2. *Longer vs Shorter Total Treatment Time.* There is no established optimal length of treatment for an IRT protocol. We have generally used 7–10 hours for groups, and much less for individual treatment. For non-PTSD patients, as little as 1 hour might be needed for a chronic nightmare patient receptive to this form of therapy.
3. *More vs Less Exposure Component to Therapy.* This is a major area of interest because it was always assumed that IRT was really some form of covert exposure therapy, and undoubtedly it does create an opportunity for indirect exposure in that it engages a patient to at least think about the nightmare problem, but the IRT program initially developed by Kellner and Neidhart and continued by Krakow and Hollifield [22] de-emphasizes exposure as much as possible. On the other hand, Davis and Wright [23] have been developing an IRT variation with a greater exposure component.
4. *Treating Chronic vs Acute Nightmares.* It is very difficult to conduct research on acute nightmare patients, especially as nightmares would be expected to resolve spontaneously in a large number of cases. We recently

published a case report on 11 US combat soldiers who were treated with IRT while serving in Iraq, of whom 7 responded with marked reductions in nightmares [24]. Future research needs to look at this area, because it raises the interesting question: Would early treatment of nightmares, a major re-experiencing phenomenon of PTSD, lead to some decreased risk for developing chronic PTSD?

5. *Treatment Delivery Formats: Personal Encounter, Postal, Audiotape & Workbook.* There has been some development of IRT formats beyond traditional clinical sessions. Marks [25] has been working with a postal version, which has been studied in a randomized controlled trial. Krakow has been working with an audio series and treatment workbook version, which has not been studied.

PROOF OF CONCEPT/SUPPORTING DATA/EVIDENCE BASE

Several review articles have appeared in the scientific literature in the past few years that either suggest or endorse IRT as a first-line therapy for the treatment of chronic nightmares. These articles, in various formats, list the evidence in a host of IRT studies by the various research groups who have undertaken such efforts. The five main reviews published between 2006 and 2008 were by Lancee et al. [26], Wittmann et al. [27], Lamarch and De Koninck [28], Spoormaker et al. [29], and Maher et al. [30]. However, to our knowledge, our single RCT on the use of IRT in adolescents reflects the only controlled study in this age group, and this study was a non-randomized controlled trial due to the logistical issues inherent in the collaboration between New Mexico and Wyoming researchers. Moreover, of 30 participants assigned to treatment and control groups, 11 dropped out or did not provide data, thus the results were based on 19 individuals (9 treatment, 10 controls). Statistically significant treatment effects for nightmares and nights per week of nightmares were very large, but there were no significant effects for changes in sleep or PTSD scores as seen in adult studies. Overall, the data support IRT for the treatment of nightmares in adolescents, but, given that this study appears to be the only controlled study conducted, replication is essential.

REFERENCES

[1] L. Terr, Nightmares in children, in: C. Guillemmault, (Ed.), Sleep and Its Disturbances in Children, Raven Press, New York, NY, 1987, pp. 231–242.

[2] A. Vela-Bueno, E.O. Bixler, B. Dobladez-Blanco, et al., Prevalence of night terrors and nightmares in elementary school children: A pilot study, Res. Commun. Psychol. Psychiatry Behav. 3 (1985) 177–188.

[3] G. Klackenberg, A prospective longitudinal study of children. Chapter XIV, Further studies of sleep behavior in a longitudinally followed up sample, Acta Paediatr. Scand. 224 (1971) 161–185.

[4] J. Simonds, H. Parraga, Sleep behaviors and disorders in children and adolescents evaluated at psychiatric clinics, Dev. Behav. Pediatr. 1 (1984) 6–10.
[5] L. Yang, C. Zuo, L.F. Eaton, Research note: sleep problems of normal Chinese adolescents, J. Child Psychol. Psychiatry 1 (1987) 167–172.
[6] E. Hartmann, The Nightmare: The Psychology and Biology of Terrifying Dreams, Basic Books, New York, NY, 1984.
[7] M. Schredl, R. Pallmer, A. Montasser, Anxiety dreams in schoolaged children, Dreaming 4 (1996) 265–270.
[8] J. Vignau, D. Bailly, A. Duhamel, Epidemiologic study of sleep quality and troubles in French secondary school adolescents, J. Adolesc. Health 21 (1997) 343–350.
[9] K. Lee, G. McEnany, D. Weekes, Gender differences in sleep patterns for early adolescents, J. Adolesc Health 24 (1999) 16–20.
[10] D. Sandoval, B. Krakow, R Schrader, et al., Adult nightmares sufferers: can they be identified and treated in childhood?, (Abstr) Sleep Res. 26 (1997) 256.
[11] R. Manni, M.T. Ratti, G. Marchioni, et al., Poor sleep in adolescents: a study of 869 17-year-old Italian secondary school students, J. Sleep Res. 6 (1997) 44–49.
[12] A.P. Mannarino, J.A. Cohen, A clinical-demographic study of sexually abused children, Child Abuse Negl. 10 (1986) 17–23.
[13] B. Krakow, D. Sandoval, R. Schrader, et al., Treatment of chronic nightmares in adjudicated adolescent girls in a residential facility, J. Adolescent Health 29 (2) (2001) 94–100.
[14] G. Halliday, Direct psychological therapies for nightmares: a review, Clin. Psychol. Rev. 7 (1987) 501–523.
[15] L. Handler, The amelioration of nightmares in children, Psychotherapy: Theory, Research, and Practice 9 (1972) 54–56.
[16] N. Cavior, A. Deutsch, Systematic desensitization to reduce dream anxiety, J. Nerv. Ment. Dis. 161 (1975) 433–435.
[17] E.M. Palace, C. Johnston, Treatment of recurrent nightmares by the dream reorganization approach, J. Behav. Ther. Exp. Psychiatry 3 (1989) 219–226.
[18] X. Pellicer, Eye movement desensitization treatment of a child's nightmares: a case report, J. Behav. Ther. Exp. Psychiatry 1 (1993) 73–75.
[19] I. Wile, Auto-suggested dreams as a factor in therapy, Am. J. Orthospsychiatry 4 (1934) 449–453.
[20] B. Krakow, R. Kellner, D. Pathak, et al., Imagery rehearsal treatment for chronic nightmares, Behav. Res. Ther. 7 (1995) 837–843.
[21] B. Krakow, A. Zadra, Clinical management of chronic nightmares: imagery rehearsal therapy, Behav. Sleep Med. 4 (2006) 45–70.
[22] B. Krakow, M. Hollifield, L. Johnston, et al., Imagery rehearsal therapy for chronic nightmares in sexual assault survivors with posttraumatic stress disorder, JAMA 286 (2001) 537–545.
[23] J.L. Davis, D.C. Wright, Exposure, relaxation, and rescripting treatment for trauma-related nightmares, J. Trauma Dissociation 7 (2006) 5–18.
[24] B. Moore, B. Krakow, Imagery rehearsal therapy for acute posttraumatic nightmares among combat soldiers in Iraq, Am. J. Psychiatry 164 (2007) 683–684.
[25] S. Grandi, S. Fabbri, N. Panattoni, et al., Self-exposure treatment of recurrent nightmares: waiting-list-controlled trial and 4-year follow-up, Psychother Psychosom. 75 (6) (2006) 384–388.
[26] J. Lancee, V.I. Spoormaker, B. Krakow, J. van den Bout, A systematic review of cognitive-behavioral treatment for nightmares: toward a well-established treatment, J. Clin. Sleep Med. 4 (5) (2008) 475–480, Review.

[27] L. Wittmann, M. Schredl, M. Kramer, Dreaming in posttraumatic stress disorder: a critical review of phenomenology, psychophysiology and treatment, Psychother Psychosom. 76 (1) (2007) 25–39, Review.

[28] L.J. Lamarche, J. De Koninck, Sleep disturbance in adults with posttraumatic stress disorder: a review, J. Clin. Psychiatry 68 (8) (2007) 1257–1270, Review.

[29] V.I. Spoormaker, M. Schredl, J. van den Bout, Nightmares: from anxiety symptom to sleep disorder, Sleep Med. Rev. 10 (1) (2006) 19–31 Epub 2005 Dec 27. Review.

[30] M.J. Maher, S.A. Rego, G.M. Asnis, Sleep disturbances in patients with post-traumatic stress disorder: epidemiology, impact and approaches to management, CNS Drugs 20 (7) (2006) 567–590, Review.

RECOMMENDED READING

B. Krakow, Sound Sleep, Sound Mind, Wiley & Sons, Inc., Hoboken, NJ, 2007.

B. Krakow, J. Krakow, Turning Nightmares into Dreams, New Sleepy Times, Albuquerque, NM, 2002.

B. Krakow, E.J. Neidhardt, Conquering Bad Dreams & Nightmares, Berkley Books, New York, NY, 1992.

B. Naparstek, Staying Well with Guided Imagery, Warner Books, New York, NY, 1995.

Chapter 36

Moisture Alarm Therapy for Primary Nocturnal Enuresis

William J. Warzak

Munroe-Meyer Institute for Genetics and Rehabilitation, Department of Pediatrics, University of Nebraska Medical Center, Omaha, Nebraska

Patrick C. Friman

Director of Boys Town Center for Behavioral Health, University of Nebraska Medical Center, Boys Town, NE

PROTOCOL NAME

Moisture alarm therapy for primary nocturnal enuresis.

GROSS INDICATION

Nocturnal enuresis, or enuresis, is a very common parasomnia affecting 5–7 million children annually. It is largely an inherited condition wherein children involuntarily pass urine while asleep. The moisture alarm is the single best evidence-based intervention to treat this disorder.

SPECIFIC INDICATION

Alarm treatment is indicated for children with *primary* enuresis (children have not been fully continent for at least 6 months) and *secondary* enuresis (children who have been continent for at least 6 months but relapsed). Alarm treatment is especially indicated for children who are monosymptomatic (incontinent only while sleeping at night). Most alarm trials have been restricted to children 5 years of age and older [1].

CONTRAINDICATIONS

A small subsample of enuretic children exhibit clinical features suggestive of lower urinary tract dysfunction. These children are more likely to be wet during the day (i.e., have daytime incontinence) and exhibit other symptoms such as increased/decreased voiding frequency, voiding postponement, holding maneuvers, or staccato stream. Because alarm treatment is not typically indicated

Behavioral Treatments for Sleep Disorders. DOI: 10.1016/B978-0-12-381522-4.00036-5

for these children, identifying them is critical, underscoring the importance of obtaining a medical examination prior to the inauguration of alarm treatment.

RATIONALE FOR INTERVENTION

Nocturnal enuresis affects 15–20 percent of 5-year-old children, with as many as 10 percent of those children remaining wet at 10 years of age. Prevalence rates tend to be somewhat higher for boys than girls throughout. By 12 years of age, approximately 8 percent of boys and 4 percent of girls continue to be enuretic [2]. Treatment is often deferred until age 6 or 7, because enuresis shows a steady decline with age and has an annual spontaneous remission rate of approximately 15 percent [3]. In addition, younger children may be less motivated to participate in treatment. After the age of 6 or 7, however, numerous reasons for treatment arise. For example, nocturnal wetting episodes inexorably interfere with participation in recreational activities (such as sleepovers, overnight trips, and camp), thus imposing an obstacle to important social and developmental experiences. Chronic bedwetting also can result in sleep disruption for the child and other family members [4]. In addition, incontinence is a leading cause of child abuse [5]. Finally, for all of the above reasons, a child with enuresis may develop an unhealthy low self-regard that interferes with effective psychosocial development.

There are a number of medications used for treatment of enuresis (e.g., desmopressin, tolterodine, imipramine, and oxybutinin), none of which are indicated as front-line treatment for several reasons. For example, medication yields much lower levels of success than that produced by the moisture alarm. Additionally, the effects, when produced, typically occur only while the medication is taken, and dissipate when medication is discontinued. Perhaps most importantly, each medication produces problematic side effects, and occasionally significant health risk. For example, the Food and Drug Administration has recently ruled that the intranasal form of desmopressin is inappropriate as a treatment for enuresis because of its relationship to cardiac risk in a small number of patients. Nevertheless, although not indicated as a primary intervention, medicine should be considered if alarm therapy is unsuccessful.

STEP BY STEP DESCRIPTION OF PROCEDURES

1. *Selecting the right time to begin.* Most typically developing children will acquire some measure of voiding control between the ages of 3 and 4, and by 5 years of age many children will have achieved nocturnal and daytime continence. Nevertheless, 15–20 percent of these children will be enuretic, and many professionals, if not parents, may choose not to intervene at this age, especially if the child is not deemed to be at risk. However, children who continue to wet the bed after 7 years of age should be considered candidates for intervention.

2. *Preliminary evaluation by a physician.* Before treatment begins, the child should be evaluated by a physician. The evaluation should include a brief neurologic exam, urinalysis, and perhaps a urine culture, to exclude factors that might suggest symptoms of lower urinary tract dysfunction, or identify co-morbid conditions, such as diabetes insipidis, spina bifida, or spinal cord trauma, that might influence treatment outcome. In addition, sleep disorders that may affect enuresis, such as sleep apnea, obstructive tonsils, mouth breathing or snoring, need to be evaluated as possibly contributory to enuresis.
3. *Education and demystification.* Children and their parents are often the victims of misinformation regarding enuresis. It is often helpful to identify other members of the child's family that exhibited enuresis in childhood. In addition, it may be helpful to inform the child that there are many children their own age, some of whom may be their classmates, who also wet the bed. Children and their parents also should be assured that enuresis is often a heritable condition, and is not the result of psychological attributes such as laziness or stubbornness. Furthermore, the biobehavioral nature of enuresis is such that it is not possible for enuretic children to control their condition independently, and therefore punishment of wetting episodes is never appropriate. Finally, parents and children should be informed that the alarm may not be effective for several weeks. One method for tracking slow progress is to measure the size of the urine spot (which typically shrinks during treatment) and monitor the amount the child voids in the toilet following alarm onset (which typically increases over time of treatment).
4. *Interview by behavioral health staff.* Following the medical exam, the behavioral health professional should conduct a thorough evaluation that obtains information on all conditions that are relevant to alarm treatment. These conditions include any that could complicate or contraindicate treatment. At a minimum, the evaluation should include the following.
   - Age of daytime dryness may shed light on the developmental status of the child, and this, in turn, may affect training expectations.
   - Family history of bed-wetting may influence expectations of when the child may achieve dryness given no intervention.
   - Severity and frequency of the bed-wetting certainly affects expectations regarding successful treatment in the short-run, with more frequent wetting and multiple wettings per night being adverse predictors of success.
   - Daytime symptoms of dysfunctional voiding may considerably alter treatment planning. A history of difficult or painful urination, hesitancy, urgency, or daytime wetting suggests non-monosymptomatic enuresis, and may indicate additional assessment and treatment procedures over and above the moisture alarm. Similarly, symptoms such as giggle

incontinence, stress incontinence (i.e., incontinence upon physical exertion), post-void dribbling, overactive bladder, and Hinman syndrome indicate additional assessment and potential referral to a urologist.
- Current medications also may affect elimination. The use of enuresis-related medications (and their history of use), such as desmopressin (DDAVP), imipramine (Tofranil), oxybutin (Ditropan), and tolterodine (Detrol), should be ascertained. Other medications that may indirectly affect enuresis by contributing to constipation, or altered sleep–wake cycles, also should be identified.
- Co-morbidities (e.g., ADHD, diabetes insipidus) often influence treatment, if only because significant health issues complicate structured routines.
- Constipation or bowel irregularity is common among enuretic children. Constipation can interfere with bladder function by impinging on the bladder and/or by inhibiting its natural expansion as it fills.
- School issues may influence the ultimate success of treatment for enuresis or constipation. For example, if school schedules preclude sufficient opportunities to drink during the school day, the student may compensate by drinking more fluids during the afternoon and evening hours, thereby contributing to urine formation in the evening or after bedtime.
- Food sensitivities may affect a variety of children. These do not include allergies, but rather reactions to substances within foods that can affect urodynamics. Examples include caffeine and tryptophan.
- Compliance issues are crucial. Levels of compliance should be obtained for all children considered for alarm therapy. Children who are not under effective instructional control are poor candidates for the moisture alarm. For these children, it may be more effective to implement compliance training prior to implementing a full treatment plan including the moisture alarm.
- Motivation to participate in alarm procedures is important to achieving success. An older child's motivation to be dry often increases as the social limitations imposed by enuresis increase. However, younger children whose social functioning has not yet been significantly affected by the limitations imposed by enuresis may benefit from structured programming to increase compliance. An optimal motivational system would provide rewards for compliance with alarm procedures rather than for dry nights, which result from a combination of factors, many of which are beyond the child's control.

5. *Moisture alarm procedural checklist.* Successful implementation of alarm therapy requires consideration of supplies and procedures.

Important Supplies

- An alarm that has a salient wake-up cue. Auditory alarms have the most supportive data but vibrating alarms have been shown to be effective, and may be preferred when incontinent children share a bedroom. Alarms are widely available online from $50.00–$100.00 (e.g., www.bedwettingstore.com).

- Alarm batteries (and extra set of batteries).
- Clips and fasteners to attach the alarm to the child's undergarment.
- T-shirt to control wires, if any, from the moisture sensors to the alarm.
- Snug-fitting cotton panties or briefs are preferred.
- Mattress cover.
- Nightlight in the bathroom.
- Parents may need a baby monitor if their bedroom is far removed from their child's.

Important Procedures

- Reassure the child that the procedure is safe and will not hurt.
- Carry out a trial run prior to bedtime to demonstrate how the alarm works and feels (i.e., model the entire procedure and then have the child imitate the procedure).
- Start each night with a clean bed.
- Ensure double voids before sleep. Parents should have the child void during the pre-bedtime routine, and have them void one more time before actually going to bed.
- Place sensor with consideration of boys' and girls' physiology.
- Give the child responsibility for clean-up, as necessary. Parents must convey to their child that the child's assistance is a matter of responsibility, and is not intended as punishment.
- Data collection is completed by the child (with parental assistance as needed) each morning.
- Deliver reinforcers, rewards, etc., contingent upon compliance with alarm procedures.

Procedural Sequence

1. Prepare the child for bed consistent with proper sleep hygiene, including double voiding.
2. Attach the alarm appropriately to the child's undergarment as directed by the manufacturer.
3. Turn on baby monitor, if applicable.
4. When the alarm sounds, if the child has not awakened, a parent/guardian should immediately wake the child. For example, the parent may call the child's name, shake him or her until awake, or wipe the child's face with a damp washcloth. Regardless, the goal is to have the child awaken, toilet him- or herself, and participate in clean-up procedures independently.

5. Wakefulness may be demonstrated by having the child count backwards from 10 or answer a question of the parent's choosing.
6. Upon awakening, the child should disconnect the alarm, walk to the bathroom, void in the toilet, and complete cleanliness hygiene.
7. Following the bathroom visit, the child should mark his or her calendar to indicate a wetting episode, assist with bedclothes clean-up as stipulated by the parent, reattach the alarm, and return to bed.
8. Upon awakening in the morning, parents should provide the agreed-upon reward for participation in alarm procedures, as appropriate.

POSSIBLE MODIFICATIONS/VARIANTS

There are treatment packages that incorporate the above components as well as a number of additional features, such as cleanliness training, positive practice, awakening schedules, etc. The two foremost packages are Dry Bed training [6] and Full Spectrum Home Training [7]. Both of these packages require considerably more effort than the moisture alarm alone, and a discussion of them is beyond the scope of this chapter. Nevertheless, they provide additional resources to the child and family having difficulty achieving night-time continence.

Children who relapse at the conclusion of treatment are often successful if provided a renewed alarm trial. In addition, these children may benefit from overlearning – a procedure in which success with the alarm is followed by a 2-week fluid challenge, typically 8 oz of water at bedtime, followed by alarm trials until dry nights are re-established. Dry bed criterion is typically 14 consecutive dry nights.

Treatment failures may result from numerous causes, some of which are matters of adherence. Perhaps the most common cause of failure is premature termination of the alarm procedure. There is ample literature to suggest that the alarm often requires a 10- to 12-week course of treatment, and parents need to be apprised of this. Other sources of failure arise within the context of matching procedures to children, and these may be addressed with modifications of the standard procedure. For example, it is not uncommon for children to sleep through the alarm, and some enuretic children may actually have a higher auditory arousal threshold than non-enuretic children. Parents should be prepared to awaken the child upon onset of the alarm. They may need to incorporate an auditory monitoring device, such as a baby monitor, if the parental bedroom is too far away for parents to hear the alarm. Other children are comfortable with the procedure at home, but are confronted with obstacles to implementation if they attend a sleep-over – in which case, a sleeping bag with a liner and a change of clothes stored in the bottom of the bag may be an appropriate stop-gap procedure for the night.

Finally, water restriction, possibly the most widely used method for managing enuresis (by parents and professionals), is unpleasant, and possibly even harmful to the child. There is no evidence that restricting fluids prior to bed (unless a child clearly over-indulges) has any positive effect on treatment. In fact, there is evidence that many of these children are insufficiently hydrated, and fluid restriction at bedtime, after dinner, etc. merely compounds that problem.

PROOF OF CONCEPT/SUPPORTING DATA/EVIDENCE BASE

The diversity of research methods used to evaluate the moisture alarm contrasts sharply with the singularity of the findings they produce. Regardless of method, case report, case study, controlled group trial, or comparative group trial, research on alarm treatment routinely yields successful outcomes, perhaps in part because it teaches specific continence skills. Results from case reports and studies range as high as 100 percent successful with 0 percent relapse, and results from controlled trials range as high as 80 percent successful and as low as 17 percent for relapse. More generally, the collective evaluation research on alarm treatment shows that its success rate is higher and its relapse rate is lower than any other method [4,8–10]. On the strength of this body of research, prominent enuresis investigators have argued that alarm-based treatment meets the rigorous "Chambless" criteria [11] for effective treatment of enuresis [12]. In conclusion, the moisture alarm is a robust and routinely effective intervention, and should be the first-line treatment for most children with monosymptomatic enuresis.

REFERENCES

[1] C.M.A. Glazener, J.H.C. Evans, R.E. Peto, Alarm interventions for nocturnal enuresis in children, Cochrane Database of Systematic Reviews (Issue 2) (2005). Art. No.: CD002911. DOI: 10.1002/14651858.CD002911.pub2.

[2] R.T. Gross, S.M. Dornbusch, Enuresis, in: M.D. Levine, W.B. Carey, A.C. Crocker, R.T. Gross, (Eds.), Developmental-Behavioral Pediatrics, W.B. Saunders, Philadelphia, PA, 1983, pp. 575–586.

[3] W.I. Forsythe, A. Redmond, Enuresis and spontaneous cure rate: study of 1129 enuretics, Arch. Dis. Child. 49 (1974) 259–269.

[4] P.C. Friman, W.J. Warzak, Nocturnal enuresis: a prevalent, persistent, yet curable parasomnia, Pediatrician 17 (1) (1990) 38–45.

[5] R. Helfer, C.H. Kempe, Child Abuse and Neglect, Ballinger, Cambridge, MA, 1976.

[6] N.H. Azrin, T.J. Sneed, R.M. Foxx, Dry-bed training: rapid elimination of childhood enuresis, Behav. Res. Ther. 12 (3) (1974) 147–156.

[7] J.P. Whelan, A.C. Houts, Effects of a waking schedule on the outcome of primary enuretic children treated with full-spectrum home training, Health Psychol. 9 (1990) 164–176.

[8] P.C. Friman, Encopresis and enuresis, in: M. Hersen, D. Reitman, (Eds.), Handbook of Assessment, Case Conceptualization, and Treatment, Vol 2, Children and Adolescents, Wiley, Hoboken, NJ, 2007, pp. 589–621.

[9] P.C. Friman, Evidence based therapies for enuresis and encopresis, in: R.G. Steele, T.D. Elkin, M.C. Roberts, (Eds.), Handbook of Evidence-based Therapies for Children and Adolescents, Springer, New York, NY, 2008, pp. 311–333.

[10] A.C. Houts, J.S. Berman, H. Abramson, Effectiveness of psychological and pharmacological treatments for nocturnal enuresis, J. Consult. Clin. Psychol. 62 (1994) 737–745.

[11] D.L. Chambless, S.D. Hollon, Defining empirically supported therapies, J. Consult. Clin. Psychol. 6 (1) (1998) 7–18.

[12] M.W. Mellon, M.L. McGrath, Empirically supported treatments in pediatric psychology: nocturnal enuresis, J. Pediatr. Psychol. 25 (2000) 193–214.

RECOMMENDED READING

P.C. Friman, M.L. Handwerk, S.M. Swearer, et al., Do children with primary nocturnal enuresis have clinically significant behavior problems? Arch. Pediatr. Adolesc. Med. 152 (1998) 537–539.

G.A. Gimpel, W.J. Warzak, B.R. Kuhn, J.N. Walburn, Clinical perspectives in primary nocturnal enuresis, Clin. Pediatr. 37 (1998) 23–29.

K. Hjalmas, T. Arnold, W. Bower, et al., Nocturnal enuresis: An international evidence based management strategy, J. Urol. 171 (2004) 2545–2561.

W.J. Warzak, Psychosocial implications of nocturnal enuresis, Clin. Pediatr. 32 (July Special Edition) (1993) 38–40.

N.M. Wolfish, R.T. Pivik, K.A. Busby, Elevated sleep arousal thresholds in enuretic boys: clinical implications, Acta Paediatr. 86 (1997) 381–384.

Chapter 37

Promoting Positive Airway Pressure Adherence in Children Using Escape Extinction within a Multi-Component Behavior Therapy Approach

Keith J. Slifer

Pediatric Psychology Program, Department of Behavioral Psychology, Kennedy Krieger Institute, Baltimore, MD

Departments of Psychiatry and Behavioral Sciences and Pediatrics, Johns Hopkins University School of Medicine, Baltimore, MD

PROTOCOL NAME

Promoting positive airway pressure adherence in children using escape extinction within a multi-component behavior therapy approach.

GROSS INDICATION

Continuous Positive Airway Pressure (CPAP) and Bi-level Positive Airway Pressure (BiPAP) are types of mechanical respiratory assistance prescribed for individuals with breathing disorders. Examples of such disorders in children include hypoventilation, hypercarbia, obstructive sleep apnea, and central apnea. PAP has been used successfully in infants and children; however, behavioral tolerance and adherence with these devices pose a significant challenge in pediatrics. When PAP is not successful with children, the vast majority of the time it is because of poor behavioral tolerance and therefore poor adherence. Behavior therapy protocols have been used to increase child tolerance of and adherence to PAP therapy, and there is published preliminary evidence to support effectiveness of these protocols with preschool and school-aged children.

SPECIFIC INDICATION

There are specific pulmonary indications for using these different breathing therapies, but for the purposes of this chapter dealing with children's

Behavioral Treatments for Sleep Disorders. DOI: 10.1016/B978-0-12-381522-4.00037-7

adherence with these technologies, they will be referred to as Positive Airway Pressure (PAP). While these devices were originally used in intensive care and acute care hospital settings, they are now routinely prescribed by pulmonologists for home management of some types of breathing disorders during hours of sleep, in individuals of all ages.

Behavior therapy to increase cooperation and adherence with PAP regimens is indicated for children of all ages, including those with intellectual and developmental disabilities. However, there is some preliminary evidence that behavior therapy for PAP tolerance and adherence is more easily accomplished with children who are older and cognitively are more typically developing. In infants, young children, and those with intellectual or developmental disabilities the behavior therapy is focused on the caregiver – child dyad, and its success is dependent upon the caregiver's ability and motivation to modify his or her own behavior patterns. There is no published evidence to suggest that behavioral therapy is more effective for any particular type of breathing disorders or specific medical diagnoses or syndromes.

CONTRAINDICATIONS

There is no research evidence to support any particular contraindications for behavior therapy. However, clinical judgment and experience suggest that children who are medically too fragile to tolerate increased levels of physical exertion and arousal are not good candidates for this type of behavior therapy. Using carefully graduated exposure to the PAP equipment and routine decreases physical arousal and exertion that may be experienced during behavior therapy. Nonetheless, emotional arousal and physical exertion may not be completely avoidable. This is especially true during escape prevention (escape extinction) procedures, when crying and some degree of physical resistance may occur. Therefore, the child's ability to tolerate the amount of arousal and physical exertion that typically occur during a crying spell or tantrum must be verified with the child's pediatrician or pulmonologist in order to safely employ the escape extinction component of the behavior therapy protocol described below.

Another contraindication would be if the child has severe aggressive or self-injurious behavior. In such cases, the behavioral protocol below should be employed only with the assistance of a behavioral psychologist or behavior analyst who has expertise in managing these types of behavior problems.

In some cases, overall parenting skills may be limited by cognitive difficulties or other psychosocial factors that interfere with learning or implementing the behavioral protocol. These caregivers may also have great difficulty managing their children in a variety of home and community settings, suggesting that more fundamental behavioral parent training may be needed before expecting them to implement a PAP adherence protocol.

Finally, if the parent or caregiver is opposed to behavior therapy that may cause temporary increases in child distress, then success with a behavioral protocol may not be possible.

RATIONALE FOR INTERVENTION

PAP has been used successfully in infants and children; however, behavioral tolerance and adherence with these devices pose a significant challenge in pediatrics. When PAP is not successful with children, the vast majority of the time it is because of poor behavioral tolerance and therefore poor adherence. This is particularly the case for preschool-aged children, and those with developmental disabilities, anxiety, or behavior problems. These children commonly resist (verbally, emotionally, and physically) attempts to put on the mask by crying, head turning, and using their hands to cover their faces or push away the mask. Many develop conditioned anxiety because the sight, sound, and physical sensation of PAP become associated with discomfort from the pressure of the mask, the airflow into the nostrils, and physiologic arousal from struggling to resist the mask. Children learn very quickly that these behaviors often result in discontinuation of the caregiver's efforts to apply the mask. In this way, these escape/avoidance behaviors are strengthened through negative reinforcement (they make the non-preferred sensations go away).

A multi-component behavior therapy protocol can be used to increase child tolerance of and adherence to PAP therapy. This behavior therapy approach is based on the concept of escape extinction, which involves ensuring that the mask is placed by the caregiver despite the child's escape/avoidance behaviors. If the child manages to displace or remove the mask, it is immediately replaced by the caregiver and only removed after a pre-designated period of adherence, and only removed by the caregiver at the appropriate time. The objective is to remove any negative reinforcement of escape/avoidance behaviors. However, escape extinction procedures should be embedded within the positive context that can be created by also using distraction, counter-conditioning, stimulus fading for graduated exposure to the mask/air pressure, and differential positive reinforcement to shape cooperation and adherence. Without these other techniques to create a positive context, escape extinction alone would be simply coercive and unpalatable to most caregivers. There is published preliminary evidence to support the effectiveness of these behavioral protocols with preschool and school-aged children.

In order to increase adherence with PAP, children must learn to relax and tolerate the novel and non-preferred stimulation involved with wearing the mask and experiencing air pressure into the nostrils and airway. When a child experiences uncomfortable stimulation, he or she will instinctively attempt to withdraw from it, to escape its proximity, and to avoid it in the future. If the experience is very intense during a single exposure, or is repeated often, the child is likely to develop conditioned anxiety (conditioned autonomic nervous system arousal) when exposed to sights, sounds, or smells that have been associated with the uncomfortable stimulation. The child may develop a conditioned avoidance response such that whenever the stimuli associated with PAP are encountered (sight of the mask or machine), he or she becomes physiologically aroused and attempts to physically avoid or escape the situation. Children may exhibit a variety of escape-avoidance motivated behaviors when they are anticipating an uncomfortable sensation. These behaviors may include crying, head turning, pushing away, running, hiding, hitting, kicking, spitting, etc. Many caregivers respond to these behaviors by attempting to comfort, coax, or reason with the child to calm him or her and obtain cooperation. Caregivers often learn to avoid the child's distress and disruptive behavior by removing and/or protecting the child from the threatening situation. In this way, both child and parent behavior is motivated and shaped by escape and avoidance.

Caregivers who are attempting to implement PAP typically react to child distress by trying to calm the child using verbal explanations, coaxing, apologies, expressions of affection, and removing the mask. This only strengthens the distress and, escape and avoidance behaviors. With repetition of this parent–child interaction pattern the child develops a varied and persistent repertoire of distress and escape behavior in response to the mask, and caregivers give up on implementing the PAP regimen.

Thus, the goals of behavior therapy to enhance adherence with PAP are to decrease or eliminate the escape/avoidance function of distress behavior, and to positively reinforce approaching, wearing, and, ultimately, sustained adherence with the mask and air pressure for the prescribed duration of the PAP regimen.

As will become clear in reading the step by step procedures presented below, the multi-component protocol is time- and procedure-intensive, and for many children and their caregivers will require the assistance and guidance of a specialized professional. This can be costly in terms of time and resources devoted to behavior therapy. These costs are justifiable in relation to either the negative health and cognitive consequences of a lifetime with sleep-disordered breathing, and PAP non-adherence. They also are justifiable when compared to the alternative, more invasive medical intervention for obstructive sleep apnea: surgical placement of a tracheostomy tube. This surgery is associated with all the risks of complications that accompany any major surgery. It might also not be effective for a child with behavior problems that may be as likely to disrupt or remove the breathing tube as they are to remove a PAP mask. In such cases, behavior therapy may be required anyway to prevent the child removing the tracheostomy tube. On the other hand, once a child and caregivers have successfully participated in behavior therapy for PAP adherence, behavior therapy can be discontinued and the PAP integrated into the child's life like other daily care activities (bathing, toileting, brushing teeth). In short, PAP becomes part of the child's bedtime routine.

STEP BY STEP DESCRIPTION OF PROCEDURES

The PAP adherence training protocol is implemented using a combination of behavior therapy techniques. These include: (1) conducting a task analysis of the regimen, (2) providing distraction from uncomfortable sensations using preferred activities, (3) counter-conditioning emotional arousal by providing preferred activities to induce a relaxed, positive state, (4) maintaining the child's positive state while gradually exposing him or her to the steps in the task analysis and the associated sensations, (5) differential reinforcement of partial adherence by providing contingent praise and positive events (including mask removal by the therapist after a given interval of child adherence), and (6) placing escape/avoidance behavior on extinction (by interrupting, blocking or redirecting these behaviors).

Measurement of PAP Adherence

Adherence with PAP therapy can be assessed and recorded using a task analysis format, which breaks down the child behavior required for adherence into sequential observable steps. Koontz and colleagues [1] published a task analysis of PAP that can be used to record child adherence for each step that the child completes or tolerates. Using this task analysis set up as a data sheet, one can score each step completed (e.g., within 10 seconds of a verbal prompt, with or without assistance, and without escape-avoidance behavior; see Table 37.1). Using this information, the percentage of steps of the task analysis that are completed by the child can be calculated (number of steps completed divided by the total number of steps in the task analysis, multiplied by 100). This type of measurement can be used during and across behavior therapy sessions to document the child's success and progress. After the child is able to tolerate the mask and air pressure for more than a minute without distress, adherence data can be recorded in terms of minutes or hours of use. If staff resources are available, this can be accomplished by keeping 24-hour written records based on observation of the child at regular time intervals (e.g., every 30 minutes) and recording whether or not the child is asleep or awake, the mask is in place, and the device is operating properly. In most cases, this level of direct observation will not be possible. For example, in the home a parent cannot stay up all night to observe and record every 30 minutes. Alternatively, the parent can record: (1) what time the mask was placed, (2) what time the child fell asleep with the mask on, (3) what time the child awakened, and (4) whether or not the mask was still in place. Based on this information, the duration of PAP adherence can be quantified. Parents may choose to set an alarm clock and check their child at planned intervals throughout the night. Parents can be alerted to mask removals by the monitor alarm that is available on many PAP machines, or the low oxygen saturation limit alarm on a child's pulse oximeter. In this way, each time the mask is dislodged or removed the parent can be alerted, intervene to replace the mask, and record the time of these events. For parents who are heavy sleepers, the monitor or oximeter alarm can be amplified using a commercially available baby monitor with the microphone placed in the child's room and the speaker located on the parent's night stand. Finally, many PAP machines are equipped with a Smart Card (Respironics, Inc., Murrysville, PA; www.respironics.com) or

TABLE 37.1 PAP Task Analysis

Step	Tolerance/ Cooperation? ✓	Attempts to Avoid or Escape? ✓	Crying or Negative Vocalization? ✓
1. The child sits on the bed or stretcher.			
2. The child cooperates with having the PAP cap placed on the back of the head.			
3. The child lies in the supine position on the bed/stretcher.			
4. The child remains supine and calm while the mask (not attached to the hose or cap) is placed in position on the face for 5 seconds.			
5. The child remains supine and calm while the mask (not attached to the hose or cap) is placed in position on the face for 10 seconds.			
6. The child remains supine and calm while the mask (not attached to the hose or cap) is placed in position on the face for 1 minute.			
7. The child remains supine and calm while one side of the mask is attached to the cap. **Prior to next step, the mask will need to be connected to the tube and the tube will need to be connected to the machine.			
8. The child remains supine and calm while the mask (attached to the hose and one side of the cap) is placed in position on the face and while the air is turned on for 3 seconds.			
9. The child remains supine and calm while the mask (attached to the hose and one side of the cap) is placed in position on the face and while the air is turned on for 5 seconds.			
10. The child remains supine and calm while the mask (attached to the hose and one side of the cap) is placed in position on the face and while the air is turned on for 10 seconds.			

11. The child remains supine and calm while the mask (attached to the hose and one side of the cap) is placed in position on the face and while the air is turned on for 1 minute.
12. The child remains supine and calm while the mask is placed in position on the face and is connected to the cap on both sides.
13. The child remains supine and calm while the mask (attached to hose and both sides of the cap) is placed in position on the face and while the air is turned on for 1 minute.
14. The child remains supine and calm while the mask (attached to hose and both sides of the cap) is placed in position on the face and while the air is turned on for 5 minutes.
15. The child remains supine and calm while the mask (attached to hose and both sides of the cap) is placed in position on the face and while the air is turned on for 10 minutes.
16. The child remains supine and calm while the mask (attached to hose and both sides of the cap) is placed in position on the face and while the air is turned on for 15 minutes.

Reprinted with Permission from: K.L. Koontz, K.J. Slifer, M.D. Cataldo, & C.L. Marcus, Improving pediatric compliance with positive airway pressure: The impact of Behavior Intervention. Sleep, 26 (8) (2003) 1010–1015.

similar electronic monitoring device, which may provide more accurate, objective adherence data. These devices automatically record data on when the PAP is running, the mask is in place, and the machine is functioning properly, indicating that the child is wearing the mask. However, these monitoring devices may not be available for all machines, and may not be covered by some health insurance providers. Another limitation of this technology is that it requires a computer and specific software to download and analyze the data. Therefore, in most cases these data would only be available when the Smart Card or its equivalent is taken to the physician's office or clinic, and professional time is available to analyze and interpret the data.

Initial Behavioral Assessment

Before initiating behavioral treatment the child should be observed during one or more attempts to don the PAP mask at either naptime or bedtime, and initial adherence data recorded. These assessments should only progress through the PAP task analysis to the point where the child exhibits obvious distress and attempts to avoid or escape the mask or equipment. It is not necessary or wise to persist with these trials without behavioral intervention, because doing so will only reinforce the child's distress and escape behavior.

Reinforcer or Stimulus Preference Assessment

Before attempting to implement the behavior therapy protocol, it is important to obtain information about the child's favorite activities that might be used for relaxation, distraction, and motivation (e.g., snacks, bubbles, videogames, movies, singing, small rewards, etc.). This can be accomplished by interviewing the parent, having the parent or caregiver complete a reinforcement questionnaire [2], or conducting a more formal assessment where potentially reinforcing stimuli are presented in pairs to the child and the child's hierarchy of choices is systematically determined [3–5]. The most highly preferred items are then either provided non-contingently (delivered independent of the child's behavior) to distract or relax the child during exposure to the PAP mask and air pressure, or presented contingent upon (immediately following and in response to) positive behavior such as direction following, cooperation, and coping with presentation of the PAP equipment and its accompanying sensations.

Summary of Protocol Procedures

The PAP adherence training protocol is implemented by conducting a task analysis of the regimen, providing distraction from uncomfortable sensations, counter-conditioning emotional arousal using preferred activities, gradually exposing the child to the steps in the task analysis and associated sensations, providing differential reinforcement for cooperation and mask tolerance via contingent praise, positive events, and mask removal by the therapist after a given interval of child adherence. The one component that is most critical to successful intervention is placing escape/avoidance behavior on extinction by interrupting, blocking, or redirecting these behaviors.

Specific Behavior Therapy Procedures

Behavior therapy for PAP adherence requires behavioral rehearsal sessions during which the PAP equipment and mask are presented one step at a time according to the sequence outlined in the PAP task analysis. If a child has difficulty progressing from one step to the next, the steps shown in the task analysis (see Table 37.1) may be further subdivided into smaller components or briefer exposure durations.

When first attempting to place the mask on the child, he or she may cry, scream, block the placement of the PAP mask, or otherwise try to escape. If the child begins to show these behaviors at the sight or mention of the PAP machine, or even more remotely related stimuli in the environment, then conditioned anxiety is thought to have developed. During counter-conditioning, the child's conditioned anxiety is treated by carefully planned, graduated exposure to the mask, equipment, and air pressure while the child participates in a distracting, pleasurable activity. The activity must be one that produces an emotional state that is incompatible with anxiety (i.e., pleasure, relaxation). When the child appears relaxed and to be enjoying the activity, gradual exposure to PAP equipment is accomplished by slowly increasing the child's proximity to the equipment and the duration of contact with the mask, air pressure, etc. Initially, this may involve simply looking at or touching the mask, wearing the cap without the mask attached, feeling the airflow with hands or face, talking into the hose with active airflow, and so forth. During these exposures, escape prevention must be used in conjunction with the counter-conditioning procedures described above. By blocking escape behavior, the caregiver enables the child ultimately to experience each step of the task analysis while also having positive experiences (e.g. distraction, relaxation). As the child experiences a reduction of anxiety and exhibits fewer avoidant behaviors, compliant behaviors can be strengthened using differential reinforcement. Preferred items or events are provided in response to the child's efforts at cooperating with and tolerating the mask and air pressure, but not in response to distress, avoidance, or escape behavior. The therapist can use a visible timer, such as a kitchen timer, to set the exposure time for each trial. If the child is compliant during the set exposure interval, then compliance is negatively reinforced because the exposure is terminated when the timer bell rings. It is especially important that the exposure ends when the bell rings, and not contingent on escape behavior. After the child has successfully tolerated exposure at the current duration, then the exposure can be increased by moderately increasing the interval set on the timer. In a similar fashion, the child progresses through successive steps of the task-analyzed regimen, receiving praise and other reinforcing events after completing each step. The achievement of adherence at each level of the task analysis increases the frequency with which the child experiences success without feeling overwhelmed by anxiety or discomfort, and increases the probability that the child will cooperate with future increases in duration and difficulty.

During the escape prevention (escape extinction) procedure, the therapist (and, subsequently, the caregiver) blocks or prevents the child's avoidance or escape from the PAP stimuli through brief verbal prompting, re-direction to a specific activity, and, if necessary, physically blocking escape and gently guiding the child to remain in the situation (e.g., gently guiding hands down from the mask). The child's attempts to block or remove the mask must be interrupted each time, and the mask must be immediately replaced every time the child dislodges or removes it.

The procedures described above are presented at a rate that challenges the child to develop coping skills, but does not over-arouse him or her. This creates a neutral, safe environment for learning. It allows the child to experience immediate success with initial steps in the PAP routine, and to develop positive momentum for greater probability of adherence during subsequent sessions when duration of exposure, proximity to equipment, and discomfort are increased. The use of a preferred activity during exposure provides an antecedent intervention that enhances the child's relaxation and willingness to approach the therapist and training environment, rather than trying to avoid or escape them with disruptive behavior. The therapist ignores negative vocalizations, but intermittently reassures the child (e.g., "you can do it, you will be OK"). After the child is able comfortably to tolerate each step of the task analysis during behavioral rehearsal sessions, treatment efforts focus on increasing the duration of wearing the PAP, and generalizing the treatment effects to the child's home environment during hours of sleep.

Caregiver Training and Procedures for Adherence Promotion

Parents and other available caregivers should be involved in the behavior therapy sessions as directed by the behavior therapist. Initially, this will involve helping to engage the child in a preferred, distracting activity while the therapist conducts brief exposures to the mask, tubing, etc., and providing praise, affection, or other positive reinforcement to the child in response to his or her cooperation as prompted by the therapist. When the therapist judges the child to be ready to have the mask attached, the caregiver can assist with placing and securing the mask, straps and cap on the child's head, and, when prompted by the therapist, can remove or assist with removing theses items.

As therapy sessions progress, caregivers receive training using demonstrations, verbal and written instructions, role-play, in vivo behavioral rehearsal with the child, and provision of corrective verbal feedback. As they demonstrate proficiency with implementing the behavioral protocol in session, the caregiver can gradually take over increasing responsibility for conducting the session. The number of caregiver training sessions will vary, depending on the caregiver's availability for training, learning abilities, and beliefs about the importance of the PAP regimen and the need for training.

Once deemed by the therapist to be sufficiently trained, the caregiver must be assisted in developing a consistent bedtime routine lasting 20–30 minutes, including soothing activities (reading stories, calming music, etc.) and always culminating with donning the PAP mask and lying down in bed to go to sleep. Initially, the caregiver can be given "homework" assignments to complete with the child (e.g., each evening at bedtime set a timer for 5 minutes, put the mask on your child, block mask removal or replace mask as necessary, remove the mask when the timer alarms). While continuing to reinforce the child's and caregiver's performance in sessions, the duration of mask wearing at home can be systematically increased until the child reliably falls asleep with the mask in place, with airflow at the pulmonologist-prescribed settings.

IMPORTANT CAUTION: The child should never wear the mask with tubing attached unless the tubing is connected to the PAP machine with the airflow turned on as prescribed by the child's physician. Breathing through the tubing without the airflow on can potentially increase the child's blood carbon dioxide saturation to a dangerous level.

POSSIBLE MODIFICATIONS/VARIANTS

There are few medical alternatives to PAP for these children. Undergoing a tracheostomy is the most likely if the breathing disorder is severe and surgical interventions (tonsillectomy and adenoidectomy) have failed to resolve the problem. However, tracheostomy has significant risks, and child adherence may still be required for success and safety (e.g., the child must not dislodge the tracheostomy tube or connection with the source of oxygen, and must tolerate routine tracheostomy care).

It is recommend that when physicians prescribe PAP or similar regimens for children, the family should be referred to a behavior therapist that can train the child to cope with the equipment and assist the caregiver in identifying and overcoming barriers to consistent regimen adherence.

Caregiver consistency and patience are important for long-term adherence. When behavioral training is implemented, there is often considerable variability in the number of minutes or, ultimately, hours the child can tolerate the PAP. Some children do not show an immediate and sustained improvement in adherence. This may be due to the difficulty of training all of the child's caregivers to ensure that the behavioral intervention is implemented consistently. Even well-trained caregivers may be more or less diligent about implementing the behavioral procedures from day to day, because caregiver resources and emotional reserve may fluctuate. The quality of the child's sleep also can vary for reasons not directly related to the breathing problems and PAP (e.g., diet, exercise, illness, environmental disturbance, change of routine, emotional state). When the child does not sleep soundly, and there are awakenings or partial arousals during the night, the child may become confused or more aware of discomfort from the mask or airflow, and may reflexively grab and dislodge the mask. Therefore, the child should be taught to tolerate the mask when fully awake. Although attempting to place the equipment by stealth once the child is asleep may be successful at times, this approach is usually ineffective in the long term. If children are not trained to tolerate the mask when fully awake, they are more likely to awaken during the night and immediately remove the mask, which is perceived as an aversive foreign object.

Other possible reasons for adherence problems also should be considered. Use of PAP pressures that are too high can increase discomfort and arousal from sleep due to ear pain, headache, difficulty exhaling, and dry eyes (air leaking from the mask into the eyes). Pressures that are too low to overcome the obstructed breathing problem can cause a feeling of suffocation while wearing the mask. The behavior therapist should consult with the prescribing pulmonologist to ensure appropriate pressure settings have been determined during PAP titration in a sleep laboratory. Repeat sleep studies may be helpful once the patient is cooperating with the PAP routine, because the first assessment of pressure requirements may have been based on a suboptimal evaluation with a marginally cooperative child. A repeat sleep study allows for fine-tuning of mask fit and pressure settings. If nasal or sinus irritation develops from dry airflow, PAP machines can be outfitted with humidifiers, which may improve adherence.

Of course, it is preferable to avoid the development of escape-motivated distress behavior in response to PAP. Therefore, proactive consultation between the behavior therapist, respiratory therapist, physician and/or nurse should occur to ensure that a proper mask, cap, and other necessary equipment are selected in the first place. Working together, they can introduce the child and family to the PAP sensations and routine in a systematic and non-traumatic manner. Whenever possible, children should be properly trained prior to attempting polysomnography in order to prevent the development of conditioned anxiety and escape behavior that would subsequently interfere with PAP adherence.

Clinical experience with these children and families indicates that child cooperation and long-term adherence are dependent on caregiver behavior. If the child dislodges the mask in the night, whether intentionally or unintentionally, the caregiver must discover the problem and replace the mask. Otherwise, negative reinforcement of escape behavior will occur (pushing the mask out of place or removing it relieves the child's immediate discomfort). As discussed above under "Measurement of PAP Adherence", caregivers should be assisted with establishing a way to monitor PAP status during the night. Even when using a PAP machine equipped with an alarm that sounds if the mask is removed or not properly positioned, the alarm may not be loud enough to awaken an exhausted and soundly sleeping caregiver. Caregivers should be encouraged to use a high-quality baby monitor to amplify the alarm and monitor the sounds of the child stirring or awakening during the night. Alternatively, some caregivers may choose to set an alarm clock to awaken at intervals to check and if necessary replace the mask. Parents of young children often have their children sleep in or near the parent's bed to facilitate monitoring. Even in the best of cases with the most highly motivated parents, the process of establishing long-term PAP adherence is imperfect and takes time.

Caregivers who experience guilt or conflict over enforcing an intervention that causes short-term discomfort for important long-term health benefits will have difficulty obtaining PAP adherence with their child. Parents may worry that a child with a breathing or heart condition will be irreversibly harmed if stressed by a tantrum or physical prompting. Such fears should be validated with the child's physician to avoid behavior therapy if it is contraindicated, or to reassure the parent if there is no contraindication.

If a caregiver does not comprehend or believe the seriousness of the child's breathing problems, he or she may regard PAP as optional, and not believe it is necessary to replace the mask each time it is removed. Such a caregiver's understanding of the risks of untreated breathing problems and the benefits of PAP should be addressed through a joint meeting with the physician and behavior therapist.

In cases where the caregiver is not fully committed or is unable to invest the time and energy required to assure adherence throughout the night, more modest intermediate goals might be set. Mask removal may be primarily motivated by escape from discomfort. Therefore, the caregiver should select an interval for PAP use that realistically can be enforced. For example, the caregiver may begin by implementing the behavioral procedures for only 30 minutes, with emphasis on the rule that only the caregiver applies and removes the mask. If the child attempts to remove the mask, the attempt is blocked. If the mask is successfully removed, it is replaced. If the child wears the mask for the established interval, a special positive reinforcer can be awarded. Increasing the duration of enforcement should only occur when both caregiver and child have mastered the current duration. In this way, both experience success and a positive interaction, rather than failure and conflict. This approach may not be feasible with some types of breathing problems. For example, if the child's medical condition is so acutely tenuous that less than complete adherence during hours of sleep would be dangerous, then more invasive medical interventions would be necessary if the parent were unable to enforce adherence throughout the night.

PROOF OF CONCEPT/SUPPORTING DATA/EVIDENCE BASE

There is extensive evidence from the applied behavior analysis literature that some child behavior problems are maintained by their escape function, and that these behaviors can be reduced using an escape extinction intervention. For example, this approach has been used to successfully treat self-injury [6], food refusal [7], distress during dental procedures [8], and distress during EEG examinations [9].

A 1995 study examining the safety and efficacy of CPAP with children found that when CPAP was not effective, it was because of poor adherence in 92 percent of unsuccessful cases [10]. In that same year, the first article describing successful behavioral intervention to increase compliance with nasal CPAP in children was published [11]. In that study, four children ranging in age from 3 to 12 years of age with diagnosed syndromes (Hunter's, Hurler's, Treacher Collins, Down) involving maxillofacial abnormalities were provided with behavioral intervention to facilitate their compliance with CPAP. Three of the four children had mental retardation (MR), and the youngest child (age 3) had severe MR. The patients and their parents attended training sessions, and the parents learned to coach their children during exposure to and wearing the PAP. The parents participated in a behavioral skills training program using this approach. Subsequently, all four of the children began wearing CPAP during sleep at home, and continued doing so at 3-month follow-up. At 9-month follow-up, three of the four were still successfully using CPAP.

Although other publications have reported use of educational and behavioral interventions to facilitate PAP adherence, these articles lack an adequate description of the intervention procedures that were utilized [12,13].

Two other published studies have described and demonstrated behavioral methods for increasing children's adherence with PAP therapy [1,14]. The first study was a non-experimental case series clinical report of outcome data that supported the utility of behavior analysis and therapy for improving PAP adherence and facilitating effective clinical management of OSA [1]. Although that report included some children with developmental disabilities, the children who achieved the greatest increases in mean hours per night of PAP adherence (i.e., >5.0 hours/night) were those with higher levels of estimated cognitive functioning. In only one case was a mean increase in adherence of greater than 5 hours per night achieved with a child with mental retardation (MR). For one other child with mild MR and three children with moderate to severe MR, the mean increase in hours of adherence per day ranged from 4.0 to 5.0. However, that study was based on a non-experimental analysis of retrospective clinic data.

Slifer and colleagues [14] conducted a prospective study using repeated measures of cooperation and adherence and single subject experimental design. Their study provides additional preliminary evidence that the "package" of procedures described in this chapter appears to be effective for desensitizing preschool children with developmental delay, behavior problems, and serious health conditions to PAP.

The four children were referred because of their severe behavioral reactions to the PAP mask and airflow during initial attempts to conduct polysomnography or to initiate PAP therapy. The four children were between 3 and 5 years of age, and had a variety of health impairments (obesity, cor pulmonale, diabetes, reactive airway disease, lung hypoplasia, status post-craniopharyngioma resection). Using the same behavior therapy protocol as presented in this chapter, all four children tolerated PAP while sleeping for age-appropriate durations. Home follow-up data were obtained for three of the children that indicated the parents were able to continue the protocol with maintenance of therapeutic benefits.

REFERENCES

[1] K.L. Koontz, K.J. Slifer, M.D. Cataldo, C.L. Marcus, Improving pediatric compliance with positive airway pressure therapy: the impact of behavioral intervention, Sleep 26 (2003) 1–6.

[2] D. Phillips, S.C. Fischer, R. Singh, A children's reinforcement survey schedule, J. Behav. Ther. Exp. Psychiatry 8 (1977) 131–134.

[3] W.W. Fisher, C.C. Piazza, L.G. Bowman, A. Amari, Integrating caregiver report with a systematic choice assessment to enhance reinforcer identification, Am. J. Ment. Retard. 101 (1996) 15–25.

[4] J. Northup, T. George, K. Jones, et al., A comparison of reinforcer assessment methods: the utility of verbal and pictorial choice procedures, J. Appl. Behav. Anal. 29 (1996) 201–212.

[5] G.M. Pace, M.T. Ivancic, G.L. Edwards, et al., Assessment of stimulus preference and reinforcer value with profoundly retarded individuals, J. Appl. Behav. Anal. 18 (1985) 249–255.

[6] B.A. Iwata, GM Pace, M.J. Kalsher, et al., Experimental analysis and extinction of self-injurious escape behavior, J. Appl. Behav. Anal. 23 (1990) 11–27.

[7] C.C. Piazza, M.R. Patel, C.S. Gulotta, B.M. Sevin, On the relative contributions of positive reinforcement and escape extinction in the treatment of food refusal, J. Appl. Behav. Anal. 36 (2003) 309–324.

[8] P.M. O'Callaghan, K.D. Allen, S. Powell, F. Salama, The efficacy of noncontingent escape for decreasing children's disruptive behavior during restorative dental treatment, J. Appl. Behav. Anal. 39 (2006) 161–171.

[9] K.J. Slifer, K. Avis, R. Frutchey, Behavioral intervention to increase compliance with electroencephalogram (EEG) procedures in children with developmental disabilities, Epilepsy Behav. 13 (2008) 189–195.

[10] C.L. Marcus, J.L. Carroll, O. Bamford, et al., Supplemental oxygen during sleep in children with sleep-disordered breathing, Am. J. Respir. Crit. Care Med. 152 (1995) 1297–1301.

[11] J.C. Rains, Treatment of obstructive sleep apnea in pediatric patients. Behavioral intervention for compliance with nasal continuous positive airway pressure, Clin. Pediatr. 34 (1995) 535–541.

[12] V.G. Kirk, A.R. O'Donnell, Continuous positive airway pressure for children: a discussion on how to maximize compliance, Sleep Med. Rev. 10 (2006) 119–127.

[13] E.C. Uong, M. Epperson, S.A. Bathon, D.B. Jeffe, Adherence to nasal positive airway pressure therapy among school-aged children and adolescents with obstructive sleep apnea syndrome, Pediatrics 120 (2007) 1203–1211.

[14] K.J. Slifer, D. Kruglak, E. Benore, et al., Behavioral training for increasing preschool children's adherence with positive airway pressure: a preliminary study, Behav. Sleep Med. 5 (2007) 147–175.

RECOMMENDED READING

American Academy of Pediatrics, Section on Pediatric Pulmonary, Subcommittee on Obstructive Sleep Apnea Syndrome. Clinical practice guideline: diagnosis and management of childhood obstructive sleep apnea syndrome, Pediatrics 109 (2002) 704–712.

A.C. Halbower, E.M. Mahone, Neuropsychological morbidity linked to childhood sleep-disordered breathing, Sleep Med. Rev. 10 (2006) 97–107.

A.C. Halbower, M. Degaonkar, P.B. Barker, et al., Childhood obstructive sleep apnea associates with neuropsychological deficits and neuronal brain injury, PLoS Med. 3 (2006) 1391–1402.

K.L. Koontz, K.J. Slifer, M.D. Cataldo, C.L. Marcus, Improving pediatric compliance with positive airway pressure therapy: the impact of behavioral intervention, Sleep 26 (2003) 1–6.

A.J. Lipton, D. Gozal, Treatment of obstructive sleep apnea in children: do we really know how? Sleep Med. Rev. 7 (2003) 61–80.

C.L. Marcus, G. Rosen, S.L. Davidson-Ward, et al., Efficacy and compliance with positive airway pressure therapy in children with obstructive sleep apnea, Pediatrics 117 (2006) 442–451.

K.J. Slifer, D. Kruglak, E. Benore, et al., Behavioral training for increasing preschool children's adherence with positive airway pressure: a preliminary study, Behav. Sleep Med. 5 (2007) 147–175.

GLOSSARY

The recommended behavioral intervention protocol involves several basic behavior principles and intervention strategies, which are defined below.

Contingent or contingency This refers to an "if – then" relationship between behavior and stimulus. For example, in contingent reinforcement, the reinforcing stimulus is presented by the therapist only if the target behavior occurs, and therefore is always delivered after the target behavior is observed.

Non-contingent This refers to the absence of an "if – then" relationship between behavior and stimulus. Thus, in non-contingent reinforcement the reinforcing stimulus is presented independent of the individual's behavior.

Positive reinforcement This involves providing a preferred item or activity contingent on a target behavior that is to be strengthened.

Negative reinforcement This involves removing an aversive or non-preferred item or activity contingent on a target behavior that one wishes to strengthen.

Differential reinforcement This involves providing a reinforcer in response to behavior one wishes to increase, but not in response to behavior one intends to decrease.

Counter-conditioning This involves modifying conditioned anxiety by carefully planned, graduated exposure to the anxiety-causing or non-preferred stimulus while the patient is participating in a distracting, relaxing, or otherwise pleasurable activity.

Shaping This involves using differential reinforcement to teach successive approximations of a target behavior.

Escape extinction (escape prevention) This consists of blocking the patient's escape from a feared or non-preferred stimulus, thereby weakening the escape behavior that has been maintained by negative reinforcement.

In vivo behavioral rehearsal This refers to giving the child the opportunity to practice "in real life" the skills necessary to cope and cooperate with the behavioral demands of the problem situation. This practice is done under conditions that are the same as or closely match the actual problem situation. Thus, real PAP equipment is used, rather than toys or imagined equipment.

Chapter 38

Using Motivational Interviewing to Facilitate Healthier Sleep-Related Behaviors in Adolescents

Melanie A. Gold
Division of Adolescent Medicine, Department of Pediatrics, University of Pittsburgh School of Medicine, Pittsburgh, PA
Student Health Services, Division of Student Affairs, University of Pittsburgh Student Health Service, Pittsburgh, PA

Ronald E. Dahl
Department of Psychology, University of Pittsburgh, Pittsburgh, PA

PROTOCOL NAME

Using motivational interviewing (MI) to facilitate healthier sleep-related behaviors in adolescents.

GROSS INDICATION

This intervention is indicated to increase motivation and facilitate effective behavior change relevant to behavioral aspects of sleep among adolescents.

SPECIFIC INDICATION

Motivation is a crucial component to many types of behavior change in adolescents; however, to date there is no empirical evidence to indicate that MI is effective for specific sleep disorders.

CONTRAINDICATIONS

There is no evidence to suggest that MI is contraindicated for any specific sleep disorders or types of adolescent patients.

Behavioral Treatments for Sleep Disorders. DOI: 10.1016/B978-0-12-381522-4.00038-9

RATIONALE FOR INTERVENTION

Clinicians who care for adolescents with sleep disorders are constantly addressing behavioral issues. Whether trying to motivate changes in sleep habits and schedules, modifying late-night social activities, avoiding caffeine, tobacco, drug or alcohol intake, altering behaviors that negatively affect sleep, or trying to improve treatment adherence in patients with narcolepsy or sleep apnea, clinicians often struggle with how best to help adolescents make positive changes in their sleep-related behaviors. Simply giving advice or education alone is rarely an effective method for facilitating behavior change, particularly when there may be ambivalence or resistance to change (which is quite common among adolescents). Adolescents often perceive advice as akin to being lectured, and may quickly "tune out" the clinician. In some cases, hearing an adult authority figure advocating what an adolescent "should" do can simply activate unspoken counter-arguments in the adolescent, or stir up feelings of doubt as to whether the clinician's perspective or advice has any relevance.

An alternative approach to facilitating behavior change that has proven effective in motivating effective behavior change in adolescents is called motivational interviewing (MI). MI is a clinical approach that is patient-centered, directive, and seeks to enhance *intrinsic* motivation to change by exploring and resolving ambivalence that is rooted in that individual's natural motivations, and that supports the individual's goals, values, and beliefs. For example, in working with an adolescent struggling with daytime sleepiness stemming from erratic and late-night schedules on school nights, it is not useful simply to instruct the adolescent about the importance of earlier and more regular bedtimes. An MI approach might explore how the adolescent feels when he or she wakes up in the morning, what it is like dealing with parental anger about missing the school bus from oversleeping, or the adolescent's desire to look more attractive by eliminating dark circles under his or her eyes, while at the same time acknowledging the adolescent's ambivalence about going to bed earlier and curtailing enjoyable late-night activities such as social interaction via Internet or cell phones.

In general, MI does not focus on directing the adolescent behavior toward goals established by the clinician, parent, or teacher (such as the need to change habits, behaviors, learn new skills, reshape cognitions, etc.). Instead, the approach begins by focusing on the adolescent's current interests and concerns, and aims to develop discrepancies between present behavior and important personal goals, values, and beliefs. MI focuses on responding to adolescents in ways that help resolve their own sources of ambivalence to behavior change, reduce resistance, and help move the adolescent to self-motivated positive changes in sleep-related behaviors.

There are three key elements that are critical components of the spirit of MI: collaboration, evocation, and autonomy.

Collaboration refers to a partnership between the clinician and the adolescent that views the adolescent as an expert about his or her own experiences, values, beliefs, and goals (related both to sleep and to other aspects of the adolescent's life).

Evocation refers to the clinician's use of open-ended questions and reflections to assist the adolescent in identifying personal intrinsic motivation for change. In MI, it is the adolescent's task to articulate and resolve ambivalence about change, and the clinician's role is to help the adolescent examine his or her internal conflicts about values, goals, beliefs, and behaviors as they pertain to making behavior change around sleep.

Autonomy refers to emphasizing that it is the adolescent's responsibility to change his or her behavior (or not), and to decide if, how, and when sleep-related changes will occur. In support of autonomy, MI proposes that the clinician does not attempt to directly persuade an adolescent to make behavioral change (since this is an ineffective way of resolving ambivalence or facilitating change, and only serves to raise resistance to behavior change).

PRINCIPLES OF MI

Clinicians can incorporate MI in their sleep medicine consultations by becoming skilled in communication strategies that have been shown to promote rapport and resolve ambivalence that is an expected and normal component of sleep-related behavioral change. The four principles of MI are: (1) to express empathy, (2) to develop discrepancy, (3) to roll with resistance, and (4) to support self-efficacy in each adolescent patient encounter.

Express Empathy

Facilitate behavior change by expressing empathy and accepting adolescent beliefs and behaviors. This is usually a much more effective approach than applying pressure through persuasion. Direct persuasion and pressure to change or "finger-wagging" usually elicits resistance, especially among adolescents, and particularly among those with an oppositional or defiant temperament. MI creates a non-judgmental environment that allows the adolescent to talk openly about his or her sleep-related behaviors, lifestyle, and beliefs. It is valuable to practice reflective listening as a way to communicate empathy and understanding. When an adolescent describes a behavior with a negative health impact, it can be helpful to temporarily hold off on voicing clinical concerns (or a judgmental facial expression or tone of voice). Instead, it is more helpful to first encourage an alliance with the adolescent by accurately reflecting the viewpoint expressed by the adolescent and resisting the urge to give advice until it is requested (or at least ask for the adolescent's permission before offering an alternative point of view).

Develop Discrepancy

This is done by gently eliciting and reflecting inconsistencies between the adolescent's current status and his or her stated goals (or between the adolescent's current behavior and his or her stated values). For example, if an adolescent with narcolepsy indicates a goal to obtain a driver's license but has not been responsible in taking his or her medications or following a regular sleep–wake schedule, the clinician might gently reflect on this discrepancy (relevant to the adolescent's goals and values). Adolescents who are conscious of these inconsistencies will usually attempt to make changes when they become aware of the consequences of current behavior. Ask the adolescent's permission to offer objective information about any discrepancies, and, when permission is granted, provide information in a non-judgmental, factual way. Always then elicit feedback from the adolescent about what he or she thought of the information.

Roll with Resistance

Roll with resistance by recognizing that it is normal for adolescents to feel ambivalent about making sleep-related behavioral change. Resistance usually occurs when the adolescent feels pushed to do something that he or she is not yet ready to do. Signs of resistance include arguing, interrupting, denying there is a problem, ignoring the clinician, missing appointments, presenting too late for an appointment, or failing to complete requested tasks. Overt compliance with covert defiance is another form of resistance, signaled when the visit goes "too smoothly" and the adolescent seems to be agreeing too easily to make behavioral changes. In MI, arguing and persuasion in the face of ambivalence are deemed counterproductive. These approaches, along with labeling the adolescent with his or her behavior ("an insomniac") can be expected to elicit a defensive response and increase resistance. When you see or hear signs of resistance, shift to a new strategy.

Support Self-Efficacy

Change is most likely to occur when the adolescent has recognized that he or she has a problem, and believes in his or her ability to do something about it. One powerful facilitator of change is communicating optimism about the motivated adolescent's ability to succeed at a desired change. When you believe an adolescent is ready to change, support self-efficacy by expressing your optimism. Point out, with permission, that change is not an all-or-nothing venture. Suggest that the adolescent's past successes and failures were learning opportunities. Help the adolescent to identify a range of effective alternatives for achieving his or her desired goals.

STEP BY STEP DESCRIPTION OF PROCEDURES

In the sleep medicine context, clinicians can use open-ended questions and reflective listening to engage adolescents in a conversation about sleep-related behavior change with the intent of maintaining their health and/or decreasing risks related to inadequate or poor-quality sleep. MI increases the adolescent's receptivity and decreases resistance to behavioral changes. Developing good rapport often begins with the clinician verifying his or her understanding of the adolescent's perspective by paraphrasing and summarizing what has been said. The clinician should not offer information or advice without first requesting and receiving permission to do so, and should always seek feedback on any information or suggestions provided.

Strategies for Establishing Rapport

Reflective listening, open-ended questions, affirmations, and summaries are four key MI strategies used to build rapport early in a sleep medicine consultation. Some of the more commonly employed reflective styles and tools to decrease resistance are described in Table 38.1.

1. *Reflective listening* calls for a warm, non-judgmental restatement, clarification, enhancement, or expansion of what the adolescent has said.
2. *Open-ended questions* encourage adolescents to talk about thoughts and feelings related to their sleep behaviors and impacting on their daily level of functioning; questions are phrased to prompt the adolescent to elaborate. With younger adolescents, it may help to begin with a limited number of choices. For example: "Would you like to talk about what it is like trying to get up for school when you are feeling so tired in the morning, or about what is going on at home that makes it difficult to go to bed at a regular time on school nights?" However, it is usually best to end with an open-ended question, like "... or maybe there is something else you would rather discuss? What do you think?"
3. *Affirmations* express appreciation. For example, "I really appreciate your being so honest with me about why you have been going to bed at 3 am", or "That's an excellent idea!" Affirmations should be genuine and used sparingly; overuse sounds inauthentic and condescending.
4. *Summaries* bring together thoughts or feelings that the adolescent has shared. If appropriate, the clinician can talk about how the adolescent's perceptions fit together. There are three types of summaries:
5. *Collecting summaries* are used during the process of exploration and gather together the adolescent's statements into a summary – for example: "There are several social advantages to staying up late at night texting and on the Internet."
6. *Linking summaries* tie together what has just been stated with something previously expressed in order to develop discrepancy – for example: "You like staying up late at night, and at the same time you really dislike feeling so sleep-deprived."
7. *Transitional summaries* prepare for a shift in focus (as when ending an encounter) by pulling together essential points to decide on the next step – for example: "From what you have said so far, you want to think about possible ways that you could get more sleep and get to school on time while maintaining your social connection with your friends. What ideas do you have about how to do that?"

TABLE 38.1 Strategies to Increase Receptivity and Decrease Resistance to Making Behavior Changes Related to Improved Sleep

Strategy	Description	Examples
Reflections		
Simple reflection	Repeat what the adolescent just said, staying close to his or her words.	**Adolescent**: You say that I have to make all these changes to get enough sleep, but I don't think I need it to feel better. **Clinician**: You're not sure that this is really necessary.
Reflection of meaning	Reflect implied or underlying cognitive content in what was just said.	**Adolescent**: I'm not an insomniac! **Clinician**: That label really doesn't fit you.
Reflection of feeling	Reflect implied or underlying affective or emotional content in what was said.	**Adolescent**: I'm no insomniac! **Clinician**: It makes you *angry* when you think someone sees you that way.
Double-sided reflection	Used when both sides of ambivalence have been expressed: reflects the two perspectives, usually starting with the side favoring the *status quo* (not changing) and ending with the side favoring change.	**Adolescent**: Sometimes I get mad at myself for staying up until 2 am playing computer games or listening to music on week nights because I can't get up for school in the morning, but I always catch up on my sleep over the weekends, so I know I am ultimately getting enough sleep. **Clinician**: You don't believe that getting 4 hours of sleep on the week day nights is much of a problem, and at the same time it bothers you when you stay up too late and can't get up in time for school.
Amplified reflection	Used when only the negative side of ambivalence is expressed: exaggerate or intensify what was said to lead the adolescent to correct the distortion. (This requires a light touch so as not to sound condescending or sarcastic. It is effective only when the adolescent has some ambivalence about the negative side.)	**Adolescent**: I'm not sure I really need to go through all this treatment to get more sleep. **Clinician**: Your life is really fine right now, just the way it is.

Decreasing resistance		
Shifting focus	Temporarily shift attention away from contentious area to common ground.	**Adolescent**: You say that I have to make all these changes so I can get more sleep, but I don't think I need to. I am functioning just fine the way things are right now. **Clinician**: You're confident that you don't need more sleep. Tell me about that.
Emphasizing personal choice and control	Assure that any decision about whether or not to change is the adolescent's choice; only he or she can take action toward change.	**Adolescent**: You say that I have to make all these changes so I can get more sleep, but I don't think I need to. I am functioning just fine the way things are right now. **Clinician**: Whether or not you make any changes in your sleep or other activities is completely up to you. I definitely would not want you to feel pressured to do anything against your will.
Reframing	Restates what was said from a new perspective and invites the adolescent to consider this viewpoint.	**Adolescent**: Every time I talk to my parents they bug me about my staying up late and falling asleep in class. Why won't they get off my back and leave me alone? **Clinician**: Your parents worry about you, and it feels more like nagging than a way of expressing the concern they have for you.
Agreement with a twist	Combines a reflection and a reframe; requires a light touch and sensitivity so it does not sound like sarcasm or criticism.	**Adolescent**: Every time I talk to my parents they bug me about my staying up late and falling asleep in class. Why won't they get off my back and leave me alone? **Clinician**: You really do wish they would leave you alone, even if it meant that they had to stop caring about what happens to you.
Coming Alongside (e.g., siding with the negative)	A last resort: agreeing with expressions of negativity. Extreme exaggeration intended to bring the adolescent back to a more open posture.	**Adolescent**: I'm really not sure I want to go through all this stuff you want me to do to fix my sleep issues. **Clinician**: This treatment approach may be more than you can handle right now. Maybe this isn't the right time for a change.

Additional MI Strategies for Encounters in Sleep Medicine with Adolescents

Several MI strategies that enhance rapport and/or build motivation for change adapt well to the sleep medicine context. Generally, only one or two of these strategies would be used in a single consultation or follow-up visit.

Asking Permission

Before offering specific information or advice about sleep issues, find out whether that information or advice will be welcomed by the adolescent. Ask: "Would you like to know more about why your sleep patterns on weekends influence your sleep on school nights?" or "Would it be ok if I told you what I thought about this?" This step is critical. If the adolescent declines, move to another topic by saying "I respect the fact that you told me you are not interested in hearing about sleep schedules ... It is up to you to decide what we talk about. What *would* you like to discuss or learn about?"

Elicit–Provide–Elicit (Ask–Tell–Ask)

Before launching into a lecture about the definition of a sleep disorder, the importance of sleep, or what measures adolescents can take to improve the quality and quantity of their sleep, first elicit what the adolescent already knows about the topic and/or options for behavior change. Many adolescents already have the needed information (which can save the clinician time by avoiding providing information that is not needed). In addition, adolescents may already have excellent ideas about what to do to improve their sleep. In this case, the clinician can affirm the adolescent's resourcefulness and follow the adolescent's lead by supporting his or her ideas for behavior change. Adolescents are more likely to make behavioral changes that they have suggested themselves rather than those suggested by others. When the clinician has elicited that the adolescent already has the needed information or ideas regarding making behavior change, shift the focus from providing information or framing a realistic plan to discussing how he or she can implement these ideas successfully. When gaps in knowledge are identified, or the adolescent does not have specific ideas regarding possible behavior changes, it can be helpful to provide information and advice. Always ask permission prior to giving information or advice, and, most importantly, after doing so, elicit the adolescent's reaction to what you have said by asking "What do you make of this information/these options? How does this help you or change things?" Not all information or advice provided by clinicians to adolescents will be viewed as useful or acceptable, and it is critically important for the clinician to know how the adolescent has received the clinician's recommendations.

Decisional Balance

Ask the adolescent presenting for a sleep consultation to talk about the advantages and disadvantages of the change he or she is considering, or that others want them to make. Ask about the "good" and "not so good" things about change, rather than asking about the "good" and the "bad" aspects of change. For adolescents who are not interested in change (pre-contemplation), ask about the "good" and "not so good" things of maintaining the status quo or keeping the situation the same. For adolescents in pre-contemplation to make change, summarize the two sides of change, presenting the adolescent's argument for change second, then ask an open-ended question prompting talk about the change or a commitment to change. The dialogue below might be useful for an adolescent who is not interested in changing his sleep patterns:

I would like to better understand what you see as the "good things" about staying up late at night on the week nights. What do you enjoy or like about it? What else?

Ask until no further "good things" arise, then continue:

What is the other side of that? What are the "not-so-good things" about staying up late at night on the week nights? What else?

Again, ask until no further "not-so-good things" arise. Then reflect both sides by summarizing:

So the good things about staying up on the week nights are ... and the not-so-good things are ...

Finally, ask the adolescent to assess:

What do you make of this? How does this fit with how you see staying up late at night and how does it fit in with your future goals?

Decisional balance conversations elicit discrepancy between current behavior and future goals, values, and beliefs. Discrepancy is uncomfortable and adolescents do not like feeling internally discrepant, and will thus work to resolve inconsistencies by changing their behavior to fit their goals, values, perceived identity, or beliefs.

Importance and Confidence Rulers

It is often helpful to assess early on whether to focus on the *importance* of changing a sleep-related behavior or the adolescent's *confidence* in his or her ability to change that behavior. Importance and confidence rulers are useful tools in this regard. To do so, ask the adolescent "On a scale from 0 to 10 where 10 is the most important and 0 is the least important, what number would you give for how important it is to you to [behavior change related to sleep]?" "Why did you choose a [current number] instead of a [lower number]?" Then elicit all the reasons by asking "What else?" and reflecting what was said until the adolescent says, "That's it"; then ask "What would need to happen to make it a [higher number]?" Then ask "On a scale from 0 to 10 where 10 is the most confident and 0 is the least, what number would you give for how confident you are that you could [behavior change] if you wanted to? Why is it a [current number] instead of a [lower number]? What would need to happen to make it a [higher number]?"

While many adolescents will respond readily to a question such as "How important is it to you to go to sleep each night at the same time right now?" or "How confident are you that you could go to sleep each night at the same time if you wanted to right now?", this approach may be too abstract for younger adolescents. If this is the case, importance and confidence rulers, as illustrated below, can be quickly drawn on paper as visual aids. Ask the adolescent to point to a number on the scale that indicates how important (or how confident) he or she feels about making a specific sleep-related behavior change.

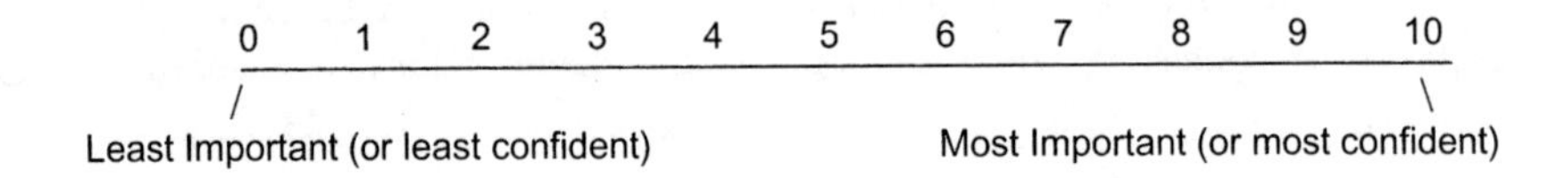

The focus of the conversation will depend on the rating levels for importance and confidence. If one number is distinctly lower than the other, focus on the *lower* number first. If importance is low (≤ 5), or if both importance and confidence levels are about the same, focus on importance. If both are very low (≤ 3), explore feelings about talking about the behavior. If both are high (8–10), explore what is preventing the adolescent from changing the behavior.

FIGURE 38.1 Importance and Confidence rulers.

Some adolescents have difficulty assigning values to numbers without a visual aid. In these instances, it may be helpful to draw two separate visual scales, one each for importance and confidence (Figure 38.1). For example, if a clinician wants to assess an adolescent's perceived importance and confidence to go to sleep at the same time each night, the clinician can say:

I would like to know how you feel right now about going to sleep at the same time each night. It is up to you to decide what time that might be. I have two questions for you using these two rulers [see Figure 38.1]. First, how important is it to you to go to sleep at the same time each night on this Importance Ruler, where 10 is the most important and 0 is the least important?"

Wait for the adolescent's response and then say:

Ok, here is the second question: if it was really important to you, how confident or sure are you that you could go to sleep at the same time each night on this Confidence Ruler, where 10 is the most confident and 0 is the least confident?

Wait for the adolescent's response. If the adolescent says Importance is a 3 and Confidence is an 8, focus on importance, and ask:

What made you choose a 3 and not a lower number like a 1 or a 2? What makes going to sleep at the same time each night this important?

Reflect reasons given and ask for elaboration ("Tell me more about that.") Then ask for more reasons by saying "What else makes it important?", and keep asking for reasons why importance is a 3 and not lower until the adolescent says "That's it". Then summarize what the adolescent said by saying "So what makes this important right now is……". Do not allow the adolescent to tell you why the number is a 3 and not a higher number. You want the adolescent to talk about reasons for going to sleep at the same time each night, not the barriers to doing so. Then ask "What would have to happen to make going to sleep at the same time each night a little bit more important to you?" Reflect and ask for elaboration by saying "what else" and reflecting until the adolescent says "That's it". Then summarize by saying "So what makes going to sleep at the same time each night important is ... and going to sleep at the same time each night would be even more important if ..." End the conversation with an open-ended question like "So what do you think you are going to do about going to sleep at the same time each night in the future?"

FRAMES

Miller and Sanchez [1] identified essential components of an effective brief intervention, summarized by the acronym "FRAMES", which overlap substantially with the key elements of MI. The clinician can conduct a short, FRAMES-based conversation after completing the history and physical examination. The example below describes a clinician's encounter with a 17-year-old patient who has been staying up until 3 am watching movies, and who presents with her parents who complain that she has been late for school every morning this past month, she is sleeping through her afternoon classes and performing poorly on exams given at the end of the day, and most recently she was in a motor vehicle accident coming home from school Monday afternoon because she felt asleep at the wheel.

(F)eedback: (review current status)

You told me you have been late for school nearly every day this month. Your parents told me you have been doing poorly on your exams, and you said that you get irritable and get into fights with your friends when you are tired.

(R)esponsibility: (emphasize personal choice)

It's up to you to decide when or if you are ready to change your sleeping behaviors.

(A)dvice: (recommend change)

Is it OK if I share with you what I think is important for you to do right now for your health? [Wait for affirmation; proceed if received] The best thing you could do right now is to get your sleeping back to a healthier schedule and stop staying up until 3 am. What do you think of that suggestion?

(M)enu: (present alternative strategies or options)

I realize that stopping watching movies late at night might be very hard. You might have some ideas about ways to help yourself get back on a healthier sleep schedule, and I could also suggest some options if you were interested. [Start with the adolescent's ideas; if none emerge, offer suggestions after obtaining permission to share suggestions.]

(E)mpathy:

I imagine even thinking about making this change may be hard.

(S)elf-efficacy: (reinforce hope and optimism)

Let's look at your past successes in other areas to see how you might apply what you learned from those experiences to this situation related to changing your sleep. I'm confident that together we can come up with a way that will work for you when you decide you want to do something about your sleeping.

Behavior Change Plan

A sleep behavior change plan is especially appropriate when the adolescent is considering making an imminent change in behavior. Some adolescents can develop a behavior change plan on their own; others are more successful with guidance. A typical behavior change plan includes the following components:

- The changes I want to make are:
- The most important reasons to make these changes are:
- The specific steps I plan to make in changing are:
- Some people who can me support are:
- They can help me by:
- I will know my plan is working when:
- Things that could interfere with my plan (barriers) and possible solutions include:

POSSIBLE MODIFICATIONS/VARIANTS

Developmental modifications include using the "open–closed–open" sandwich, in which an open-ended question is followed by several closed-ended questions, ending with another open-ended question; using fewer open-ended questions in general; as well as using more affirmations, and more reflections of emotion.

With younger adolescents, it may help to begin with a limited number of choices when using open-ended questions – for example, asking "Would you like to talk about things that interfere with getting enough sleep, the advantages of getting more sleep, or discuss weekend and weekday schedules today?", while always ending with an open-ended question like "or maybe there is something else you would rather discuss? What do you think?"

Younger adolescents may respond better to reflections of emotion than to reflections of meaning.

PROOF OF CONCEPT/SUPPORTING DATA/EVIDENCE BASE

To date, there are no published studies demonstrating that MI is effective at facilitating specific adolescent behavioral changes related to sleep behaviors. However, there is clear evidence for positive MI effects in other areas of difficult-to-change adolescent health behaviors, particularly with respect to alcohol, tobacco, and other drug use in youth [2–9]. Although not as well studied as adolescent substance use, there also have been studies showing encouraging results examining MI and adolescent behavior changes in relation to eating disorders, diabetes care, improving nutrition, weight loss, and decreasing risky sexual behaviors in adolescents [10–15]. One study also described using a motivational enhancement therapy to improve adherence to CPAP in adult patients with sleep apnea [16].

Currently, two NIH-funded research studies of behavioral treatment of sleep problems in children and adolescents are in progress, which include an MI component as part of a larger multi-modal behavioral treatment called "Sleeping Tigers" [17]. Although preliminary experiences using MI in these studies have been encouraging, data collection is still in progress, and no empirical data analyses have yet been conducted to formally evaluate effectiveness.

REFERENCES

[1] W.R. Miller, V.C. Sanchez, Motivating young adults for treatment and lifestyle change, in: G.S. Howard, P.E. Nathan (Eds.), Alcohol Use and Misuse by Young Adults, University of Notre Dame Press, Notre Dame, IN, 1994.

[2] P.M. Monti, A. Spirito, M. Myers, et al., Brief intervention for harm reduction with alcohol-positive older adolescents in a hospital emergency department, J. Consult. Clin. Psychol. 67 (6) (1999) 989–994.

[3] A. Spirito, P.M. Monti, N.P. Barnett, et al., A randomized clinical trial of a brief motivational intervention for alcohol-positive adolescents treated in an emergency department, J. Pediatr. 145 (3) (2004) 396–402.

[4] J.S. Baer, D.R. Kivlahan, A.W. Blume, et al., Brief intervention for heavy-drinking college students: 4-Year follow-up and natural history, Am. J. Public Health 91 (8) (2001) 1310–1316.

[5] K.S. Ingersoll, S.D. Ceperich, M.D. Nettleman, et al., Reducing alcohol-exposed pregnancy risk in college women: Initial outcomes of a clinical trial of a motivational intervention, J. Subst. Abuse Treat. 29 (2005) 173–180.

[6] D.R. Foxcroft, D. Ireland, G. Lowe, et al., Primary prevention for alcohol misuse in young people, Cochrane Database of Syst. Rev. (Issue 3) (2002). Art. No.: CD003024. DOI: 10.1002/14651858.CD003024.

[7] M. Dennis, S.H. Godley, G. Diamond, et al., The Cannabis Youth Treatment (CYT) Study: main findings from two randomized trials, J. Subst. Abuse Treat. 27 (3) (2004) 197–213.

[8] S. Gates, J. McCambridge, L.A. Smith, et al., Interventions for prevention of drug use by young people delivered in non-school settings, Cochrane Database Syst. Rev. 25 (1) (2006 Jan). CD005030.

[9] J. McCambridge, J. Strang, The efficacy of single-session motivational interviewing in reducing drug consumption and perceptions of drug-related risk and harm among young people: results from a multi-site cluster randomized trial, Addiction 99 (2004) 39–52.

[10] A. Richards, K.K. Kattelmann, C. Ren, Motivating 18- to 24-year-olds to increase their fruit and vegetable consumption, J. Am. Diet. Assoc. 106 (9) (2006) 1405–1411.

[11] S.M. Kiene, W.D. Barta, A brief individualized computer-delivered sexual risk reduction intervention increases HIV/AIDS preventive behavior, J. Adolesc. Health 39 (2006) 404–410.

[12] S. Channon, V.J. Smith, J.W. Gregory, A pilot study of motivational interviewing in adolescents with diabetes, Arch. Dis. Child 88 (2003) 680–683.

[13] S. Berg-Smith, V. Stevens, K. Brown, et al., A brief motivational intervention to improve dietary adherence in adolescents, Health Educ. Res. 14 (1999) 399–441.

[14] K. Resnicow, R. Davis, S. Rollnick, Motivational interviewing for pediatric obesity: conceptual issues and evidence review, J. Am. Diet. Assoc. 106 (12) (2006) 2024–2033.

[15] L.A. Kotler, G.S. Boudreau, M.J. Devlin, Emerging psychotherapies for eating disorders, J. Psychiatr. Pract. 9 (6) (2003) 431–441.

[16] M.S. Aloia, J.T. Arnedt, R.L. Riggs, et al., Clinical management of poor adherence to CPAP: motivational enhancement, Behav. Sleep Med. 2 (4) (2004) 205–222.

[17] R.E. Dahl, A.G. Harvey, Disordered sleep in an adolescent, in: C.A. Galanter, P.S. Jensen, (Eds.), DSM-IV-TR Casebook and Treatment Guide for Child Mental Health, American Psychiatric Publishing, Washington DC, 2009.

RECOMMENDED READING

Articles

T.H. Bien, W.R. Miller, J.S. Tonigan, Brief interventions for alcohol problems: a review, Addiction 88 (1993) 315–336.

S.J. Erickson, M. Gerstle, S.W. Feldstein, Brief interventions and motivational interviewing with children, adolescents, and their parents in pediatric health care settings: a review, Arch. Pediatr. Adolesc. Med. 159 (12) (2005) 1173–1180.

M.A. Gold, K. Delisi, Motivational interviewing and sexual and contraceptive behaviors, Adolesc. Med. State Art. Rev. 19 (1) (2008) 69–82.

M.A. Gold, P.K. Kokotailo, Motivational interviewing, Adolesc. Health Update, Am. Acad. Pediatr. 20 (1) (2007) 1–10.

P.K. Kokotailo, M.A. Gold, Motivational interviewing with adolescents, Adolesc. Med. State Art. Rev. 19 (1) (2008) 54–68.

H.A. Sindelar, A.M. Abrantes, C. Hart, et al., Motivational interviewing in pediatric practice, Curr. Opin. Pediatr. Pract. 34 (9) (2004) 317–348.

Books

H. Arkowitz, H.A. Westra, W.R. Miller, S. Rollnick, Motivational Interviewing in the Treatment of Psychological Problems, Guildford Press, New York, NY, 2008.

C. Dunn, S. Rollnick, Lifestyle Change, Mosby/Elsevier Limited, Philadelphia, PA, 2003.

W.R. Miller, S. Rollnick (Eds.), Motivational interviewing and the stages of change, in: Motivational Interviewing: Preparing People for Change, 2nd ed., Guilford Press, New York, NY, 2002, pp. 201–206.

S. Rollnick, P. Mason, C. Butler, Health Behavior Change: A Guide for Practitioners, Churchill Livingstone, London, UK, 1999.

S. Rollnick, W.R. Miller, C.C. Butler, Motivational Interviewing In Health Care: Helping People Change Behavior, Guilford Press, New York, NY, 2008.

Websites

www.motivationalinterview.org – a website with superb references for training opportunities, video-tapes, DVDs, books, research articles, and motivational interviewing network trainers.

M.A. Gold, Case commentary: Gynecological care for adolescents. Virtual Mentor. 2003;5(5) – a case commentary illustrating how to integrate the Transtheoretical Model and Motivational Interviewing into practical approaches to providing reproductive health care to a female adolescent. Available at: http://virtualmentor.ama-assn.org/2003/05/ccas1-0305.html. Accessed May 2, 2003 (can also can find link at: http://virtualmentor.ama-assn.org/2003/05/toc-0305.html).

VHS VIDEOTAPES AND DVDS

W.R. Miller, S. Rollnick, Motivational Interviewing: Professional Training Series. T.B. Moyers, director. Albuquerque, NM: University of New Mexico; 1998 – a series of six videotapes or two DVDs, produced at University of New Mexico, and intended to be a resource in professional training. It offers 6 hours of explanation and practical modeling of skills. The tapes include clinical demonstrations of the skills of motivational interviewing, showing 10 different therapists working with 12 clients. Links to order these tools are posted at www.motivationalinterview.org/training/videos.htm or can be ordered from Vanessa Montoya/Delilah Yao, UNM/CASAA, MSC11 6280, 1 University of New Mexico, Albuquerque, NM 87131-0001 USA, Phone: 505-925-2332, Fax: 505-925-2379, Email: dyao@unm.edu.

Index

D

E

J

L

M

CPSIA information can be obtained at www.ICGtesting.com
Printed in the USA
LVOW091934250412

279204LV00006B/4/P